COMMON PROBLEMS IN

PAIN MANAGEMENT

COMMON PROBLEMS IN
PAIN MANAGEMENT

THERESA FERRER-BRECHNER, M.D.
Adjunct Professor of Anesthesiology
University of California
Director, Pain Management Center
UCLA School of Medicine
Center for Health Sciences
Los Angeles, California

YEAR BOOK MEDICAL PUBLISHERS, INC.
CHICAGO ● LONDON ● BOCA RATON ● LITTLETON, MASS.

1   2   3   4   5   6   7   8   9   0   R   Y   94   93   92   91   90

Library of Congress Cataloging-in-Publication Data

Common problems in pain management / [edited by] Theresa Ferrer-Brechner.
        p.   cm.
    Includes bibliographical references.
    Includes index.
    ISBN 0-8151-3347-2
    1. Pain—Treatment.   2. Intractable pain—Treatment.   3. Cancer
pain—Treatment.   I. Ferrer-Brechner, Theresa.
    [DNLM: 1. Pain—therapy.   WL 704 C734]
    RB127.64   1990
616'.0472—dc20   90-12544
DNLM/DLC   CIP
for Library of Congress

Sponsoring Editor: Susan M. Gay
Associate Managing Editor, Manuscript Services: Deborah Thorp
Production Project Coordinator: Karen Halm
Proofroom Supervisor: Barbara M. Kelly

COMMON PROBLEMS IN ANESTHESIA SERIES

CONTRIBUTORS

VERNE L. BRECHNER, M.D.
Professor Emeritus, Department of Anesthesiology, UCLA; Saint Johns Hospital, Santa Monica, California

LIDO CHEN, M.D., M.P.H.
Associate Professor, University of California Irvine; Director of the Pain Management Center and Attending Anesthesiologist, University of California Irvine Medical Center, Orange, California

DENNIS W. COOMBS, M.D.
Professor of Anesthesiology, Dartmouth Hitchcock Medical Center; Director of Pain Management Services, Mary Hitchcock Memorial Hospital, Hanover, New Hampshire

DAVID H. CLEMENTS, M.D.
Associate Professor, Department of Orthopedic Surgery, Temple University School of Medicine, Philadelphia, Pennsylvania

LUIS A. CUEVA, P.T., D.D.S.
Arizona Head and Neck Treatment Center, University Medical Center, University of Arizona; VA Hospital, Tucson Arizona

LAURA DARKE, PH.D.
Assistant Professor of Anesthesiology, UCLA Pain Management Center, UCLA School of Medicine, Los Angeles, California

JOSETTE FAST, B.S., P.T.
Senior Physical Therapist of Chronic Pain Management, Department of Rehabilitation Services, UCLA Medical Center, Los Angeles, California

THERESA FERRER-BRECHNER, M.D.
Adjunct Professor of Anesthesiology and Director of the Pain Management Center, UCLA School of Medicine, Center for Health Science, Los Angeles, California

JAMES R. FRICTON, D.D.S., M.S.
Associate Professor, Department of Diagnostic and Surgical Sciences, University of Minnesota School of Dentistry; Co-Director, TMJ and Craniofacial Pain Clinic, University of Minnesota Center for Health Sciences, Minneapolis, Minnesota

AVROM GART, M.D.
Assistant Professor of Anesthesiology, UCLA Pain Management Center, Los Angeles, California

STEVEN B. GRAFF-RADFORD, D.D.S.
Assistant Professor, Director of Education, UCLA Pain Management Center; Cedars-Sinai Hospital, Los Angeles, California

MARK GREENBERG, M.D.
Staff Anesthesiologist, Santa Monica Hospital Medical Center, Santa Monica, California

CHANG-ZERN HONG, M.D.
Assistant Professor, University of California Irvine; Clinical Director, Department of Physical Medicine and Rehabilitation, University of California Irvine Medical Center, Orange, California

BERNADETTE JAEGER, D.D.S.
Associate Professor, Department of Anesthesiology, UCLA School of Medicine and Section of Gnathology, UCLA School of Dentistry; Director, Head and Neck Pain Program, Department of Anesthesiology, Pain Management Center, UCLA Center for Health Sciences, Los Angeles, California

LINDA D. KAMES, PSY.D.
Assistant Clinical Professor, Department of Anesthesiology, UCLA, Los Angeles, California
Assistant Clinical Professor, Department of Anesthesiology, UCLA, Los Angeles, California

GEORGE KROL, M.D.
Associate Professor, Department of Radiology, Cornell University Medical College; Associate Attending Physician, Medical Imaging, Memorial Sloan-Kettering Cancer Center, New York, New York

MICHAEL H. LEVY, M.D., PH.D.
Assistant Professor of Medicine, Temple University School of Medicine; Co-Director, Pain Management Center, Fox Chase Cancer Center, Philadelphia, Pennsylvania

ALLAN NUTKIEWICZ, M.D.
Assistant Professor, Division of Neurosurgery, UCLA, Los Angeles, California

RUSSELL K. PORTENOY, M.D.
Assistant Professor of Neurology, Cornell University Medical College; Director of Analgesic Studies, Pain Service, Department of Neurology, Memorial Sloan-Kettering Cancer Center, New York, New York

ANDREA RAPKIN, M.D.
Assistant Professor, Director of Ambulatory Care, Department of Obstetrics and Gynecology, UCLA, Los Angeles, California

JOHN C. ROWLINGSON, M.D.
Professor of Anesthesiology; Director, Pain Management Center, University of Virginia School of Medicine, Charlottesville, Virginia

I. JON RUSSELL, M.D., PH.D.
Associate Professor of Medicine, University of Texas Health Science Center; Director, Brady-Green Clinical Research Center, Bexar County Hospital District, Medical Center Hospital, San Antonio, Texas

VED P. SACHDEV, M.D.
  Clinical Professor and Vice Chair, Neurosurgery, Mount Sinai Medical Center, New York, New York

MICHAEL S. SIMMONS, D.M.D.
  Assistant Clinical Professor, Department of Anesthesiology, UCLA School of Medicine, Pain Management Center; Lecturer, UCLA School of Dentistry, Los Angeles, California

WILLIAM K. SOLBERG, D.D.S., M.S.D.
  Professor of Dentistry, School of Dentistry, UCLA; Attending Dentist, UCLA Medical Center, Los Angeles, California

FREDERICK M. STAMPLER, PSY.D.
  Adjunct Assistant Professor, Department of Anesthesiology, UCLA School of Medicine, Los Angeles, California

NARAYAN SUNDARESAN, M.D.
  Associate Professor of Neurosurgery, Mount Sinai Medical School; Associate Attending Surgeon, Mount Sinai Hospital, New York, New York

KATHERINE KIDDER WALDMAN, O.T.R.
  Director, Occupational Therapy, Pain Consortium of Greater Kansas City, Kansas

STEVEN D. WALDMAN, M.D.
  Associate Clinical Professor of Anesthesiology, University of Missouri; Director, Pain Consortium of Greater Kansas City, Kansas

RONALD F. YOUNG, M.D.
  Professor of Surgery/Neurosurgery and Chief of Neurosurgery, University of California Irvine Medical Center, Orange, California

To my lovely daughters,
Aileen and Lonella,
for understanding their
always-busy mother.

PREFACE

With the advent of a multidisciplinary approach to difficult pain problems, textbooks on the topic of pain have mushroomed in the last 10 years. A majority of these textbooks have been excellent in presenting academic and organized clinical information, advancing our understanding and appropriate management of the patient with difficult pain problems. However, there has been a need to tie this knowledge to our daily practice in a quick and concise way, without having to rummage through reams of available information.

The purpose of this textbook is just to provide exactly that: to present information from clinical experts that can be immediately applied in the management of a particular problem seen in everyday practice. Each chapter starts with a case presentation, followed by a clinical expert's discussion, providing a trainee or a non–pain specialist a basic understanding of the problem and a clinical expert's view of management. We are all aware that there are several approaches to difficult pain management; the editor and contributing authors do not mean to imply that the recommendations presented here are the only correct approaches.

The cases selected are based on the clinical experience of the editor over several years. The cases are meant to illustrate the more common problems referred to a pain management center because they have proven extremely difficult for the average physician to manage; by no means are they comprehensive. To facilitate a quick reference guide, sections have been divided into anatomic areas: head and neck, upper extremities, chest, abdomen, back, and lower extremities. A special section on cancer pain and psychological issues is also included. To emphasize the need for an interdisciplinary approach, the first two chapters present the general principles of evaluation and management of difficult pain problems.

The contributions of the authors are deeply appreciated. They are all busy clinicians and researchers who took precious time to provide a concise description of each case and useful methods of management. Although approaches may be biased according to areas of expertise, specialty, and work environment, contributors approached each case with utmost thought based on their vast clinical experience.

Although this book was prepared for clinicians interested in pain management, and residents and fellows in training for most specialties, clinicians in the community who are struggling with difficult pain patients, and perhaps even the patients themselves, may find this book helpful.

I would like to acknowledge the secretarial support of Edward Daniels, who single-handedly typed all of the manuscripts.

THERESA FERRER-BRECHNER, M.D.

CONTENTS

1

Basic Considerations in Evaluation of Chronic Pain

Theresa Ferrer-Brechner, M.D.
Laura Darke, Ph.D.

Physical evaluation of pain can range from being simplistic to complicated. During pain of acute duration, the cause of pain is easily definable and can be disease focused, and is not within the scope of this book. For more difficult acute pain problems with inpatients (such as severe postoperative pain, trauma pain, sickle cell crisis), it is important to immediately evaluate if the patient is grossly undermedicated or if analgesics are not being given on a regular basis, to maintain a constant and reasonable blood level. If undermedication is a problem, the cause should be immediately identified and corrected. Often, the reason can be bias of caregivers toward narcotic analgesics or the nurse may be too busy to attend to a particular patient. The medication chart, usually not included with the patient's chart, should be reviewed daily to determine the exact dosage and frequency of medications. For the evaluation and treatment of acute pain, anesthesiology-based acute pain services have been recently established.[1]

However, when pain becomes prolonged beyond the identified course of the disease, evaluation of pain becomes extremely complicated, requiring the concerted efforts of physicians, psychologists, and physical therapists. Physical evaluation should include not only traditional history and physical examination, but also other nontraditional methods of evaluating patients with pain complaints (Table 1–1). The aim of such an evaluation is to determine if both sensory or physical and affective or emotional factors are influencing the pain experience.[2]

1

TABLE 1–1.

Specialized Evaluation of Chronic Pain

Physician	Physical Therapist	Psychologist
Determination of physical mechanism of pain (nociceptive, deafferentation, or sympathetically mediated)	Physical/functional capacity	Psychosocial functional capacity
Pharmacologic history	Examination of myofascial structures and joints	Operant factors Litigation Medications Family
Examination of myofascial structures and joints		Psychopathology requiring attention before treatment Pain language

PHYSICAL ASSESSMENT OF CHRONIC PAIN

The pathophysiology of pain can be clarified by a thorough neurological exam, myofascial and joint examination and, if necessary, a differential nerve blocking procedure. Neurological examination can determine if pain is nociceptive, deafferentation, or sympathetically mediated in nature. Nociceptive pain is usually caused by irritation of peripheral nerve endings (e.g., somatic nerve impingement in the paravertebral area), while deafferentation pain occurs when there is eventual partial to complete neural damage (e.g., postherpetic neuralgia), usually characterized by lack of pinprick sensation in the area of pain complaint. Sympathetic mediated pain is characterized usually by burning pain in a hyperesthetic cold extremity and is caused by sympathetic hyperreflexia (e.g., reflex sympathetic dystrophy). Myofascial pain syndromes are characterized by existence of identifiable triggers in muscle bands, which replicate the pain complaint. Diagnostic injection of local anesthetic into the area of the trigger immediately removes the pain. Examination of various muscle groups requires special training, since myofascial examination was not part of medical school training. For more information, see Simon and Travell's descriptions of myofascial triggers and their respective pain radiation.[3] The characteristics of these pain mechanisms are listed in Table 1–2.

Differential nerve blocking can be helpful in determining whether pain is somatic nerve-mediated, sympathetic mediated, or centrally mediated.[4] Examples of useful diagnostic nerve blocks for chronic pain include differential epidural block, autonomic blocks, paravertebral somatic nerve blocks, facet nerve blocks, and myofascial trigger point injections. Appropriate semiquantitative pain scales measuring both magnitude and multidimensional aspects of pain, as well as neurologic assessment, should be performed before and after the diagnostic procedure. Evidence of an existing neural blockade must be demonstrated before a conclusion is made as to whether the nerve block has an effect on the pain experience. If a somatic nerve block is being performed, a sign of decreased response to pinprick sensation must be demonstrable along the dermatomal distribution of nerves being blocked before concluding the block's effect on the pain experience. For sympathetic block, it is necessary to demonstrate a temperature rise of at least 2°C or a decreased psychogalvanic response.

The total pain experience can be the result of one or a combination of these different mechanisms. It is important to identify the predominant mechanism so that specific appropriate physical treatments can be applied in conjunction with the pain program.

TABLE 1–2.

Physical Mechanisms of Chronic Pain

Mechanism	Characteristics	Examples
I Nociceptive	Dermatomal distribution No sensory or motor loss Shooting pain	Bone lesions Borderline disc protrusion
II Deafferentation	Sensory loss in area of pain Dysesthesia/hyperesthesia Shooting or burning pain	Postherpetic neuralgia Postthoracotomy Postmastectomy pain
III Sympathetic mediated	No sensory loss Hypersthesia Decreased temperature Burning pain	Reflex sympathetic dystrophy
IV Myofascial	Trigger points in muscle bands Stimulation of triggers replicates pain Injection of triggers stops pain Perpetuating factors: posture, stress, etc.	Quadratus lumborum trigger points producing low back pain Splenius capitus trigger points producing frontal headache
V Visceral	Deep, gnawing pain Constant or colicky Accompanying GI symptoms	Pancreatitis pain Gastric carcinoma

PSYCHOLOGICAL ASSESSMENT IN CHRONIC PAIN PATIENTS

The rationale for psychological assessment of chronic pain patients is based on the notion that chronic pain problems are extremely complex with many perpetuating factors. Psychological and behavioral factors play an important role in perpetuating chronic pain problems.

For example, affective disturbances (e.g., depression, anxiety, anger) and heightened stress levels can serve to enhance the patient's perception of pain.[5] Also, certain personality styles contribute to extreme somatic focusing and excessive use of medical systems.[6]

Behavioral styles can also play a role in perpetuating pain problems.[7] Excessive inactivity or "downtime" can be problematic for a number of reasons. First, inactivity can lead to muscle degeneration and a number of other medical problems. In addition, when inactive lifestyle patterns persist for long periods of time, the patient's "wellness" behaviors tend to diminish or fade from the patient's behavioral repertoire. The opposite behavioral problem involves excessive problems with pacing. These patients tend to "work to tolerance" and then collapse.

When a pain problem persists for a long period of time, pain behavior is susceptible to all known learning principles. The principles of operant conditioning are especially important in the development of chronic pain. Any behavior that is reinforced either by the application of a positive reward (positive reinforcement) or the removal of an aversive stimulus (negative reinforcement) will, through trials of learning, tend to increase in frequency. The positive rewards for emitting pain behaviors are many, varied, and often very personal. They include: attention, nurturance, massage, money, litigation, "special patient" status, etc. The negative reinforcers are also often complex and include avoidance of work and responsibilities, avoidance of complex psychological problems, etc.

It is also important to remember that *any intervention that reduces pain will serve as a negative reinforcer.* This has very important implications for the management of chronic pain. In general, any intervention that has been reinforcing in that it has reduced pain (visits to doctors, medications, massages, etc.) need to be placed on a "time-contingent" schedule to avoid being paired with extreme pain behaviors.

The patient and his or her family will often have a number of questions regarding the purpose of the psychological evaluation. It is helpful to explain to the patient that the reason he or she is being seen by a psychologist is not because the team considers the patient to be "crazy," but rather because chronic pain problems often have an important impact on life functioning; disrupt everyday activities; result in secondary psychological problems; have been associated with failure and frustration with the medical system; and that these and other per-

TABLE 1–3.

Common Psychological Assessment Tools for
Chronic Pain Patients

MMPI
Structured interview with patient and significant other
Additional data
  Behavioral observation
  Other self-report measures
  UCLA Pain Profile
    Pain diaries
    McGill Pain Questionnaire
    Beck Depression Inventory
    Chronic Illness Problem Inventory
    Visual analogue scales

sonality and behavioral issues interact with physical problems in a very complex way.

Psychological assessment of chronic pain patients is different from traditional psychological assessment in many important ways. The focus is on aiding medical management and *not* on obtaining diagnostic labels. This type of assessment is structured or semistructured in format and is designed to answer specific behavioral questions and yield specific behavioral recommendations.

The common assessment instruments utilized by psychologists at the UCLA Pain Management Center are listed in Table 1–3, and the written outline for the psychological evaluation is listed in Table 1–4.

Each of these headings will be explained in some detail. The *mental status examination* is given to any patient where it is expected that there may be significant problems with cognition, psychosis, or suicidal and homicidal ideation. The mental status examination includes assessment for orientation (to person, place, and time), short- and long-term memory, mood and affect, thought process, insight and judgment, and suicidal or homicidal ideation. If no problems

TABLE 1–4.

Content of Psychological
Evaluation Report

Mental status examination
Current psychological functioning
Psychosocial factors
Factors impacting on pain treatment
Recommendations

are noted in this area, this section will usually read: "within normal limits" or "WNL."

The next section of the written report focuses on *current psychological functioning*. This section provides a behavioral description of the pain problem and its impact on the patient's life. The emphasis is on behavioral assessment of antecedents and consequences of pain behaviors. For example, what activities or behaviors tend to trigger the pain problem and what tends to occur after the pain is in progress? Testing results (e.g., MMPI, Beck, CIPI) are also discussed and explained with emphasis on implications for chronic pain management. Reactive psychological problems, as well as premorbid psychological issues are also addressed in this section.

The section dealing with *psychosocial factors* is included to give the pain management team information regarding: educational and occupational status (level of sophistication), marital status and living situation (level of support), degree of life stress, historical factors relevant to the pain problem, and financial factors such as disability or litigation status.

Factors impacting on pain management treatment are so important and relevant to treatment decisions that this section is broken into several content areas:

Operant Factors.—These include all reinforcement issues that are found to be relevant to maintaining the chronic pain problem. These may include excessive marital or family attention contingent on pain behavior, disability or litigation, avoidance of work, sex, or complex psychological issues.

Respondent Factors.—These include all factors which automatically or through conditioning *trigger* the pain response. These may include known organic factors, stress factors, or certain behavioral activities.

Emotional Factors.—These include all reactive or endogenous affective factors that may play a role in perpetuating the pain problem. Depressive reactions are a common and understandable consequence of many pain problems, yet the severity of the depression may require treatment to focus on both pain and depression.

Compliance Factors.—A prediction of compliance based on an assessment of patient motivation level, insight and judgment, level of distress, adequate intellectual ability, and logistical factors such as distance and travel.

Medication Factors.—These include medication behaviors, family history of drug or alcohol problems, relevant historical factors, a statement of addiction-proneness, and alcohol/recreation drug use.

Somatic Factors.—These include a brief statement on the patient's utilization of the medical system, past medical treatments, patient's history of seeking invasive medical procedures, historical reactions to medical procedures, etc.

The *recommendations* section of the written report is the most important in that it is often the focus of the pain manager's attention. The section should be structured and focused and should, at minimum, include a statement on:

1. Treatment contracting, with specific suggestions for establishing behavioral goals, setting limits and contingencies, and establishing "exit strategies."
2. Suggestions for behavioral management of problematic behavioral patterns.
3. Suggestions for appropriate psychological and behavioral interventions such as pain class or individual relaxation training, hypnosis and imagery, biofeedback, marital and family intervention, cognitive behavioral interventions, etc.
4. Suggestions for further psychiatric evaluations for psychotropic intervention.
5. Contraindications to somatic or invasive procedures.
6. Suggestions for other outside referrals for further assessments (e.g., cognitive or neuropsychological assessments) or interventions (long-term psychotherapy, marital/family therapy, etc.).
7. Suggestions for inpatient pain programs when behavioral or psychological factors are especially severe.

EVALUATION OF PAIN LANGUAGE

Assessment of pain experience includes daily diaries that give an insight to the precipitating factors increasing pain, pattern of medication intake, and changing levels of pain intensity, as well as activity level on an hour-to-hour basis. An example of a pain diary is in Figure 1–1.

During each visit, patients can express their pain intensity levels by using a semiquantitative pain intensity visual analogue scale (VAS), which later can be plotted over a period of time.[8] In addition, the sensory and affective dimension of pain experience can also be measured during evaluation and repetitively during treatment by utilizing the McGill Pain Questionnaire (MPQ) during each visit.[9] A suggested algorithm for evaluation of chronic pain is shown in Figure 1–2.

The results of the team evaluation are best conveyed only to the managing physician, who in turn will be the primary spokesperson to the patient. This prevents any possibility of giving confusing information to the patient, and also prevents splitting of therapists. It is also important that all current or past phy-

UCLA PAIN MANAGEMENT CENTER
<u>HOURLY DIARY</u>

NAME: _____ DATE: _____

Time	Pain Rating (0–10)	Medication (Type/Amount)	Major Activity for the Hour (Be Specific)
5:00–6:00			
6:00–7:00			
7:00–8:00			
8:00–9:00			
9:00–10:00			
10:00–11:00			
11:00–12:00			
12:00–1:00			
1:00–2:00			
2:00–3:00			
3:00–4:00			
4:00–5:00			
5:00–6:00			
6:00–7:00			
7:00–8:00			
8:00–9:00			
9:00–10:00			
10:00–11:00			
11:00–12:00			
12:00–1:00			
1:00–2:00			
2:00–3:00			
3:00–4:00			
4:00–5:00			

FIG 1–1.
Example of a daily pain diary.

sicians be informed of the results of multidisciplinary/interdisciplinary evaluation. If possible, the outside physician's participation in the patient's pain treatments should be suspended while the pain evaluation and treatments are being administered.

In summary, the evaluation of difficult pain patients requires the concerted efforts of a physician, psychologist, and perhaps a physical therapist. The evaluations include physical, functional, and psychological dimensions of pain experience. Information is then filtered to the managing physician, who conveys the information to the patient.

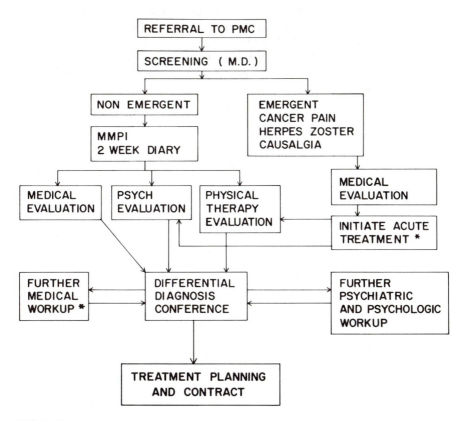

FIG 1–2.
Algorithm for evaluation of chronic pain.

REFERENCES

1. Ready BL, Oden R, Chadwick HS, et al: Development of anesthesiology based postoperative pain management service. *Anesthesiology* 1988; 68:100–106.
2. Fordyce WE: A behavioral perspective on chronic pain, in Ng LLK, Bonica JJ (eds): *Pain, Discomfort and Humanitarian Care.* New York, Elsevier/North Holland, 1980, p. 223.
3. Travell J, Simon DG: *Myofascial Pain and Dysfunction: The Trigger Point Manual.* Baltimore, Williams & Wilkins, 1983.
4. Ghia JN, Toomy TC, Mao W, et al: Towards an understanding of chronic pain mechanisms: The use of psychologic tests and a refined differential spinal block. *Anesthesiology* 1979; 50:20–25.
5. Romand JM, Turner JA: Chronic pain and depression: Does the evidence support the relationship? *Psychol Bull* 1985; 96:18–34.
6. Sternback RA: *Pain Patients: Traits and Treatments.* New York, Academic Press, 1974.
7. Fordyce WE, Steger JC: Chronic pain, in Pomerleau OF, Brady JP (eds): *Behavioral Medicine: Theory and Practice.* Baltimore, Williams & Wilkins, 1979.
8. Wallenstain SL, Heidrich G, Kaiko E, et al: Clinical evaluation of mild analgesics. The measurement of clinical pain. *Br J Clin Pharmacol* 1980; 10(suppl):3195–3275.
9. Melzack R: The McGill Pain Questionnaire: Major properties and scoring methods. *Pain* 1975; 1:277–299.

2

Basic Considerations in the Treatment of Chronic Pain

Theresa Ferrer-Brechner, M.D.
Laura Darke, Ph.D.

Treatment programs for difficult chronic pain problems require the concerted efforts of multidisciplinary health care professionals. Often, the pain management team needs to meet on a regular basis to ensure that the program is being carried out as planned. An interdisciplinary or multidisciplinary team is ideal but may prove too costly or difficult to coordinate under some circumstances. If a primary physician needs to coordinate a pain program, without the luxury of a multidisciplinary team, it is important to remember several ingredients that promote success: (1) establish a program contract, outlining goals and behavioral requirements for the patient; (2) inform all previous physicians and present consultants that you will assume the total responsibility of all pain medications and pain treatments; (3) inform all consultants that results of all evaluations are to be conveyed to the pain manager instead of to the patient; (4) establish a treatment program where all interventions and doctor's visits are arranged on a time contingent rather than a pain contingent basis over the specified period of time, for example, 6 to 8 weeks.

Treatment begins with the "treatment planning meeting." During this meeting, information obtained from the consultants or pain management team is presented to the patient by the primary physician or pain manager. Utilizing a primary physician as the only person giving information to the patient prevents confusion and an opportunity for the patient to "split" therapists. On the other hand, with cases where psychological information may make feedback a difficult or sensitive situation, it may be wise to also include a psychologist during this treatment planning meeting.

The types of treatment currently available for chronic pain fall primarily into five major categories (Table 2–1). A patient's individual program usually includes medical, cognitive/behavioral, and physical therapy interventions. Medical interventions include: pharmacologic tailoring, neurostimulation, and neural blocking procedures.

TABLE 2–1.

Five Categories of Chronic Pain

Medical interventions
  Pharmacologic therapy
    Systematic withdrawal from narcotic analgesics and
      sedatives
    Tricyclic antidepressants
    Anticonvulsant drugs for deafferentation pain
Neurostimulatory techniques
  Central stimulation
  Spinal cord stimulation
  Peripheral stimulation
Neural blocking
  Sympathetic blocks
  Epidural blocks
  Somatic nerve block
  Facet nerve block
  Trigger point injections
Psychological interventions
  Cognitive/behavioral therapy
    Education
    Skills acquisition: coping skills, relaxation and stress man-
      agement skills, appropriate patient behaviors, etc.
    Treatment of affective disturbances
    Operant reconditioning/behavior modification
Adjunctive Interventions
  Physical Therapy/Rehabilitation
    Education (i.e., perpetuating factors)
    Activation programs
    Stretching and strengthening programs
    Posture and body mechanics programs
    Joint mobilizations

MEDICAL INTERVENTIONS

Pharmacologic Therapy

Chronic (nonmalignant) pain patients are often referred to a pain center because their physicians no longer feel comfortable managing the complicated poly-pharmacy that is common in this group. In part, this polypharmacy problem results because physicians continue to treat chronic pain patients as if they had acute pain, and because patients with persistent pain visit many physicians and clinics who easily prescribe analgesics as a stop-gap measure. Prescription of centrally acting narcotic analgesics is contraindicated in patients with chronic nonmalignant pain because tolerance is inevitable, drug dependence will ensue with continued use, and side effects such as sedation, dysphoria, sleep distur-bance, or even psychosis may eventually occur.

If a patient comes to the pain center with complicated polypharmacy, im-mediate detoxification is necessary before any pain program can be effective. The steps for detoxification/substitution, as described by Halpern, consists of the following: (1) determination of 24-hour dosage of drug(s) taken while in a hospital environment for 1–2 days (or 1–2 weeks in an outpatient setting) in order to obtain a "drug profile"; (2) substitution of short-acting narcotic anal-gesics and sedatives for long-acting narcotics, such as methadone, and long-acting sedatives, such as phenobarbital; (3) combination of all substituted med-ication in a masking vehicle, such as cherry syrup ("pain cocktail").[1] While keeping the volume constant, the active medications are decreased 15–20% per week. If insomnia occurs, a tricyclic antidepressant may be added at bedtime.

Pharmacologic control of chronic nonmalignant pain is often best achieved by utilizing non-narcotic medications. Tricyclic antidepressants can block the re-uptake of serotonin and norepinephrine, thereby increasing their availability. Potentiation of adrenergic, serotonergic, and opiate pathways has been theoret-ically linked to a clinical tricyclic effect. Hameroff, in a well-designed study, evaluated the clinical effect of doxepin hydrochloride on measurable aspects of chronic neck and back pain and related depression. In a double blind technique, comparison of doxepin and a placebo over a six-week period indicated that the doxepin group had lower pain severity, decreased percentage of time pain was perceived, decreased pain associated with activity, decreased muscle tension, and improved sleep. These changes occurred between the fourth and sixth week of treatment. However, blood levels of beta endorphin and enkephalin did not differ between the doxepin-treated and placebo-treated group.[2]

The use of tricyclics has also been advocated for neuralgia and diabetic neuropathy. The analgesic effect of tricyclics have been shown to be independent of their antidepressant action and, therefore, may be related to their serotonergic action. Anticonvulsants have been used successfully in treating orofacial pain such as tic douloureux. Anti-inflammatory agents can be used if a chronic inflammatory process is suspected in chronic pain.

Neurostimulatory Techniques

Neurostimulatory techniques for pain control include central stimulation, spinal cord stimulation, and peripheral stimulation.

Central stimulation-induced analgesia can be achieved by stimulation of the periaqueductal gray (PAG) in animals and periventricular gray (PVG) in humans. The mechanism for the induced analgesia includes stimulation of the release of naturally occurring opiate-like peptides (endorphins) into the cerebrospinal fluid, thus producing pain relief diffusely throughout the body. The endorphins are hypothesized to enhance the descending pain inhibitory system from the brain stem to the raphe magnus, dorso-lateral funiculus, and eventually in the dorsal horn of the spinal cord, suppressing the ascending pain transmission pathway.[3] The development of tolerance to repetitive stimulation, presence of cross-tolerance to morphine, and antagonism of the resultant analgesia with naloxone, an opiate antagonist, has led to the idea that PVG-PAG stimulation-induced analgesia (SPA) was due primarily to the release of endorphins. However, subsequent studies suggest that naloxone does not reliably antagonize central SPA and that CSF endorphin levels do not always correlate with pain relief after deep brain stimulation (DBS).[4-5] Even cancer patients tolerant to high dosages of narcotics responded to PVG-PAG stimulation, signifying a nonopiate mechanism.[6]

Stimulating electrodes are usually placed by a neurosurgeon with sterotactic techniques under local anesthesia via a burr hole.[7] Electrodes are lowered in both the periaqueductal (PAG)-periventricular (PVG) region and in the somatosensory thalamic relay nuclei. For facial pain, thalamic electrodes are usually placed in the nucleus ventralis posteromedialis (VPM), and for extremity pain, in the nucleus ventralis posterolateralis (VPL). The electrodes are externalized via a small stub wound in the scalp and then the connecting wires are internalized under the skin and connected to a receiver that is activated by an external radiofrequency transmitter. The patient is then taught to self-stimulate for 20–30 minutes, 3–4 times per day.

This type of procedure is reserved for the chronic pain patient who has undergone a thorough evaluation in a pain center, for whom other noninvasive techniques have failed to provide significant consistent pain relief. Success for this type of treatment ranges from 60% to 70%.[8]

Peripheral mechanical or electrical stimulation of peripheral nerves in the form of acupuncture, transcutaneous electrical nerve stimulation (TENS), and trigger point injections, are often used for the control of chronic pain. Possible mechanisms of action for acute pain relief include: (1) stimulation of large somatic fibers, thus inhibiting small afferent nociceptive fibers in the dorsal horn of the spinal cord; and (2) sympathetic nervous system inhibition with resultant increase in microcirculation and chemical environment of nociceptors.

Acupuncture, in modern medicine, is performed by inserting a sterile stainless steel needle into the skin and underlying muscles, either near or distal to the pain area. It has been found that classical acupuncture points correspond to well-known trigger points. Needle puncture is known to induce current injury, which may provoke strong sympathetic and parasympathetic effect. Low frequency stimulation of acupuncture sites has been shown to release endorphins and acupuncture analgesia in animals is reversed by naloxone.[9–10] Clinically, acupuncture is primarily used for patients with myofascial pain and deafferentation pain, as one of the physical modalities of a pain program.

Transcutaneous electrical nerve stimulation (TENS) can be administered as a low frequency (2–20 Hz) high intensity stimulation, or as a high frequency (20–100 Hz) low intensity stimulation. Newer models incorporate both types of stimulations. Review of TENS therapy indicates short-term relief in 60% to 70% of chronic pain patients, but over time beneficial effects faded in 30%.[11] Unlike acupuncture, laboratory applications of TENS fail to show endorphin release.[12] TENS is theorized to induce sympathetic inhibition since vasodilation is associated with its application, thus it has been used to promote healing of ulcerative lesions.[13] In clinical practice, TENS can be a useful adjunct to a pain program, especially because the patients and their families can be taught to use this device at home, thus promoting self-management.

Neural Blocking

Permanent neuroablation by chemical or surgical techniques are invasive procedures and should be reserved primarily for terminal cancer patients. By and large, chronic nonmalignant pain should not be treated with a permanent neural interruption, since deafferentation pain can occur 4–6 months later and will be more difficult to treat. There are, however, some local anesthetic blocks that can be a useful adjunct in the management of chronic pain, such as epidural steroid block for nonsurgical low back pain with radiculopathy, facet nerve block with cryoprobe for facet arthralgia, sympathetic blocks for causalgia and herpes zoster, and trigger point injections for myofascial pain syndrome.[14–15] The number of nerve blocks must be limited in number (usually 6–8), and discontinued if it reinforces pain behavior and increases pain reports. It should also conform with a behavioral approach, thus, given time contingently, continued administration being dependent on increased activity, decreased medication, and decreased pain reports.

For cancer pain, therapeutic nerve block is indicated, especially when there is progressive disease and narcotic analgesic therapy is beginning to induce more side effects than analgesia. Since the early 1900s, neurolytic blocks have been commonly used by anesthesiologists for the management of localized cancer related pain. Various neurolytic substances have been injected into accessible plexuses and nerves in an attempt to permanently block afferent nociceptive fibers.

Trigger point injections have been done with saline, 0.5% procaine or 0.5% lidocaine in volumes of 0.5–2 cc. Studies show that procaine has less long-term muscle injury than lidocaine, making it a more ideal agent. A vapo-coolant spray, followed by muscle stretch, can be used for myofascial therapy. This can be combined with trigger point injections and physical therapy for maximum effect. For a review on management of myofascial pain with trigger point injection, spray and stretch, refer to Simon and Travell.[16]

PSYCHOLOGICAL INTERVENTIONS

Cognitive/Behavioral Therapy Education

One of the most important functions of a psychologist in a pain management setting is to educate the patient. Formal didactic programs can be done at either an individual or "pain class" level. Such programs educate patients regarding the complexity of chronic pain problems and the importance of perpetuating factors. Factors that perpetuate a patient's chronic pain problem may be behavioral, physiological, postural, affective, operant, and so on. When the patient becomes aware of the unique set of perpetuating factors that are maintaining or exacerbating the pain problem, he or she can then play an active role in the pain management program.

Skills Acquisition

The psychologist also serves to teach the patient a number of skills that will be important for the patient to self-manage the pain problem. These include coping skills, relaxation and stress management skills, appropriate patient behaviors, hypnosis, biofeedback, and activity management skills. Most of these skills are aimed at enhancing the patient's control over his or her sympathetic nervous system responses and increasing the patient's perceived control or self-efficacy.

Treatment of Affective Disturbances

When affective disturbances are severe, they need to be treated either before initiating the pain program or concomitant with the pain program. For example, when depressive reactions are extreme, there is often evidence of poor pain discriminability, which may preclude the efficiency of several somatic procedures. Vegetative symptoms associated with affective disorders can worsen pain problems by disturbing sleep, decreasing daytime activity levels, and enhancing pain perception. Anxiety and phobic reactions also may need to be managed before invasive procedures are attempted. Psychiatric consultations may become necessary when affective disturbances are severe or complex.

Operant Reconditioning/Behavior Modification

In a majority of cases, chronic pain patients have experienced systematic and repetitive reinforcement following emission of pain behaviors. These reinforcers are many, varied, and extremely personal, and include: attention from loved ones and the medical community, rest, medications, avoidance of work and other responsibilities, disability compensation, and litigation. At the same time, wellness behaviors have often been ignored or actively punished. Thus, many patients have been influenced by this operant conditioning, and behavior modification is necessary. In essence, the behavioral patterns of "sick behavior" must be replaced by "well behavior" through a conditioning process that establishes healthy behaviors. This is necessary if the patient's life style is to be constructively altered. Vocational activities that reinforce increased activity, discontinue rewards for "sick behavior" both at home and in the medical setting, establish new behavior patterns, and provide family education to change the patient's home social environment, are all necessary for a successful pain rehabilitation program. For a detailed review of the basic principles of behavior modification, refer to Fordyce.[17] The basic ingredients include: (1) alterations of pain behaviors; (2) establishment of rest made contingent on work, instead of pain, and incremental quotas of exercise are used to increase activity; (3) medication consumption is switched to a time contingent rather than pain contingent basis, and then systematically reduced; (4) social/interpersonal responses to pain behaviors are altered by systematic training of professional staff and family members; (5) promotion of re-engagement in work or other meaningful activities.

Behavioral treatments of chronic pain has been reviewed by Linton.[18] This critical exam of various published studies since 1982 indicates that an operant program is effective in increasing activity levels and decreasing medication consumption. Less impact is seen in reported levels of pain and mood. Relaxation techniques, such as biofeedback, produce mixed results. However, when relaxation was used as a coping strategy, it was helpful in controlling pain ratings, but not necessarily in increasing activity. The treatment gains tend to be maintained at follow-up and patients tend to continue utilizing techniques, although at lower rates than recommended, at the end of the program. The clinical implications of this review indicate that the clinician should match treatment methods to patients' needs, based on their evaluation. If the goal is to decrease pain intensity reports, relaxation with coping strategies may be considered. If it is important to increase activity and decrease medication, then an operant program dealing with these behaviors is in order. Whether or not this is done on an inpatient or outpatient program is dependent on the severity of inactivity, medication intake, and expected degree of compliance.

ADJUNCTIVE INTERVENTIONS

Physical therapy/rehabilitation interventions should include education regarding perpetuating factors, progressive activation, stretching and strengthening, and training in posture and body mechanics.

There are two types of physical therapy interventions that are indicated for chronic pain patients. One is the traditional "hands-on" physical therapy that may include ultrasound, massage, and joint mobilization. During the physical therapy evaluation, determination is made whether or not hands-on physical therapy is indicated. If it is indicated, the treatments should be time contingent (2–3 times per week), and of short duration (4–6 weeks). Care should be taken that the patient's pain behavior is not reinforced by passive treatments and that increased functionality occurs with treatment.

The second type of physical therapy is a "hands-off" program where the emphasis is on patient participation and a graduated increase in physical therapy activities (bicycle exercises, home exercises, etc.), as proposed by Fordyce. A quota for home exercises is given to the patient on a weekly basis. For myofascial pain, a spray and stretch program can be taught to the patient and a significant other. Usually, the home program consists of spray with a vapocoolant material followed by stretching for 6 seconds, 6 times per session. A total of 6 sessions per day is usually recommended.

REFERENCES

1. Halpern LM: Substitution-detoxification and its role in the management of chronic benign pain. *J Clin Psychiatry* 1982; 43:8, 10–14.
2. Hameroff SR, Cork RC, Weiss JL, et al: Doxepin effects on chronic pain and depression: A controlled study, in Fields HL, et al (eds): *Advances in Pain Research and Therapy.* vol 9, New York, Raven Press, 1985, pp 761–771.
3. Sherman JE, Liebeskind JC: An endorphinergic-centrifugal substrate of pain modulation: Recent findings, current concepts and complexities, in Bonica JJ (ed): *Pain* vol 58, Association for Research in Nervous and Mental Disease, New York, Raven Press, 1980, pp 190–204.
4. Carstens E, Guinan MJ, MacKinnon JD: Naloxone does not consistently affect inhibition of spinal nociceptive transmission produced by medial diencephalic stimulation in the cat. *Neurosci Lett* 1983; 42:76–80.

5. Amano K, Kitamura K, Kawamura H, et al: Alterations on immunoreactive betaendorphin in the third ventricular fluid in responses to electrical stimulation of the human periaqueductal gray matter. *Appl Neurophysiol* 1980; 13:150–158.
6. Young R, Brechner T: Electrical stimulation of the brain for relief of intractable pain due to cancer. *Cancer* 1986; 57:1266–1272.
7. Young RF, Feldman RA, Kroening R, et al: Electrical stimulation of the brain in the treatment of chronic pain in man, in Kruger L, Liebeskind JC (eds): *Advances in Pain Research and Therapy,* vol 6, New York, Raven Press, 1984, pp 289–303.
8. Hosobuchi Y: The current status of analgesic brain stimulation. *Acta Neurochir [Suppl] (Wien)* 1980; 30:219–227.
9. Sjolund B, Terenius L, Eriksson M: Increased cerebrospinal fluid levels of endorphins after electropuncture. *Acta Physiol Scand* 1977; 100:382–383.
10. Pomeranz B, Chiu D: Naloxone blockade of acupuncture analgesia: Endorphin implicated. *Life Sci* 1976; 19:1757–1762.
11. Loeser JD, Black RG, Christman A: Relief of pain by transcutaneous stimulation. *J Neurosurg* 1975; 42:308–314.
12. Chapman CR, Benedetti C, Colpitts YH, et al: Naloxone fails to reverse pain thresholds elevated by acupuncture: Acupuncture analgesia reconsidered. *Pain* 1983; 16:13–31.
13. Kaada B: Vasodilation induced by transcutaneous nerve stimulation in peripheral ischemia (Reynaud's phenomenon and diabetic polyneuropathy). *Eur Heart J* 1982; 3:303–314.
14. Benzon HT: Epidural steroid for low back pain and lumbosacral radiculopathy. *Pain* 1986; 24:277–295.
15. Brechner T: Percutaneous cryogenic neurolysis of the articular nerve of Luschka. *Reg Anaesth* (Suppl. I) 1981; 6:18.
16. Travell JG, Simon DG: *Myofascial Pain and Dysfunction: The Trigger Point Manual.* Baltimore, Williams & Wilkins Co., 1983.
17. Fordyce WT: A behavioral perspective on chronic pain, in Ng LLK, Bonica JJ (eds): *Pain, Discomfort and Humanitarian Care,* New York, Elsevier/North Holland, 1980, p. 233.
18. Linton SJ: Behavioral remediation of chronic pain: A status report. *Pain* 1986; 24:125–141.

PART I

Head and Neck Pain

3

Atypical Odontalgia

Steven B. Graff-Radford, D.D.S.
William K. Solberg, D.D.S., M.S.D.

A 56-year-old woman was referred to the UCLA Clinical Research Center for evaluation of tooth pain of unexplained origin. This pain began 7 years prior to the visit following a routine dental scaling. The patient described the pain as initiating in a maxillary first molar tooth, and although nothing abnormal was discovered on the radiogram taken at the time, the tooth was endodontically treated without success. The patient continued complaining of a steady, continuous, dull, and throbbing pain in the region of the maxillary posterior teeth, which prompted the dentist to endodontically treat the second premolar. This treatment was also ineffective as was a subsequent root canal treatment performed on the second molar three years later. The patient was at this time desperate, and found a dentist who extracted three teeth at her insistence although no local abnormality could be detected. A neurologist was consulted who felt the condition was dental and referred her back to her dentist. The pain was somewhat aggravated by cold, and could not be alleviated. Detailed physical examinations of the intraoral and extraoral structures provided no clue to etiology. Thermographic study revealed a region of increased heat emission in the area of the maxillary molars. Sensory neural blockade proved equivocal, but a stellate ganglion block decreased the pain by 75% for 5 hours. The patient was treated with up to 100 mg of amitriptyline and reported a 75% reduction in pain. One milligram of fluphenazine was added, which enhanced the relief to +80%. The patient has managed to stop the fluphenazine and decrease the amitriptyline to 50 mg, and maintains the 80% pain reduction. She reports that further reduction of medications increases the pain.

DISCUSSION

Toothache is often referred to as the severest and most common orofacial pain problem.[1] Typically, the dentist is equipped to quickly remove the causative factor of acute dental pain. When the local cause is not obvious, the problem is far less readily treated and often involves numerous unnecessary invasive treatments and consultation from various disciplines. This form of pain where there is no obvious organic cause has been referred to as atypical odontalgia (AO).[2]

Atypical odontalgia is a poorly understood phenomenon associated with persistent pain in apparently normal teeth and surrounding alveolar bone.[3] It derives its name from the broad category "atypical facial pain," which serves as a wastebasket for any facial pain the clinician is unable to diagnose.[4] Atypical odontalgia presents clinically in a manner similar to pulpal pain and regrettably, it is usually diagnosed only after failure of numerous invasive dental treatment. These treatments may occasionally eliminate the pain for a short period of time, thereby adding to the confusion. Numerous other terms have been used to describe this problem, including vascular toothache, phantom tooth pain, migrainous neuralgia, atypical facial pain, atypical facial neuralgia and dental causalgia.[4-8] The only inclusionary criterion positive to all these problems is the location of the pain. Therefore, it is at this point that a diagnosis is made, primarily by exclusion.

Clinical Characteristics.—The clinical features have been described by numerous investigators, but without concern for using the same parameters. The characteristics of 37 AO patients studied by the authors are summarized in Tables 3–1 to 3–3. AO appears to be a problem primarily affecting females in the fourth and fifth decade. The pain is an aching, burning, or throbbing sensation of moderate intensity and localized most often to a maxillary molar or premolar tooth.

TABLE 3–1.

Descriptive Data From 37 Patients With Atypical Odontalgia

Age	47.6 + 12.5 yr	—
Duration since onset	2.5 + 2.7 yr	—
Sex (%)	86.5 F	
	13.5 M	
Pattern of occurrence	Continuous	

TABLE 3–2.
Character of Pain in 37 Patients With Atypical Odontalgia*

Word	Patients Choosing Word (%)	McGill Category
Aching	41.6	Sensory
Burning	36.1	Sensory
Exhausting	36.1	Affective
Radiating	33.3	Miscellaneous
Nagging	33.3	Miscellaneous
Throbbing	30.6	Sensory
Tender	27.8	Sensory

*Most frequent word chosen on the McGill Pain Questionnaire.

Pathophysiology.—Several theories have been proposed to explain the mechanism of AO. The most often written about are psychological disorders, deafferentation, and vascular mechanisms.[3–8] There is little objective evidence supporting any of these mechanisms. By and large the proof for psychogenic pathophysiology is derived from clinical interview. In an attempt to determine the role of psychopathology, the authors administered the Minnesota Multiphasic Personality Inventory to 19 AO patients and 19 age, sex, and duration of pain-matched headache patients. There was no significant difference between the

TABLE 3–3.
Distribution of Pain in 37 Patients With Atypical Odontalgia

Tooth site (% of 101 teeth):
Molars	41.6
Premolars	28.7
Canines	19.9
Anteriors	19.8

No. of teeth involved (%):
1	37.8
2	24.3
3–5	24.3
6	13.5
Mean + SD	2.7 + 2.01

Symmetry (% of 37 patients):
		Maxilla(e)	Mandible	Maxilla/Mandible
Unilateral	81.1	62.2	16.2	2.7
Bilateral	18.9	5.4	2.7	10.2

Dermatomal distribution (%):
V2	67.6
V3	18.9
V2 and V3	13.5

mean profiles of these two groups, nor was there any elevation in mean of any scale. Approximately 40% of each group did show elevation in scale 2 (depression). It can therefore be concluded that a psychological pathogenesis is unlikely, although just as in any chronic pain problem, operant pain and behavioral factors have an impact on all pain no matter what the etiology.

A vascular or neurovascular mechanism similar to that described for migraine is unlikely considering the continuous nature of the pain. However, the results of 23 thermograms revealing asymmetry in 100% of the cases may suggest that the vascular tree is involved if only secondary to another mechanism. Further controlled trials using other toothaches of known etiology are necessary before a definitive statement can be made about thermography.

The third mechanism often described as the pathogenesis of AO is deafferentation. Most patients with AO relate the onset of their pain to minor tooth trauma or dental pulp extirpation. There is also an associated increased sensitivity to pressure over the painful region (hyperesthesia), and from preliminary studies, there is an equivocal response to local anesthetic blockade, but a seemingly impressive reduction in pain with sympathetic blockade. The proposed hypothesis by Roberts[9] fits well with the clinical findings in AO and may suggest that its pathogenesis is related to sympathetically maintained pain.

Differential Diagnosis.—There are three broad categories for pains that present in the teeth. These are secondary to pulpitis, referred toothache of known origin, and AO. Pulpitis is an inflammatory process involving the neurovascular structures of the tooth. It is diagnosed with the following inclusionary criteria: 1) association with local cause (carious lesion, trauma to tooth); 2) dental radiograph free of periapical changes; 3) intermittent or continuous pain; 4) provocable pain; 5) anesthetic block that abolishes pain. Other toothaches of known origin are referred from the musculoskeletal system, from pre- or trigeminal neuralgia, traumatic neuralgia, neuritis, sinus disease, periapical or periodontal abscess, vascular headache, myocardial infarct, or secondary to a psychogenic process. AO is therefore differentiated from the other tooth pains with the following inclusionery criteria:[1] 1) no obvious local cause; 2) no abnormality on x-ray; 3) continuous or almost continuous pain; 4) pain present longer than 4 months; 5) associated hyperesthesia; 6) somatic block equivocal.

TREATMENT

Atypical odontalgia is nonresponsive to analgesics, sedatives, surgery, and other dental intervention. There is support, however, that serotonergic antidepressant medications help reduce the pain associated with AO. The mode of action of these medications is probably related to their analgesic effects and not the antidepressant effects since these patients are not depressed in general. This effect has been demonstrated by the authors on 25 AO subjects using an average dose of 80 mg amitriptyline. A 75% average pain reduction was observed in this group using a visual analogue scale. There is a possibility that combining amitriptyline and low dose phenothiazine may be additive in their effects on deafferentation pains. The potential side effects of the phenothiazines of tardive dyskinesia may outweigh the benefit. This and other drug therapies such as the use of anticonvulsants have not been studied conclusively. The anticholinergic side effects of amitriptyline at the doses prescribed for AO are well tolerated and patients feel that the worst side effect, dry mouth, is tolerable.

CONCLUSION

Dental pain is usually associated with a local pathological process. Diagnosis can be confirmed by the temporary abolition of pain with local anesthetic block. Treatment involves the elimination of the peripheral cause. Conversely, AO probably represents a pain that may begin secondary to peripheral trauma, but is perpetuated by the central and/or sympathetic nervous systems. It is therefore best managed at this time by therapies that work centrally and not at peripheral modalities that may worsen the disease process.

REFERENCES

1. Solberg WK, Graff-Radford SB: Orodental considerations in facial pain. *Semin Neuro* 1988; 8:318–323.
2. Rees RT, Harris M: Atypical odontalgia: Differential diagnosis and treatment. *Brit Jour Oral Surg* 1978; 16:212–218.
3. Graff-Radford SB, Solberg WK: Atypical odontalgia, *Calif Dent Assoc* 1986; 14:27–32.
4. Reik L: Atypical odontalgia: A localized form of atypical facial pain. *Headache* 1984; 24:222–224.
5. Brooke RI: Atypical odontalgia. *Oral Surg* 1980; 43:196–199.
6. Brooke RI: Periodic migrainous neuraliga: A cause of dental pain. *Oral Med* 1978; 46:511–516.
7. Marbach J, Hulbrock J, Hohn C, et al: Incidence of phantom tooth pain: An atypical facial neuralgia. *Oral Surg* 1982; 53:190–193.
8. Marbach JJ: Phantom tooth pain. *J Endodontics* 1978; 4:362–371.
9. Roberts WJ: A hypothesis on the physiological basis for causalgia and related pains. *Pain* 1986; 24:297–311.

4

Migraine Headaches

Bernadette Jaeger, D.D.S.
Luis A. Cueva, D.D.S.

A 27-year-old woman had intermittent, predominantly right-sided headaches that started when she was approximately age 13 years. The pain is located in the temple region and starts as a dull ache. As the headache progresses it takes on a throbbing, pounding quality. Sometimes it will switch to the left side. The patient denies any visual or sensory changes prior to the onset of the headache, but states that she "knows" when it will appear. Precipitating factors include wine, fasting, and stress. Associated symptoms include photophobia, phonophobia, and ptosis. Rarely there is nausea present. Rest in a dark room alleviates the pain and the patient is pain free between attacks. Currently, the headaches occur once per week and will last approximately 8 hours. On further questioning, it is found that both the patient's aunt and cousin suffer from similar headaches. Physical examination, including neurologic evaluation is within normal limits. Cervical range of motion is full; however, tenderness is noted over the right transverse process of atlas and pressure here reproduces the ipsilateral headache pain. A diagnosis of migraine without aura is made based on the history of intermittent, unilateral, throbbing headaches with a temporal pattern consistent with migraine, in the presence of a negative neurologic examination. Ergotamine inhaler is prescribed at the first sign of an impending headache, with complete remission of symptoms.

DISCUSSION

It has been estimated that 76% of Americans suffer from severe headaches.[1] Consumption of analgesics such as aspirin approaches 30,000,000 pounds an-

TABLE 4–1.

Headache Classification

1. Migraine
2. Tension-type headache
3. Cluster headache and chronic paroxysmal hemicrania
4. Miscellaneous headaches unassociated with structural lesion
5. Headache associated with head trauma
6. Headache associated with vascular disorders
7. Headache associated with nonvascular intracranial disorder
8. Headache associated with substances or their withdrawal
9. Headache associated with noncephalic infection
10. Headache associated with metabolic disorder
11. Headache or facial pain associated with disorder of cranium, neck, eyes, ears, nose, sinuses, teeth, mouth, or other facial or cranial structures
12. Cranial neuralgias, nerve trunk pain, and deafferentation pain

nually, a large percentage of which is taken for headaches. While the majority of headaches are not intense enough or sufficiently frequent to cause a person to consult a health care professional, 5%–10% of the North American population do seek medical advice intermittently for severe headaches.[2] Exactly how many of these patients actually suffer from migraine remains controversial, although a recent epidemiologic study estimates an incidence of 10%.[3] A clear understanding of the characteristics of this headache type is essential for accurate diagnosis and effective treatment.

Since all physicians may be called upon to treat patients with headache, it is important to have a simple classification that will facilitate appropriate diagnosis and therapy. Appropriate diagnosis is important in migraine since effective therapy is available. To assist in appropriate diagnosis, the International Headache Society has recently developed a new, more specific classification of headaches as compared to the original Ad Hoc Committee Classification of 1962.[4–5] The main headache categories are listed in Table 4–1.

The first four categories describe primary headache disorders, whereas categories 5–11 describe headaches secondary to some type of identifiable trauma, pathology, metabolic disorder, or substance abuse. Category 12 describes the neuropathic pains.

In order to make a diagnosis in categories 1–4, which includes migraine, one of the following must be true:[4]

1. History, physical, and neurological examination do not suggest one of the disorders listed in categories 5–11;

2. History and/or physical and/or neurological examinations do suggest such a disorder, but it is ruled out by appropriate investigations;

3. Such a disorder is present, but the headache in question did not occur for the first time in close temporal relation to the disorder.

Distinction must be made between migraine and the other different primary headache types, since the different headache types respond to different medications and treatment approaches. Location and quality of pain, associated symptoms, and temporal pattern provide the necessary clues to differentiate between these headaches.

In general, the outstanding feature of all of the migraine headaches is throbbing pain, which is usually unilateral in onset, but which may become generalized. The pain is commonly limited to the head, but it may include the face and even the neck. Photo and phonophobia, or nausea and/or vomiting are present. The pain lasts 4–72 hours and the patient is pain free between attacks with days to months of remission.[6]

In contrast, tension-type headaches are usually bilateral with a pressing, nonpulsating quality. They last 30 minutes to 7 days when episodic and may be daily without remission when chronic.[4]

Cluster headaches are also unilateral, but usually orbital, supraorbital, and/or temporal in location. The pain is severe and is associated with autonomic changes such as conjunctival injection, lacrimation, nasal congestion, miosis, ptosis, or eyelid edema on the side of the pain. The temporal pattern is unique in that the headaches, which last 15–180 minutes untreated, "cluster" together, occurring from one every other day to eight per day. The "cluster period" may last from 7 days to 1 year, and the headache typically goes into remission for weeks to years at a time.[4]

Chronic paroxysmal hemicrania is similar to cluster headaches in location and quality of pain and associated symptoms. However, the pain is always on the same side and lasts only 2–45 minutes. Attack frequency is usually five or more per day without remission.[4]

Headaches in category 4 are typically short lasting and associated with certain activities or external stimuli.[4] They include such headaches as external compression headache ("swim goggle headache"), cold stimulus headache ("ice cream headache"), benign cough headache, benign exertional headache, and headache associated with sexual activity.

Migraine headaches may be classified as noted in Table 4–2. "Migraine with aura," frequently referred to as "classic" migraine, makes up about 10% of all migraine headaches.[7] These are headaches in which transient focal neurologic symptoms (the aura) precede the headache pain by 10 to 60 minutes. Visual auras are most common and may present as flashing lights, halos, or loss of part of the visual field. Somatosensory auras are also common and consist of dysesthesias that start in one hand and spread up to involve the ipsilateral side of the face, nose, and mouth.[8] Rare cases (1%) may also have unilateral ophthalmoplegia or hemiplegia;[7] retinal migraine is preceded by monocular scotomata or blindness. These are considered to be more severe forms of "classic" migraine and may become associated with permanent neurologic cerebral damage.

While "classic" migraine is associated with clear-cut clinical symptoms, it is important to stress that the overwhelming majority of migraine attacks have vague or even absent prodromata.[7] Accordingly, this "migraine without aura" is typically referred to as "common" migraine.

Migraine is more common in women than men.[3] While migraine may appear in childhood, it usually begins before the age of 40 years. Rarely, patients develop their first symptoms in the fifth or sixth decade. Seventy percent of migraine headache patients relate a history of similar headaches in a close blood relative. External and internal stimuli believed to precipitate migraine in susceptible individuals include psychological stress, depression or anxiety, endocrine factors (such as menstruation and changes in estrogen levels), alcohol intake, diets containing tyramine, eye strain, bright lights, shifts in weather, and alterations in life style (such as prolonged fasting or oversleeping).[7]

The etiology of migraine remains a puzzle, although most experts agree that a vascular mechanism is involved. Cerebral blood flow studies have shown that migraine headaches are preceded by an initial, short-lasting increase in cerebral blood flow in the occipitoparietal area.[8] This is followed by an approximately 25% decrease in blood flow, which spreads from the occipital region forward across to the front of the brain. It is these changes that are thought to be

TABLE 4–2.

Classification of Migraine

Migraine without aura
Migraine with aura
Migraine with atypical aura
Migraine with prolonged aura
Familial hemiplegic migraine
Basilar migraine
Migraine aura without headache
Migraine with acute onset aura
Ophthalmoplegic migraine
Retinal migraine
Childhood periodic syndromes that may be precursors to or associated with migraine
Benign paroxysmal vertigo of childhood
Alternating hemiplegia of childhood
Complications of migraine
Status migrainous
Migrainous infarction
Migrainous disorder not fulfilling above criteria

responsible for the aura symptoms of "classic" migraine. The headache itself is thought to occur as a result of the dilatation of the cranial noncerebral blood vessels. This vasodilatation, initially thought to be a reactive hyperemia from cerebral hypoxia, may actually be independent of the intracerebral changes associated with the aura.[9-8]

After the headache, patients usually feel lethargic and exhausted.[7] This is the time during which the vasculature is thought to return to normal. Some patients may continue to feel a deep aching pain, resulting from prolonged contraction of head and neck muscles during the migraine attack.[7]

MANAGEMENT

Treatment of the Acute Attack

An acute attack of migraine typically will resolve within 3–4 hours if the patient can get to sleep.[10] An antinauseant and simple analgesics such as aspirin and acetaminophen with or without codeine will facilitate this. A cold pack applied to the forehead or temples may also provide symptomatic relief. Ergotamines, powerful extracranial vasoconstrictors, are contraindicated once the headache is established, since they will no longer be effective. However, if the simple steps above fail to alleviate the pain, an intravenous antinauseant (such as 10 mg metoclopramide) followed by slow intravenous administration of dihydroergotamine (0.5–1.0 mg over 3–4 minutes), may provide the desired relief.[11]

Long-Term Management

Identification and Control of Precipitating Factors

The first step in the long-term management of migraine headache is to identify and control any obvious precipitating factors. Restriction of alcohol intake and elimination of tyramine-containing foods (Table 4–3) are simple, yet often effective means of decreasing the frequency of migraine attacks. Regular meals and establishment of good sleep hygiene may also help prevent the onset of migraine. For those patients in whom stress, depression, or anxiety play a role, psychological interventions, such as stress management and relaxation training, biofeedback, or cognitive behavioral therapy may be indicated.

Choose Either an Abortive or Prophylactic Medication Regimen

Abortive Medications.—Abortive medications are appropriate when the patient suffers from less than three or four migraine headaches per month and he or she can reasonably and reliably identify when a headache is going to start. Migraine with aura easily lends itself to the use of abortive medications because patients clearly know when they are going to get a headache. Migraine without

TABLE 4–3.

Tyramine Restricted Diet*

Food Group	Foods to Avoid
Beverages	Caffeine sources such as coffee, tea, or cola-type drinks; alcoholic beverages; chocolate or cocoa drinks[†]
Meat, fish, poultry	Aged, canned, cured or processed meats; canned or aged ham; salted dried fish; chicken liver; fermented sausage; any meat prepared with tenderizer, soy sauce, or yeast extract
Dairy	Cultured dairy, such as buttermilk, sour cream, chocolate milk; cheeses such as bleu, brick, brie, or camembert types, cheddar, swiss, mozzarella, parmesan, provolone, or romano
Breads and cereals	Hot, fresh, homemade yeast breads; breads and crackers with cheese; doughnuts; sourdough breads; any breads containing chocolate or nuts
Vegetables	Lima or Italian beans, lentils, snowpeas, fava beans, pinto beans, sauerkraut, onions, olives, pickles
Fruits	Avocados, bananas ($1/2$ allowed per day), figs, raisins, papaya, passion fruit, red plums
Soups	Canned soups, soup cubes, bouillon cubes, soup bases with autolyzed yeast or MSG
Desserts	Chocolate ice cream, pudding, cookies, cakes, mincemeat pies
Sweets	Chocolate candies, chocolate syrup, carob
Miscellaneous	Pizza, cheese sauce, soy sauce, MSG in excessive amounts, yeast, seasoned salt; mixed dishes: macaroni and cheese, beef stroganoff, cheese blintzes, frozen dinners

*Adapted from Diamond S, Dalessio DJ (eds): *The Practicing Physician's Approach to Headache,* ed 4. Baltimore, Williams & Wilkins, 1986, p 50.
†While caffeine and caffeinated beverages do not contain tyramine, their consumption may aggravate hypertension and precipitate headache. Further, they will prevent sleep, which is essential for the resolution of a migraine headache.

aura may also respond to these medications if the patient is able to take the medications early enough in the headache cycle.

Abortive medications all contain the vasoconstrictor, ergotamine tartrate. Ergotamine tartrate causes constriction of the extracranial blood vessels and thus is very effective at aborting a migraine. Ergomar, Ergostat, Medihaler Ergotamine, Wigrettes, Cafergot, Cafergot-PB, or Wigraine all contain ergotamine and differ mainly in the route of administration (inhalation vs. sublingual vs. oral vs. rectal). Some of them also contain caffeine, which is actually not desirable since it may inhibit sleep and sleep may be required to completely resolve the headache.[10] When using abortive medications, patients should be advised to take the medication at the first sign of an impending headache. Depending on the type of ergotamine preparation chosen, doses are repeated at 5–15 minute intervals until the headache disappears or the maximum per headache dose for that preparation is reached.[12]

Ergot preparations are potent peripheral vasoconstrictors and should not be used in patients with significant peripheral vascular disease, hypertension, coronary insufficiency, or angina. Ergots should also be avoided in pregnancy since they are oxytocic. Even healthy patients must use caution with ergotamine preparations because overuse or abuse may lead to ergotism. This is a condition characterized by tingling, burning, and numbness in the hands and feet, a result of peripheral ischemia. People with ergotism are at risk for gangrene, and coronary and visceral arteries may also be compromised. For this reason, if a patient is experiencing more than four migraine headaches per month, it is advisable to use a prophylactic medication instead.

Prophylactic Medications.—Prophylactic medications include beta-blockers such as propranolol (Inderal), tricyclic antidepressants such as amitriptyline (Elavil), and calcium channel blockers such as diltiazem (Cardizem). Other popular medications used for the prophylaxis of migraine include methysergide (Sansert), which is a lysergic acid derivative closely related to the naturally occuring ergot alkaloids, and cyproheptadine (Periactin), which is an antihistamine with antiserotonin activity. These medications differ in their pharmacologic actions, but all are prescribed on a daily basis and are thought to prevent the onset of a migraine attack by stabilizing the vasculature.

Nonpharmacological Treatment of Migraine

There are numerous nonpharmacological treatments for migraine (Table 4–4), but few of the enthusiastic claims of treatment success cited in the literature or media are backed by scientific data. This is because it is difficult to design appropriate double blind, placebo-controlled studies when the active treatment is difficult to disguise. This is in contrast to medications, which easily lend themselves to this type of research.

TABLE 4–4.

A List of Various Nonpharmacological Therapies

Stress management and relaxation training
Cognitive and behavioral training
Biofeedback
   Temperature training
   EMG—frontalis relaxation training, relaxation techniques
Hypnosis
Meditation
Physical therapy
   Cervical mobilization or manipulation
   Soft tissue mobilization
Acupuncture/acupressure
TENS (Transcutaneous Electrical Nerve Stimulation)

Medications are valuable if the desired pain relief is achieved without any unacceptable side effects. However, patients may sometimes achieve good pain relief, while suffering from fatigue (beta blockers), dry mouth (tricyclics), flushing, muscle aches, or retroperitoneal fibrosis (methysergide), to name a few. At other times, patients may not tolerate an effective medication because of allergy, or may simply desire to achieve control over their headaches without medications. Nonpharmacological approaches may provide alternatives to medications in these situations. In addition, combinations of pharmacological and nonpharmacological approaches are often more successful than either one alone.

REFERENCES

1. Ries PW: Current Estimates From the National Health Interview Survey, United States, 1984. National Center for Health Statistics; 1986. Vital and Health Statistics, Series 10, No. 156. Dept of Health and Human Services publication (PHS)86–1584.
2. Campbell, KJ: Headache in adults: An overview. *J Cranio Dis Fac Oral Pain* 1987; 1:11–15.
3. Linet MS, Stewart WF, Celentano DD, et al: An epidemiologic study of headache among adolescents and young adults. *JAMA*. 1989, Vol. 261, 15:2211–2216.
4. Headache Classification Committee of the International Headache Society: Classification and diagnostic criteria for headache disorders, cranial neuralgias and facial pain. *Cephalalgia*. 1988, 8(Supp):1–96.
5. Ad Hoc Committee on Classification of Headache of NIH. *JAMA* 1962; 179:717–718.
6. Olesen J: Some clinical features of the acute migraine attack: An analysis of 750 patients. *Headache* 1978; 12:268–271.
7. Dalessio DJ: Migraine headaches. *Hosp Med* 1985; Mar:214–217.
8. Spierings ELH: Recent advances in the understanding of migraine. *Headache* 1988; 28:655–658.
9. Wolff HG, Tunis MM, Goodell H: Studies of headache: Evidence of tissue damage and changes in pain sensitivity in subjects with vascular headache of the migraine type. *Arch Intern Med* 1953; 92:478–484.
10. Wilkinson M: Treatment of migraine. *Headache* 1988; 28:659–661.
11. Edmeads J: Emergency management of headache. *Headache* 1988; 28:675–679.
12. Diamond S, Dalessio DJ: Migraine headache, in Diamond S, Dalessio DJ (eds): *The Practicing Physician's Approach to Headache,* ed 4. Baltimore, Williams & Wilkins, 1986, p 50.

5

Chronic Headache Related to Temporomandibular Disorder

William K. Solberg, D.D.S., M.S.D.

A 29-year-old woman presented with recurrent locking of the jaw, painful chewing, and associated temporal headache, which was worse on the left side (Fig 5–1). In addition, she complained of an almost continuous clogging sensation in the ears. She had a 7-year history of recurrent headaches and variable left-sided jaw pain. Despite these problems, she sought medical consultation infrequently. She consulted an ophthalmologist about her headaches without positive findings. She experienced more and more left jaw pain complicated by jaw locking. She routinely unlocked her jaw by learned maneuvers. She noticed that her headaches worsened with vigorous chewing. Typically, her left jaw ache progressed to a throbbing pain, and this was followed by a "headache" in the left temple. She consulted her dentist, who referred her for temporomandibular joint consultation. Figure 5–2 shows the relative importance of complaints according to a forced-decision rating by the patient. This scale indicated that the major complaints were headache and painful chewing.

DISCUSSION

The mention of temporomandibular disorder (TMD) evokes the image of a patient complaining of chewing pain accompanied by joint popping and variable limitation of mouth opening (Table 5–1). Lesser symptoms such as fullness of the ears, ringing of the ears, and dizziness are not considered genuine symptoms of

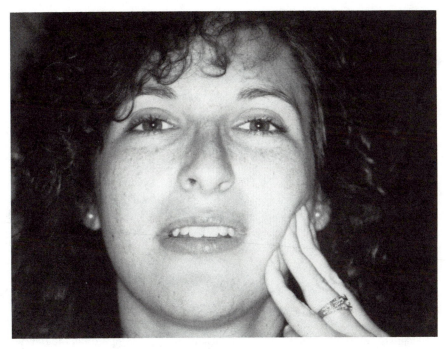

FIG 5–1.
Woman, age 29 years, with episodic left TMJ locking, painful chewing, fullness of the ears, and recurrent left temporal headache induced by use of the jaw.

TMD. Headache, on the other hand, is often among the TMD patient's chief complaints. This raises the possibility that some headaches are truly part of the so-called temporomandibular joint (TMJ) syndrome. The following case illustrated headache caused by pathology in the TMJ. The differential diagnosis of headaches associated with, but not caused by, TMD will be discussed.

The patient was married and a homemaker with two young children: one child was an infant who kept her up several times a night. She was constantly tired. She admitted to habitual bruxism, cheek biting, and habitual chewing on the left side. Jaw opening provoked pain in the left cheek and temple. Opening and closing was accompanied by brisk popping in the left TMJ. She briefly took ibuprofen, 400 mg, as needed, without benefit. Acetaminophen, 500 mg, six per day, predictably reduced her jaw aches and headaches by 75%. Both TMJs were tender, but the left TMJ was more tender. Multiple tender points and trigger points were identified in the musculature of the jaws, upper neck, and shoulder (Fig 5–3). Her slightly overdeveloped lower jaw had been orthodontically treated, and her teeth closed with acceptable fit and function.

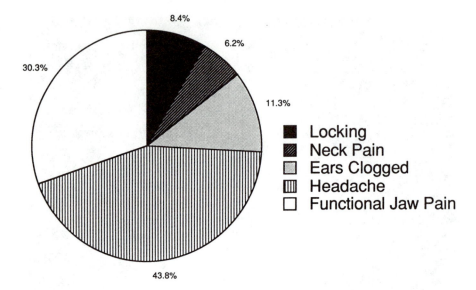

FIG 5–2.
Relative importance of complaints according to a forced-decision rating by the patient.

The following problems were identified: (1) left temporomandibular derangement with associated myofascial headache; (2) myofascial cervical pain; (3) interval headache resembling a combination of tension and migraine types; (4) disturbed sleep, primarily because of a wakeful infant; (5) fullness of the ears (clogging sensation). The following plan was adopted: (1) pain diary and treatment log; (2) scheduled reduction of analgesics; (3) six weekly physical therapy visits with the concurrent full-time use of a TMJ repositioning appliance

TABLE 5–1.

Descriptive Features of Temporomandibular Disorders*

Prevalence	5% will have clinical disorder
Onset	Ages 15–40 yr, mean age 28 yr
Gender	Women 3:1
Pain Quality	Dull, associated with jaw function
Jaw Dysfunction	TMJ clicking, locking, jaw restriction
Bite Discrepancy	May be disrupted; unlikely a primary cause
Emotional Distress	Not necessary as casual factor
Natural Course	3–5 yr
Treatment	Mean duration, 3–6 mo; mean visits, 4–6

*Unpublished data from the UCLA Temporomandibular and Facial Pain Clinic, and from Solberg WK, Woo MW, Houston JB: *J Am Dent Assoc* 1979; 98:25–34.

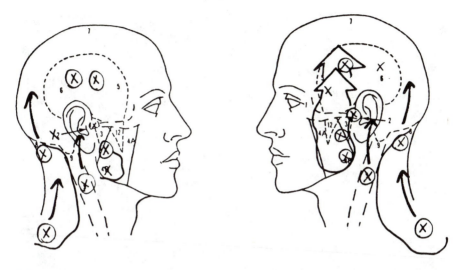

FIG 5–3.
The distribution of the pain complaint. Superimposed "Xs" identify areas of palpable tenderness. Some of these tender points referred pain back to remote areas of the head and neck. Note that the headache spread from the left jaw region in association with jaw use.

(splint); (4) home therapy program; (5) husband's agreement to care for the baby during the nights for the next 6 weeks.

The course of active treatment was 7 weeks, with all appointments programmed in advance (Table 5–2). Initially, it was apparent that some of the headaches started suddenly at the base of the neck and spread to the eyes. These headaches were infrequent, and were clearly distinguished from the primary headaches. Weeks 1 and 2 consisted of physical therapy to the neck and jaws, supplemented by a home program. In week 3, the mandibular repositioning appliance was delivered with immediate relief of jaw clicking and locking (Fig 5–4). This appliance has been described previously.[2] By week 7, all symptoms were relieved (Table 5–2). The clogged sensation in the ears changed from frequent to infrequent and finally disappeared. She now reported episodic headaches of moderate intensity, and these appeared to be provoked by fatigue. Over the next 3 months, she had two such headache attacks and they were controlled by an oral medication containing butabarbital 50 mg, acetaminophen 325 mg, and caffeine 40 mg, two capsules each attack. Figure 5–5 shows the relative treatment effectiveness according to the forced-decision rating completed by the patient. This subjective patient rating indicates that the mandibular appliance provided significant benefit.

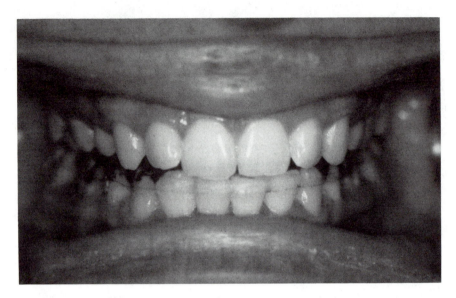

FIG 5–4.
Mandibular repositioning appliance (splint) slightly advancing the mandible, thereby preventing disc condyle interference on opening.

TABLE 5–2.
Flow Sheet Summarizing Treatment Outcome*

	Week						
	1	2	3	4	5	6	7
Left jaw, chewing pain	2	2	3	2	1	0	0
Right jaw, chewing pain	0	1	2	0	0	0	0
Bilateral neck ache	1	2	1	0	1	0	0
Unilateral headache	0	2	3	0	0	0	0
Clogged feeling in ears	+	+	+	+	+/−	−	−
Locking of left TMJ	+	+	+	−	−	−	−
Aspirin, p.o. per day	4	2	4	4	0	0	0
Ibuprofen, p.o. per day	NA	NA	NA	NA	4	2	0
Physical therapy, visits	1	1	1	1	1	0	0
Bite splint adjustments	NA	NA	1	1	1	1	0

*0 = no pain; 10 = most intense pain imaginable; NA = not applicable at this appointment; + = yes; and − = no.

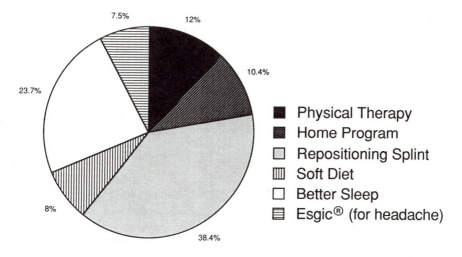

FIG 5–5.
Rating of treatment effectiveness by the patient following resolution of symptoms.

DISCUSSION

This case comprises three problems: headache associated with true TMJ arthropathy, myofascial pain of jaw and cervical muscle origin, and superimposed headache probably related to a combination of tension and migraine types. Although headache was the most acute symptom, chewing pain with jaw dysfunction was nevertheless a prominent complaint. Information leading to a clear understanding of the clogged sensation is sparse; it is probably related to muscle hyperactivity mediated by the central nervous system. This case was managed by physical and behavioral methods, and not limited to dental methods such as bite splints. Medications normally advocated for control of tension and migraine headache ultimately played a minor role.

The question has been raised whether headaches can actually be caused by TMJ arthropathy. On the basis of recent studies, recurrent headache should be added to the list of TMJ symptoms.[3–5] Pincus and Tucker found that headaches caused by TMD were more common in their neurological practice than were migraine headaches (26% and 20%, respectively).[6] Reik and Hale found a TMD-induced headache in 11% of 100 consecutive patients seen in their headache clinic.[4] Their criteria for TMJ-induced headache were: (1) continuous, unilateral, dull to throbbing pain in the ear, temple, above and behind the eye, occasionally spreading to the neck; (2) tenderness over the TMJ and associated areas, often with restricted range of jaw motion; and (3) unilateral headache without other clear cause, when face and jaw pain are present. It is the author's opinion that the primary headache in this case report fits these inclusion criteria.

DIFFERENTIAL DIAGNOSIS

Bilateral tension headache is usually unrelated to pathological changes in the TMJ. For example, tension headache with pericranial tenderness and the so-called myofascial pain-dysfunction syndrome (MPD) appear to be indistinguishable in the clinical setting with the exception that MPD pain is also distributed over the jaw muscles.[7] In addition, the pathogenesis of tension headache and TMD are described similarly, with the suspicion that they are epiphenomena of the same underlying cause, e.g., stress and other emotional factors.[7–8] Stressful events have been hypothesized to produce a biochemical change in the brain, which reduces serotonin levels.[9]

Treatments for tension headache and MPD are essentially similar: salicylates, nonsteroidal anti-inflammatory medications, soft diet, thermal modalities, jaw and neck exercises supplemented by low doses of amitriptyline or trazodone, 30–75 mg, h.s., when necessary. Bite appliance therapy and autogenic relaxation training may be used when clearly indicated. Episodic migraine headache, although unilateral, can be distinguished easily because of its intermittent frequency and because it is unaffected by jaw use. Migraine headache is sometimes superimposed on TMD symptoms, but TMD therapy does not affect outcome. Therefore, in contrast to tension headache and TMD, migraine headache and TMD share few common treatments.

SUMMARY

There are two types of headaches commonly seen in TMD patients. The first is the bilateral tension headache that is not directly caused by TMD, but is frequently lessened by TMD treatment.[10] The second type, the unilateral temporal headache that is caused by true TMJ pathology, such as the temporomandibular joint internal derangement in this case report, is decisively altered by biomechanical devices, such as bite splints and other direct therapy to the TMJs. Therefore, when a patient presents with unilateral headache and causal factors are not clear, a history and examination for TMJ pain, tenderness, joint dysfunction, and restricted jaw movement should be performed. If findings meet the criteria for TMJ-induced headache, TMJ consultation should be considered.

REFERENCES

1. Solberg WK, Woo MW, Houston JB: Prevalence of mandibular dysfunction in young adults. *J Am Dent Assoc* 1979; 98:25–34.
2. Solberg WK: Temporomandibular disorders: Management of internal derangement. *Br Dent J* 1986; 160:379–385.
3. Magnusson T, Carlsson GE: Comparison between two groups of patients in respect to headache and mandibular dysfunction. *Swed Dent J* 1978; 2:85–92.
4. Reik L Jr, Hale M: The temporomandibular joint pain-dysfunction syndrome: A frequent cause of headache. *Headache* 1981; 21:151–156.
5. Forssell H, Kangasniemi P: Correlation of the frequency and intensity of headache to mandibular dysfunction in headache patients. *Proc Finn Dent Soc* 1984; 80:223–226.
6. Pincus JH, Tucker GJ: *Behavioral Neurology* ed 2. New York, Oxford University Press, 1978.
7. Green CS, Olson RE, Laskin DM: Psychological factors in the etiology, progression, and treatment of MPD syndrome. *J Am Dent Assoc* 1982; 105:443–448.
8. Raskin NH: *Headache.* ed 2. New York, Churchill Livingston, 1988.
9. Magnusson T, Carlsson GE: Changes in recurrent headache and mandibular dysfunction after various types of dental treatment. *Acta Odontol Scand* 1980; 38:311–320.
10. Diamond S, Medina J: *Headaches. Clin Symp* 1981; 33:1–32.

6

Cluster Headache

Michael Simmons, D.M.D.

A 25-year-old man presents with a recent history of intense pain and distress. He has been suffering with headaches occurring several times a day that wake him from sleep. With onset of these strictly unilateral headaches, he is unable to get any relief with pain medications and simply paces to and fro in a room by himself until the pain dissipates, usually 40 minutes later. The headache reappears twice every 24 hours; one of which wakes him regularly from sleep. Associated with his retro-orbital pain is conjunctival injection, sweating, and nasal stuffiness on the same side.

DISCUSSION

Cluster headache is the most severely painful benign, but recurrent, headache known to man. Patients in the midst of a cluster type headache present commonly to hospital emergency rooms. Their previous experience tells them that once the attack has started, nothing short of an intravenous analgesic will even touch the agonizing pain. The patients in the grip of this pain are often seen to grasp their head and bang it severely against the wall in a mad attempt to alter the pain. It appears the only saving grace preventing often-mentioned suicidal escape is the knowledge that the headache will run its course and will leave completely, nearly as fast as its onset.

Periodic migrainous neuralgia is another of the many names given to this group of extremely painful, benign unilateral headaches that have onset primarily in males between the ages of 20–50 years, but mostly around 30 years. The

TABLE 6–1.

Synonyms for Cluster Headache

Name	Author	Year
Sphenopalatine neuralgia	Sluder	1908
Erythromelalgia of the head	Bing	1910
Periodic migrainous neuralgia	Harris	1926
Vidian neuralgia	Vail	1932
Ciliary neuralgia	Harris	1936
Histamine cephalgia	Horton	1939
Greater superficial petrosal neuralgia	Gardner	1947
Cluster headache	Kunkle	1952
Autonomic facial neuralgia	White	1955
A particular variety of headache	Symonds	1956

most common name given is cluster, because of the periodicity of their occurrence in that, when they do occur, it is in clusters of painful episodes. Other names attributed to this condition include: ciliary neuralgia by Harris, in 1936, since the pain is felt mainly in or behind the eye; and histaminic cephalgia by Horton, in 1941, since injection of histamine would cause immediate headache onset. Listed in Table 6–1 is a more complete history of the synonyms that illustrate the changing concepts of etiology through time.

Diagnosis relies upon the unilaterality and painlike quality, the periodicity and duration, and the associated autonomic phenomena. Cluster affects males more frequently than females, in a ratio of approximately 7:1, often with a history of smoking and drinking, with first occurrence in the second to third decade. It is described as throbbing and frequently as deep, boring, and very severe. The bouts or clusters may include up to eight episodes of pain per day, or as few as one episode every 2 days, each lasting 15 minutes to 3 hours. Periods of pain last 3 to 12 weeks, and can recur every 3 months. Nocturnal onset of pain that wakes subjects has been frequently reported and appears during REM sleep. Associated autonomic phenomena include ipsilateral congested nose, rhinorrhea, bloodshot eye, epiphora, lacrimation, blurred vision, facial flushing, forehead and facial sweating, miosis, and ptosis, although rarely are more than a few of these symptoms present. The International Headache Society (IHS) Ad Hoc Committee, as of 1988, requires at least one autonomic change be present for diagnosis.[1]

The differential diagnosis should include trigeminal neuralgia, temporal arteritis, myofascial pain, infection or neoplasm of the paranasal sinuses, and glaucoma. Consequently, before diagnosis is confirmed, a neurologic exam must be performed and, if indicated, neuroimaging to rule out an organic disorder. Prevalence of this headache is rare and difficult to assess due to the frequent number of misdiagnoses, but is thought to be less than 1% of the population.

For example, in the dental literature, toothaches are cited as one of the most common presentations of this disease process. Indeed, Brooke stated 100% of patients described the pain as presenting as toothache (53%) or jaw pain (47%).[2] These patients had multiple oral surgical or endodontic procedures performed which, if concurrent with the end of the cluster period, could easily be misconstrued for effective treatment and accurate diagnosis.

The pathophysiology is not known, but is thought to involve the vascular supply to the periorbital region. This is supported by the very common conjunctival injection, the provoked onset by nitroglycerine, and the relief obtained by vasoconstrictor drugs. Whether or not there is a neurogenous component precipitating the vascular changes remains to be substantiated.

In contrast to migraine, with or without aura, no specific environmental triggers for cluster headache can be elicited from the majority of patients. However, in the literature, some correlation is made by a small percentage of patients with alcohol intake and seasonal changes, especially around spring and fall. Also, in contrast to migraine, blood chemistries are somewhat altered in respect to histamine and serotonin levels. A 90% increase in plasma histamine is seen during cluster, where no change is seen in migraine. Conversely, the 80% decrease in plasma serotonin during migraine has no significant change with cluster. From a psychologic standpoint, it is reported there is no significant difference in any Minnesota Multiphasic Personality Inventory (MMPI) scores in normals and cluster patients, whereas significant differences are found in migraine, tension, and combined headache sufferers when compared to normals.

In a small percentage of patients, the periods of remission shorten and eventually disappear, and they enter a chronic phase termed secondary chronic cluster. This is differentiated from primary chronic cluster when absence of remission periods begin at onset of the first presentation. The chronic phase has a minimum of two headaches per week for more than 2 years. More recently, in 1988, the Ad Hoc Committee of the IHS has proposed the chronic disorder if no remission of two weeks occurs within 1 year.

Some variability in types of cluster include an extremely rare bilateral form. Other authors have described cluster variants such as chronic paroxysmal hemicrania, and hemicrania continua, although these are not recognized as being sufficiently validated to be included in the recent classification by the IHS Ad Hoc Committee.

MANAGEMENT

Treatment of episodic cluster, the most common form, is divided into abortive and prophylactic therapies. Abortive therapy is usually initiated with a trial of oxygen or ergotamine preparation at onset of the headache. Both of these are thought to be effective via a transient cerebral vasoconstriction. Kudrow found cessation of pain with 7 liters per minute oxygen by face mask for 15 minutes in 8 out of 10 consecutive headaches in 82% of subjects.[3] He compared this to the same group of 50 patients in the alternate phase of a crossover trial with sublingual erogtamine 2 mg at onset, followed by 1 mg repeat doses, if needed, at 15 and 30 minutes, and found 70% of the subjects with the same response. While a majority of patients respond well to oxygen and ergotamine, some patients find the headache recurs within a short time, requiring repeated administration. It is not clear what percentage of patients abort the headache, as opposed to simply delaying its onset. Cluster headache patients have been shown to have a hyperresponsiveness to oxygen therapy during a cluster headache that resulted in a greater than normal fall in cerebral blood flow with oxygen therapy. The ergotamine preparations used are limited to those that bypass the stomach, since there is gastroparesis associated with the headache. These modes would include DHE injection of 1 mg, which the patient may be taught to self-administer. Repetition of this dose, however, might pose a problem, since the patient would be in the midst of an attack. An ergotamine medihaler that gives doses of 0.2 mg is an effective means of administration, or the sublingual ergotamine, 1–2 mg at onset, with additional 1 mg doses at half-hour intervals, to a maximum of 5 mg per day or 12 mg per week. For patients that suffer nocturnal waking onset, 2 mg of ergotamine may be taken before sleep.

Sphenopalatine ganglion block with intranasal cocaine 5%, of aqueous 4% lidocaine has proved effective by applying a soaked cotton pledget on an intranasal applicator, or by administering 0.3–0.5 cc of nasal drops and lying supine with the head tilted backward toward the floor at 30° and turned to the side of the headache. Maximum administration is limited to twice in 5 hours. Since both lidocaine and cocaine are equally effective in aborting the headache, it is the local anesthetic, and not the sympathomimetic effects that are responsible. Other abortive therapies that have been successfully tried include prednisone, using a single dose of 30 mg.

Prophylactic medications used also include prednisone. Lance, recommends three 25 mg tablets daily for 3 days, reducing the dose by half a tablet every 3 days until the cluster headaches start to reappear.[4] He then stabilizes the dose at a level just sufficient to prevent attacks. As the duration of a bout ends, the treatment is gradually withdrawn. The mechanism of action of the prednisone is not known. Kudrow uses the prednisone at 50 mg daily for 5 days, then 30 mg for 5 days, then gradually reduces the medication over the next 11 days, until the lowest effective dosage is found.

A more popular prophylactic medication for episodic cluster is methysergide. Since the cluster bouts are usually shorter than three months' duration, high doses may be used with little risk of retroperitoneal fibrosis. The dose recommended by Lance starts with 1 mg three times daily, and may be increased to three times this level in order to suppress the attacks. Various authors have advocated pizotifen (pizotyline) and chlorpromazine for the suppression of cluster bouts, but success rates are not well established. Recently, the calcium channel blockers have been advocated as successful in both the episodic and chronic forms. In particular, verapamil was shown to be effective in 79% of chronic cluster sufferers, although tolerance often develops requiring increased dosage of changing to another calcium antagonist, such as nimodipine or nifedipine.

If breakthrough of a headache occurs while on the prophylactic regimen, as seen with the intake of alcohol, then ergotamine tartrate may be used abortively, in conjunction with prophylactic medications.

Chronic cluster headache represents a more difficult management problem, since it is commonly recalcitrant to the described medical management. In these cases, lithium carbonate has been documented to be effective. Kudrow prescribed doses of 300–600 mg daily, increasing to 900 mg after some weeks, if necessary, but always maintaining a weekly tested serum level of less than 1.2 mEq/L. After the first month, blood levels were tested on a monthly basis. Since the lithium carbonate has been shown to not affect cerebral hemodynamics, the mechanism of action is theorized to be via a central neurogenic effect influencing the rhythmicity of headache mechanisms somewhat like its effect on manic depressive episodes. This central effect may be related to the influence of lithium on the metabolism of cerebral amines and acetylcholine. Lithium has also been shown to stabilize serotonin neurotransmission within the CNS.

Ineffective treatments that have been attempted for both episodic and chronic cluster include histamine desensitization and biofeedback, frontal EMG and thermal, or relaxation training. Some reported success with meditative and bio-feedback treatments is mentioned by various authors, although they do not routinely recommend such treatment as effective.

Surgical treatments have been attempted for chronic cluster, but historically have proven to be largely unsuccessful. Procedures attempted include resection of the greater superficial petrosal nerve, section of the nervus intermedius, sphenopalatine ganglionectomy, and cryosurgery of the facial arteries. Alcohol injection of the gasserian ganglion and trigeminal root section have also been tried, but were gradually abandoned because of the high incidence of complications and the unreliability of the procedure. The common complications of these surgeries were neuroparalytic or postoperative herpetic keratitis and anesthesia dolorosa of the denervated area.

More recently, surgery has again come to be favored for severe intractable cluster. Onofrio and Campbell reported in 1986 on 26 patients treated with posterior fossa trigeminal sensory rhizotomy, or percutaneous radiofrequency trigeminal gangliorhizolysis at the Mayo Clinic.[5] Relief of pain was excellent in 54%, fair to good in 15%, and poor in 31%. In analyzing these results, one must take into consideration that these patients were otherwise refractory to medical treatment, were in a somewhat hopeless situation, and in certain cases, reported to be contemplating suicide. The authors state that success is evident only when corneal anesthesia or dense analgesia result. However, corneal anesthesia does not predict pain relief. The headache-free state requires total analgesia of the first and second divisions of the trigeminal nerve on the affected side, and dense or complete corneal numbness. Prior to surgical intervention, the patient may have the opportunity to feel effects of the sensory alteration by a trial of lidocaine trigeminal ganglion blockade. There is a small percentage of patients who will, however, suffer the consequences of anesthesia dolorosa as a consequence of the surgery. More recently, Mathew and Hurt have reported an excellent success rate in two-thirds of their intractable cluster cases treated with the percutaneous radiofrequency gangliorhizolysis.[6] In this study, excellence is defined as having no cluster headaches and no medications for treatment of the headaches since the surgery (between 6–63 months), on average 28 months previous.

Although trigeminal nerve, ganglion, and root procedures were performed with interruption of the pain pathways in mind, recently postulated concepts suggest that these procedures interfere with the axon reflex and release of substance P. Consequently, there is altered physiology in the development of the cluster headache, which is perhaps the reason for the successful surgical outcome.

In conclusion, the clinical profile of this syndrome is easily distinguished from other types of headaches. With careful attention to characteristics of: (1) unilaterality of pain; (2) pain intensity; (3) location; (4) accompanying autonomic phenomena, and (5) the temporal clustering pattern, one can readily diagnose its presence. A patient that presents in the midst of an attack (acute cluster), is treated with immediate injection of either DHE or meperidine (Demerol) if the headache is well established, and history of presentation indicates some time before spontaneous reprieve. In order to effect the best long-term treatment, patients must be advised that a wide range of medications may be used by clinical trial on several occasions, and response to such trials is not uncommonly inconsistent. If all medical management fails, a surgical approach is not unwarranted, and, with some risk, might afford the desired response.

REFERENCES

1. International Headache Society Ad Hoc Committee on Classification and Diagnostic Criteria for Headache Disorders, Cranial Neuralgias and Facial Pain. *Cephalalgia* 1988; (suppl 7):1–96.
2. Brooke RI: Periodic migrainous neuralgia: A cause of dental pain. *Oral Surgery* 1978; 46:511–516
3. Kudrow L: *Cluster Headache, Mechanisms and Management.* New York, Oxford University Press, 1980.

4. Lance WJ: *Mechanism and Management of Headache.* Butterworth, London 1983.
5. Onofrio BM, Campbell JK: Surgical treatment of chronic cluster headache. *Mayo Clin Proc* 1986; 61:537–544.
6. Mathew NT, Hurt W: Percutaneous radiofrequency trigeminal gangliorhizolysis in intractable headache. *Headache* 1988; 28:328–331.

7

Trigeminal Neuralgia

Ronald F. Young, M.D.

The patient was a 74-year-old woman with an 8-year history of left facial pain. The pain was described as sharp, knifelike, or electric shock–like and lasting for a fraction of a second to a few seconds at maximum. The pain had occurred intermittently in irregular bouts lasting from weeks to months, but for the preceding 3 months the patient had pain on a regular basis. The pain was located in the left upper lip and cheek and was also felt in the upper teeth. Occasionally, the patient also felt pain in the lower lip and lower teeth on the left. The pain could be triggered by talking, chewing, brushing her teeth on the left, washing the left side of her face, and occasionally, even by cold wind blowing against her face. She had been previously treated with phenytoin (Dilantin) and carbamazepine (Tegretol) but had noted significant side effects with both and was unable to take them at a level sufficient to produce effective pain control.

DISCUSSION

The patient presents with the three cardinal features of trigeminal neuralgia. These include: (1) pain located within one or more branches of the trigeminal nerve; (2) description of pain as a brief, sharp, knifelike or electrical shocklike sensation; and (3) the presence of trigger zones from which normally innocuous stimulation elicits pain. Trigeminal neuralgia is essentially a diagnosis made by careful history. When pain extends outside the distribution of the trigeminal nerve, pathologic processes other than trigeminal neuralgia should be considered. These include various forms of headache, such as cluster headaches, malignancies of the skull base, diseases of the paranasal sinuses, and dental pathology, among others. Dental disease is often confused with trigeminal neuralgia and endodontic treatment and extractions are often performed without relief of pain. Although some patients with trigeminal neuralgia have background dull, aching pain, generally the presence of pain lasting for hours, days, or weeks without interruption indicates a diagnosis other than trigeminal neuralgia. The presence of trigger zones is one of the most characteristic features of trigeminal neuralgia and the absence of trigger zones should cast significant doubt on the diagnosis. Physical examination in trigeminal neuralgia is generally considered to be normal, although careful sensory examination within the trigeminal divisions in which the patient experiences pain will often show slight decreases in sensitivity to pinprick or to tactile stimulation.

The pathological process responsible for trigeminal neuralgia is open to question, however, electron microscopic studies of the trigeminal nerve root in patients with trigeminal neuralgia show segmental demyelination. The most commonly accepted current hypothesis is that trigeminal neuralgia results from compression and irritation of the trigeminal nerve root by adjacent arterial loops. This pathologic process was originally described by Walter Dandy in the 1930s and was reemphasized by James Gardner. Peter Jannetta and Robert Rand were the first to employ the operating microscope to clearly identify the presence of arterial loops compressing the trigeminal nerve. Jannetta popularized the idea that decompression of the trigeminal nerve by microsurgically separating compressing vessels and placing a prosthetic, shock absorbing material between the vessel and the trigeminal nerve could abolish the pain of trigeminal neuralgia. Previous, so-called peripheral theories of trigeminal neuralgia had suggested that the trigeminal root might be compressed or irritated by variations in the anatomy of the petrous bone over which the trigeminal nerve root passes, or pressure by a dural band at the tentorial notch through which the trigeminal nerve root passes, or irritation or compression by the underlying carotid artery, particularly when the bony wall between the trigeminal nerve and artery is deficient. A variety of central processes within the brain stem have also been suggested as responsible for trigeminal neuralgia, but at this time there appears to be less support for a central hypothesis.

In some instances, trigeminal neuralgia may be symptomatic of intracranial lesions, which may be treated by direct surgery. Schwannomas of the gasserian ganglion, meningiomas or epidermoid lesions of the petrous bone, acoustic neuromas, aneurysms of the posterior fossa arteries, and atherosclerotic ectasia of the vertebrobasilar arteries are examples of intracranial lesions that may produce symptoms indistinguishable from so-called "idiopathic" trigeminal neuralgia. Such lesions are usually associated with more specific findings on neurological examination, such as significant facial sensory loss, hearing loss, facial weakness, and ataxia. Patients with multiple sclerosis often present with trigeminal neuralgia due to demyelinating plaques in the trigeminal root entry zone at the pons. As one embarks on treatment of trigeminal neuralgia, neuroimaging studies such as a contrast-enhanced computerized tomographic scan or magnetic resonance scan are recommended to specifically exclude primarily treatable lesions.

The clinical treatment of trigeminal neuralgia generally begins with anticonvulsant agents such as phenytoin (Dilantin) or carbamazepine (Tegretol). Trigeminal neuralgia tends to occur primarily in the older population, particularly from ages 55 or 60 and older. Such patients are particularly susceptible to the unwanted side effects of both agents, including disturbances of organic mental function, as well as difficulty with gait. Nevertheless, Dilantin and Tegretol provide at least partial relief of pain in virtually all patients with trigeminal neuralgia. These agents represent the recommended first treatment approach. Recently, it has been recommended that Baclofen (Lioresal) may also provide relief from trigeminal neuralgia. The side effects with this later agent are less, but nevertheless they do occur. When trigeminal neuralgia is no longer effectively relieved by Dilantin, Tegretol, or Lioresal, or when the side effects preclude sufficient dosage to provide relief, surgical treatment should be considered.

Although microvascular decompression of the trigeminal nerve offers the potential for relief of trigeminal neuralgia without alteration in facial sensation, the procedure represents a formidable surgical challenge in the posterior fossa. Since most patients with trigeminal neuralgia are in the elderly age group, the risk of posterior fossa craniotomy is significant. A mortality rate of at least 1% has been reported in the hands of the best neurosurgeons utilizing microsurgical techniques for this procedure, throughout the world. Additionally, the potential for injury to the cerebellum, brain stem, and adjacent cranial nerves raises the possibility of other serious, but nonfatal complications. For this reason, the percutaneous approaches for trigeminal neuralgia represent a safer and easier approach for most patients.

Radiofrequency rhizolysis of the trigeminal nerve has been utilized since the 1970s. In this technique, a radiofrequency electrode is passed percutaneously through the foramen ovale under fluoroscopic control. The procedure is carried out under local anesthesia, supplemented by intravenous barbiturates to produce brief, general anesthesia during lesioning. When the electrode is located radiographically within the trigeminal cistern, low-level electrical stimulation can be carried out with the patient under local anesthesia. Paresthesias are produced in the distribution of the trigeminal branch closest to the needle tip at extremely low stimulus voltages. When paresthesias are produced at voltages in the range of 0.1 to 0.5 volts, radiofrequency lesioning may proceed. Intravenous methohexital (Sodium Brevital) or thiopental (Sodium Pentothal) is given and the temperature of the lesioning electrode is raised to 70–85°C, usually for periods of 60 seconds. Such lesions produce analgesia, i.e., loss of pinprick sensation, but preservation of tactile sensation. The short-acting nature of the barbiturate agents described allows for examination of the patient's responses to sensory stimulation on the face and particularly on the surface of the cornea, virtually immediately after lesioning. Controlled radiofrequency lesions may thus be made, producing generally mild analgesia.

Initial relief of pain may be expected in at least 95% of patients with this technique. Excessive calcification of the skull base rarely makes penetration of the foramen ovale impossible, and at times, severe osteoporosis of the skull base makes identification of the foramen ovale fluoroscopically difficult. Recurrence of pain may occur if injury, but not destruction, of the trigeminal nerve rootlets occurs with mild radiofrequency heating. Return of pain is usually accompanied by return of sensation. The procedure may be repeated if sensation and pain recur simultaneously. The main complications of radiofrequency rhizolysis include injury to adjacent cranial nerves, particularly the third or sixth, producing diplopia and excessive injury to the trigeminal nerve, producing dense anesthesia, particularly of the cornea. Corneal anesthesia may result in delayed corneal injury, corneal ulceration, neuroparalytic keratitis and, in rare instances, blindness. Injury to vascular structures such as the carotid artery was reported in the past, but with proper fluoroscopic control of needle placement, such vascular injury should not occur. The most serious complication of radiofrequency rhizolysis is anesthesia dolorosa, which occurs in a small percentage of patients. This extremely distressing and poorly treated pain syndrome is characterized by anesthesia associated with severe, constant, burning pain, which is usually unresponsive to all forms of medical treatment.

Sten Hakinson, a Swedish neurosurgeon, reported around 1980 the treatment of trigeminal neuralgia by instillation of pure glycerol into the trigeminal cistern. Originally, Hakinson reported that trigeminal neuralgia could be relieved by this technique without producing alteration in facial sensation. Subsequent investigations, however, have shown that although glycerol does produce resolution of trigeminal neuralgia in a high percentage of patients, alterations in facial sensation do occur with glycerol. Glycerol is, in fact, a mild neurotoxin, which produces lysis of myelin and axons when applied directly to nerve root fibers.

In the author's experience, initial relief of pain with glycerol instilled into the retrogasserian cistern can be accomplished in well over 90% of patients. Failures usually occur for technical reasons, in which the glycerol is instilled adjacent to, but not within the trigeminal cistern. The sensory alterations produced by glycerol tend to be less noticeable and less long lasting than those produced with radiofrequency rhizolysis. The procedure is performed on an outpatient basis, and can be accomplished by the experienced operator in perhaps 20–30 minutes. In the author's experience in treating over 200 patients with the retrogasserian glycerol technique, long-term relief of pain can be expected in approximately 80% of patients. The procedure can be repeated if trigeminal neuralgia recurs, coincident with return of normal facial sensation. Corneal anesthesia may occur with retrogasserian glycerol, but the extent of anesthesia tends to be less than with radiofrequency rhizolysis, and the author has never observed neuroparalytic keratitis after glycerol rhizolysis.

The author generally recommends glycerol rhizolysis as the surgical procedure of choice in patients over 60 years of age. The procedure is accomplished quickly and safely on an outpatient basis. If technical problems prevent injection of glycerol into the trigeminal cistern, radiofrequency rhizolysis is recommended. For patients in good health, under 60 years of age, neurovascular decompression is an excellent procedure, since pain relief may be accomplished without sensory loss. Many younger patients, however, when presented with a comparison of the risks of the various available procedures, chose one of the percutaneous approaches, in spite of the likelihood of some loss of facial sensation.

BIBLIOGRAPHY

Dallessio D: Treatment of trigeminal neuralgia. *JAMA* 1981; 245:2519–2520.

Hakinson S: Trigeminal neuralgia treated by the injection of glycerol into the trigeminal cistern. *Neurosurg* 1981; 9:638–656.

Lunsford LD, Bennett MA: Percutaneous retrogasserian glycerol rhizotomy for tic douloureux: Part I, technique and results in 112 patients. *Neurosurgery* 1984; 14:424–430.

Sweet WH: Current concepts: The treatment of trigeminal neuralgia. *N Engl J Med* 1986; 315:174–177.

Young RF: Glycerol rhizolysis for treatment of trigeminal neuralgia. *J Neurosurg* 1988; 69:39–45.

8

Glossopharyngeal Neuralgia

Allan Nutkiewicz, M.D.

A 69-year-old male has a 3-year history of repetitive, lancinating pain in his throat that occurs when he swallows, chews, or speaks. On examination he sits forward in the chair drooling from the side of his mouth. His neurological examination is normal. Magnetic resonance imaging (MRI) of the brain is normal.

DISCUSSION

Glossopharyngeal neuralgia is characterized by paroxysms of pain in the sensory distribution of the ninth cranial nerve. The pain is typically a repetitive, lancinating series of shocks involving the region around the tonsil and posterior one-third of the tongue. The pain is always unilateral. Occasionally, the pain may radiate to the ear. In exceptional cases it may begin deep in the ear.

The pain is brought on by stimulation of the glossopharyngeal nerve sensory area. Commonly, the pain is induced by swallowing or protruding the tongue. Hence food, drink, or saliva can also produce the pain. The ear may be extremely sensitive to the touch and be a trigger point for the pain.

Remissions can last for years, but spontaneous cures have never been reported. The vast majority of cases reported are idiopathic, although recently, the same causation believed to induce trigeminal neuralgia, that is, tortuous loops of the vertebral or basilar artery resting on the glossopharyngeal-vagus complex adjacent to the brain stem, has been proposed. Some cases have been ascribed to cerebellopontine angle and nasopharyngeal tumors.

Associated with glossopharyngeal neuralgia have been episodes of cardiac arrest, syncope, and seizures. Repetitive afferent impulses from the pharynx to the hypersensitized dorsal motor nucleus of the vagus induce uncompensated parasympathetic tone to the heart leading to asystole. The increased vagal tone is also the basis for syncope and seizures. Instead of cardiac arrest, there is decreased cardiac output and cerebral hypoxia.

MEDICAL MANAGEMENT

Pain in a similar distribution, but continuous in nature, may occur as a result of tumors involving the tonsil and pharynx. These causes must be excluded. Magnetic resonance imaging of these areas, as well as the posterior fossa, are imperative in the workup of these patients.

Once the diagnosis has been made, the mainstay of medical therapy is carbamazepine (Tegretol). The medication is begun at 200 mg three times a day, and slowly increased in increments of 200 mg until the pain is controlled, or until a daily maximum of 1,200 mg in divided doses is reached. It is the rare patient who will be able to tolerate a full dose of 1,200 mg a day without complaining of a ''zombie-like'' feeling. Once this side effect has been reached, it is usually intolerable to the patient. Close monitoring of the patient's white blood count is mandatory.

If, after a good trial of carbamazepine has been tried and failed, there are second-line drugs that may be tried. These are phenytoin and baclofen. The results for these medications are significantly worse than for carbamazepine.

SURGICAL MANAGEMENT

When medical management has failed, surgery becomes the treatment of choice. Peripheral division of the branches of the ninth and tenth nerves has been attempted in the past but is significantly more dangerous than intracranial division because of the close proximity of fibers of the vagus nerve. There is also the possibility that the sectioned fibers will regenerate and that relief will be transient.

Percutaneous radiofrequency rhizotomies have been performed in the past with an unacceptably high rate of permanent injury to the vagus nerve leaving patients with vocal cord paralysis and altered swallowing mechanisms.

Intracranial microsurgical sectioning of the glossopharyngeal nerve and upper rootlets of the vagus nerve is the procedure of choice, as it leaves the patient with no discernible sequelae and permanent relief of their pain.

There has been some interest in performing only a microvascular decompression of the ninth nerve for the same reasons the decompression of the fifth cranial nerve is performed for trigeminal neuralgia. However, the risk of recurrence for this procedure is significant and, therefore, it makes little sense to subject the patient to this operation.

The reported complications of the intracranial sectioning of the ninth and upper rootlets of the tenth nerve are primarily cardiac arrythmias and are usually transient. There has been one reported episode of intraoperative hypertensive crisis with hemorrhage and death.

For patients of any age, with modern microneurosurgical techniques and experiences with neuroanesthesia, there is little justification for not offering this procedure for the permanent relief of this terribly painful and distressing condition.

BIBLIOGRAPHY

Dandy W-E: Glossopharyngeal neuralgia: Its diagnosis and treatment. *Arch Surg* 1927; 15:198–214.

Laha RK, Janetta PJ: Glossopharyngeal neuralgia. *J Neurosurg* 1977; 47:316–220.

9

Myofascial Headache

Michael Simmons, D.M.D.

A 33-year-old female secretary presents with a dull, aching headache of unknown etiology. Onset occurred spontaneously 3 years previously. Since onset she has been evaluated by a neurologist following computed tomographic (CT) scan of the brain, and found to have no abnormalities. The history reveals the headaches are mainly on the right side of the head, although when severe, they progress bilaterally. The headaches are associated with tenderness in the masseter, temporalis, and splenius capitus muscles. They are described as a constant, deep, boring pain in the temple region, lasting 3–4 days. More recently, they have become incapacitating. The diagnosis of myofascial headache is made on the basis of periodicity, location, and quality of the head pain and the ability to reduce the headache after identification and stretching of the causative muscles.

DISCUSSION

The clinician faced with a patient complaining of headache should try to immediately differentiate if there is a serious or life-threatening process causing the pain, or whether the headache is due to a benign disturbance of physiology or a symptom of a psychologic disturbance. Obviously, the former requires immediate identification and attention. Fortunately, only a small minority of headaches, 2%, have important organic causes for the complaints, such as cranial mass lesions, infections, intracranial bleeding, or CSF disturbances. The recent onset headache should always be evaluated critically with a cranial nerve examination approach and intracranial CT or magnetic resonance imaging (MRI). If the patient has no neurologic complaints, particular emphasis should be placed on extraocular movements, pupillary responses, and visual field examination, since these aspects would not present with symptoms.

Headache of long standing without neurologic symptomatology is assessed by complete history, and detail is paid to quality and location, periodicity and duration, precipitating, aggravating, and ameliorating factors. The longer standing the headache, the less likely it is life threatening.

Myofascial headache or head pain is more frequently described as dull, deep aching or pressurelike pain that may start gradually or with an abrupt onset. Generally, one side is significantly worse than the other, although the pain is not uncommonly bilateral.

Autonomic phenomena are frequently reported in conjunction with myofascial pain, as well as proprioreceptive disturbances. These may include localized vasoconstriction, sweating, lacrimation, coryza, salivation, dizziness, and tinnitus. Certain muscles, such as the trapezius and sternocleidomastoid, are more prone to involve such concomitants.

For many years, myofascial pain has been thought of as a component of pain syndromes such as MPDS (myofascial pain dysfunction syndrome), TMJ (temporomandibular joint) dysfunction, fibrositis syndrome, and also by other names such as fibrositis, fibromyalgia, muscular rheumatism, myofibrositis, myogelosis, and myalgia. It is no wonder it became a wastebasket term, especially since biopsy, x-ray, and blood tests could not verify significant alteration from the norms. Fortunately, at this time, there is a significant body of literature that defines its clinical existence, characteristics, and causative factors.[1]

Myofascial pain is that associated with trigger points in the muscle and surrounding fascia that refers either locally or distantly to a separate pain zone, known as the "zone of reference." The pattern of referred pain does not correspond to segmental dermatomal or myotomal sensory distribution. Trigger points are digitally palpable, tender taut bands felt within skeletal muscle. They are thought to form as a result of macrotraumatic muscle injury or repeated microtrauma, such as strain from chronically poor posture or parafunctional oral habits of clenching or grinding of the teeth. Muscles may be predisposed to development of trigger points with sleep disorders, stress, joint dysfunctions, or poor nutrition.

Two types of trigger points exist, latent and active. Active trigger points, when palpated, replicate the patient's pain, while latent trigger points can refer pain to a characteristic reference zone when palpated, but will not do so spontaneously.[2] The prevalence of myofascial pain has been recently quantified when 30% of patients presented to a UCLA internist with a chief complaint of pain. Of these patients, 30% had identifiable trigger points that responded well to trigger point therapy.[3] Up to one year follow-up on these patients has revealed no other findings that would explain another cause of their original pain complaint.

In the later years of life, restricted muscle function is the primary presentation of trigger points, while in the prime years, the complaint of pain is most commonly given. If specific muscle syndromes are not addressed appropriately, multiple muscle syndromes, followed by a chronic pain syndrome, may develop with their associated psychological and behavioral problems.

Myofascial pain is distinguished in the literature from the more generalized phenomena seen in primary or secondary fibromyalgia syndrome.[4-5] These latter two phenomena are currently thought to be a clinical pain disorder in which the presence of multiple fibrositic tender points are associated with characteristic symptoms of prolonged generalized muscle aching and stiffness, fatigue, and a sleep disturbance. Secondary fibromyalgia differs from the primary form in that it is associated with some other inflammatory disease, such as rheumatoid arthritis, systemic lupus erythematosus, or one of the seronegative spondarthropathies.

Myofascial headache may be recognized by the following inclusionary factors:

1. The quality of the pain is deep, dull, and aching.
2. The patient's headache or head pain can be reproduced by palpation of specific muscle zones that coincide with mapped referral patterns of myofascial trigger points.
3. The pain can be temporarily reduced by 50% or more with spray and stretch or trigger point injection techniques, as advocated by Travell and Simons.[2]

To ensure diagnosis, two exclusionary phenomena must also be taken into account. First, in order to differentiate from a vascular headache, there can be no associated visual aura. Secondly, the pain pattern must not follow any peripheral nerve distribution.

MANAGEMENT

After identifying the patient as having myofascial head pain, it is of primary importance to map all objective findings of the palpation exam with the appropriate references. Although a simple case may involve single muscle problems, there is often secondary or contributory muscles that may appear only after initial treatment of the obvious active trigger point. Since referral is usually in a cephalic direction, the tendency is to uncover contributing latent trigger points further down the patient's head and neck.

Once the primary trigger points have been mapped, the patient is given a visual analogue scale (VAS), on which to note a current pain level. This is usually a 10-cm straight line that has the two end scale markings of "no pain" and "worst pain imaginable." The patient is asked to place a slash mark on the scale at the point that corresponds to "their pain of chief complaint" at this moment. Having done this, the muscle harboring the active trigger point is sprayed with fluorimethane, generally from a caudal to cephalad direction, in a slow enough manner that allows all but running of the liquid. Repetitive sweeping strokes with the spray are made approximately 1 cm apart until the muscle has been covered. Successful application of the spray can be ensured by continuing the direction of the spray from the muscle to include the zone of reference. Immediately after a complete muscle has been swept, the patient's muscle is placed on stretch with gentle pressure. During this prolonged stretch, the skin is allowed to recover its normal temperature. The fluorimethane spray is repeated. It is important to know that the spray itself is simply a distraction technique so that the action of stretch can take place. Theoretically, the sensory pain information of the cold spray inhibits or overwhelms the neuromuscular feedback of protective muscle splinting that prevents the muscle from being passively stretched.

The skin is allowed to rewarm between successive spray patterns so that there is negligible change in muscle temperature. Repeated stretching to restore the muscle to its appropriate working length results in the elimination of the activity of the trigger point. Immediately following the stretching, the muscle is gently guided through the restored full range of motion to ensure the new range is imprinted and the patient is aware of it. The patient is given a new 10-cm pain rating scale on which to mark the current level of pain. The pre- and post-stretch subjective reports of pain are compared. These are the millimeter distances measured from the "no pain" end of the scale. If there is a significant reduction, the patient is instructed to repeat home stretches for a period of a week, and return for follow-up. While this technique is successful for muscles that can be manually placed on stretch, there are times when either a muscle cannot be stretched or it has been resistant or unresponsive to spray and stretch techniques. In these cases, an injection technique using local anesthetic, saline, or a dry needle are employed. Simply dry needling causes postoperative soreness within minutes, and occasionally the treatment is unendurably painful. Procaine 0.5% without epinephrine is the most appropriate anesthetic, since it has been shown to cause the least muscle necrosis and causes fast relief of the painful trigger point, allowing the operator to more easily perform the manual stretch.

Injection of approximately 1 cc per trigger point, spread out in a fan-shaped pattern to find additional satellite trigger points in the immediate vicinity is most effective. During the injection procedure, patients are asked to describe the sensation. Most often they will describe it as their pain, a deep, dull ache, or burning with referral to the reference zone. It is important to remember that following injection, the muscle must be stretched in order to effect treatment, and that the injection only allows for the ability to do such stretching. Post-injection treatment should include moist heat application. Steroid therapy, oral or intramuscular, is indicated only if there is a history of excessive post-injection soreness. The most important aspect of treatment of myofascial pain is the identification and removal of the perpetuating factors. This is not usually as significant if the trigger point resulted from macrotrauma, since it is unlikely that regular activities precipitate the same injury. However, if the causative factor is microtrauma, such as a daily clenching and grinding of the teeth with resultant temporalis and masseter trigger points that lead to referred headache, the trigger points will readily return. In such cases, the use of an intraoral appliance or behavioral techniques to decrease muscle tension levels may be used to reduce these habits, especially if they occur at night while asleep. During daytime activities, the patient must learn appropriate positioning of the mandible and stretching exercises to perform on a frequent and regular basis, whether or not the pain has returned. If the cause of the head pain is from posterior cervical muscle strain secondary to chronic forward head posture, then posture retraining, along with myofascial therapy, is essential for long-term success.

Chronic cases of myofascial pain often involve debilitating pain, restriction in movement, and significant changes in life style. At this point, successful treatment relies on a multidisciplinary approach. A team of practitioners should include a pain manager to coordinate and follow up with all modalities of treatment, and a psychologist to identify illness focus, contributing operants, and teach patients techniques of self-management, as well as possibly referring to psychiatric management, those patients with severe depression, anxiety, or psychoses. Another essential team member is the physical therapist, who will treat underlying joint issues that perpetuate muscle splinting, help with the home exercise program, and teach the patient and spouse techniques of self-management. Treatment contracts are helpful with this type of patient, which show time and cost of treatment, spell out the goals, and indicate how patients will be detoxified from any narcotic medications to which they may be addicted.[6]

Obviously, perpetuating factors such as sleep disturbances, depression, etc., may require medication usage, and it is not uncommon for pain specialists to advocate low dose antidepressants in particular, for their side effects of increased sleep and CNS serotoninergic pain relieving abilities.

REFERENCES

1. Fricton JR, Kroening R, Haley D, et al: Myofascial pain syndrome of the head and neck: A review of clinical characteristics of 164 patients. *Oral Surg* 1985; 60:615–623.
2. Travell JG, Simons DG: Myofascial Pain and Dysfunction, in *The Trigger Point Manual*. Baltimore, Williams & Wilkins, 1983.
3. Skootsky SA, Jaeger B, Oya RK: Prevalence of myofascial pain and recognition in general internal medicine patients. *West J Med* 1989; 151:157–160.

4. McCain GA, Scudds RA: The concept of fibromyalgia (fibrositis): Clinical value, relation and significance to other chronic musculoskeletal pain syndromes. *Pain* 1988; 33:273–287.

5. Yunus MB: Fibromyalgia syndrome: A need for uniform classification. *J Rheumatol* 1983; 10:841–844.

6. Graff-Radford SB, Reeves JL, Jaeger B: Management of chronic head and neck pain: Effectiveness of altering factors perpetuating myofascial pain. *Headache.* 1987; 27:186–190.

10

Facial Causalgia

Bernadette Jaeger, D.D.S.

A 33-year-old woman is admitted for diagnosis and treatment of an intense left-sided facial pain described as a constant burning. The burning radiates from the preauricular area to the orbit, zygoma, mandible, and occasionally to the shoulder. The pain is exacerbated by chewing, smiling, light touch over the specific facial areas, cold air, and cold liquid. Photophobia of the left eye and a constant pinching sensation over the left eyebrow and mandible are also noted. Narcotic medications fail to relieve these symptoms. The pain began one year earlier after extraction of an upper molar. An alveolar osteitis apparently developed, which was treated without relief of symptoms. Two ipsilateral mandibular teeth were extracted in an attempt to relieve the patient's pain. Alveolar osteitis again developed, and was treated without relief of pain. Examination of the patient reveals slight swelling and elevated skin temperature over the affected side of the face. The patient cannot open her mouth widely, and translation of the left condyle is limited. Intra- and extraoral palpation is not possible because the patient complains of pain at the slightest touch. Temporomandibular joint (TMJ) tomograms reveal flattening of the left condyle. Bony sclerosis in the area of the extraction sites is seen on dental and panoramic radiographs. Computed tomography (CT) of the brain, mandible, and retropharyngeal area, gallium scan, and skin tests for cocci infection are all negative. Reflex sympathetic dystrophy of the face is added to the differential diagnosis because of the burning hyperesthetic quality of the pain, onset after tooth extraction, and localized temperature elevation in the absence of infection. A left stellate ganglion block with local anesthetic completely eliminates the burning pain and hyperpathia. Relief outlasts the duration of the anesthetic. The patient undergoes a series of 15 blocks with complete resolution of her pain as measured by self-report and repeated charting of a visual analogue scale (VAS). She remains well and requires no analgesics at a 15-month follow-up.

DISCUSSION

Reflex sympathetic dystrophy (RSD), was originally described by Mitchell in 1864.[1] He called this pain "causalgia" from the Greek words 'kausos' meaning heat, and 'algia' meaning pain. This "causalgia" or "burning pain," as described by Mitchell, was a pain that appeared following a high velocity missile wound to a major peripheral nerve. Consequently, it was typically seen in the extremities. In 1947, Evans described RSD as a burning pain that also had many other features of sympathetic stimulation such as redness, swelling, sweating, and atrophic changes in the skin, muscles, and bones.[2] He noted that this syndrome could occur, not only as a result of large peripheral nerve injuries, but also following very minor injuries such as fractures or sprains. It was the same year that Bingham reported RSD or "causalgia" of the face.[3] Since that time, only 7 or 8 cases of RSD of the face have been reported in the world literature.

Reflex sympathetic dystrophy of the extremities has been extensively described, and is characterized by burning pain, hyperpathia, and allodynia, with variable degrees of vasomotor, sudomotor, and trophic changes. These temperature, color, and nutritional changes are thought to be secondary to changes in sympathetically mediated blood flow. Onset of the pain may occur immediately, or within weeks after an injury. The precipitating event may actually be overlooked because of its apparent trivial nature. Delay in recognition and treatment of RSD may result in prolonged pain and disability.

In the facial region, the diagnosis of a sympathetically mediated pain syndrome may be obscured secondary to a lack of marked vasomotor, sudomotor, and trophic changes. The apparent absence of these changes may be due to the rich anastomatic and collateral vascular supply to the face, since it appears that RSD follows the topography of the sympathetically innervated vascular system.

PATHOPHYSIOLOGY

The underlying mechanisms of RSD are unknown, yet it is clear that many of its manifestations are due to sympathetic dysregulation. Doupe et al., in 1944,[4] and Nathan in 1947,[5] proposed the formation of an artificial synapse between somatic afferent and sympathetic efferent fibers. It is thought that sensory nerves would be excited by outgoing sympathetic impulses. Livingston in 1944,[6] and Sunderland in 1976,[7] proposed that self-sustaining hyperactive foci of abnormal neuronal activity could develop in the dorsal horn of the spinal cord as the result of death and malfunctioning of these cells secondary to peripheral damage. They also felt that this "disorganized, intraspinal focus of abnormal hyperactivity" may shift with time from the cord to higher centers and further perpetuate the pain.

In 1971, Melzack proposed that part of the brain stem reticular system may exert a tonic inhibitory effect on the transmission of impulses at all synaptic levels.[8] He speculated that loss of sensory input after a nerve injury could produce a decrease in this tonic inhibition. This would produce a release of self-sustaining activity at all synaptic levels that could be repeatedly triggered by discharge from surviving nerve fibers. Devor, in 1983, proposed that the basic cause of pain in RSD was due to the development of abnormal electrogenic membrane properties in the region of demyelination and sprout outgrowth.[9] Normally, afferents in the mid-course of intact nerves are incapable of generating impulses but, after various types of nerve injury, including demyelination, an "ectopic pacemaker" capability develops. These sites are also chemosensitive to alpha adrenergic agonists and to sympathetic efferent discharge.

Another explanation for continued pain in RSD rests on the observation that central changes in the excitability of neurons may occur after the damage in the periphery. There is experimental evidence to support this. Anderson,[10] in 1971, and Westrum et al.,[11] in 1968, have shown that spontaneous neuronal hyperactivity in the spinal trigeminal nucleus of cats occurs after ipsilateral rhizotomy. Westrum et al., also demonstrated central neuronal degeneration in the trigeminal nucleus after damage to a tooth pulp or after section of the trigeminal nerve.

Thus, painful injuries may cause secondary processes, not associated with tissue damage, that produce a prolongation and spread of nociceptive input. These secondary processes may actually be self-perpetuating since they may become independent nociceptive foci that are not a part of the original site of injury.

DIAGNOSIS

The diagnosis of reflex sympathetic dystrophy depends upon relief of pain with sympathetic blockade. In the head and neck region this requires blockade of the stellate ganglion. The sympathetic fibers that serve the orofacial region arise primarily in the first and second upper thoracic spinal segments. The fibers course upward through the stellate and middle cervical ganglia to synapse in the superior cervical ganglion before leaving the sympathetic chain to run with the blood vessels supplying the facial region.

Successful blockade of the stellate ganglion should be accompanied by Horner's syndrome and skin warming. Sympathetic blockade often produces pain relief that outlasts the duration of the local anesthetic.

TREATMENT

Recommended treatment for reflex sympathetic dystrophy of the face is repeated sympathetic blockade. Early intervention is stressed, as advanced cases may require sympathectomy, or may fail to respond well to any treatment.

A stellate ganglion block is not without potential complications. An injection performed too low may cause pneumothorax. Injection of local anesthetic drugs into the vertebral artery may lead to dizziness, convulsions, and unconsciousness. If anesthetic enters the dura, the risk of a high spinal anesthetic and possible respiratory arrest exists. An injection may also puncture the pharynx if it is made too medially. The most common side effect of stellate ganglion block is anesthesia of the recurrent laryngeal nerve. This results in hoarseness and an obtunded gag reflex for several hours. Also, it is fairly common that the brachial plexus may be affected, resulting in mild sensory loss of the ipsilateral upper extremity.

In cases of bilateral facial causalgia, stellate ganglion blocks are best carried out on one side at a time on alternate days. Bilateral blockade may result in bradycardia or bilateral recurrent laryngeal nerve palsy with acute respiratory obstruction. Of interest is the presence of enkephalin in the sympathetic ganglia.[12] Based on this information, Mays et al., in 1981, experimented with morphine for stellate ganglion blocks.[13] They found that with morphine there was no Horner's syndrome and no temperature change to the face. However, it was associated with profound pain relief. In contrast, subcutaneous morphine injection provided no relief. They concluded from this that the pain relief was not due to a systemic narcotic action, but rather from a local action of the morphine at the stellate ganglion. Thus, performing stellate ganglion blocks with morphine may be a useful alternative in patients with bilateral pain.

SUMMARY

1. There is a small but treatable group of patients with facial pain that is secondary to reflex sympathetic dystrophy (facial causalgia).
2. Local anesthetic blocks of the stellate ganglion can confirm this diagnosis, and are the main form of treatment.
3. Other agents injected around the stellate ganglion, such as morphine, may also prove helpful.

REFERENCES

1. Mitchell SW, Moorehouse GR, Kenn WW: *Gunshot Wounds and Other Injuries of Nerves*. Philadelphia, JB Lippincott Co., 1864.

2. Evans JA: Reflex sympathetic dystrophy: Report on 57 cases. *Ann Intern Med* 1947; 26:417–426.
3. Bingham JAW: Causalgia of the face. Two cases successfully treated by sympathectomy. *Br Med J* 1947; 1:804–805.
4. Doupe T, Cullen CH, Chance GQ: Post-traumatic pain and the causalgic syndrome. *J Neurol Neurosurg Psychiatry* 1944; 7:33–48.
5. Nathan PW: On the pathogenesis of causalgia in peripheral nerve injuries. *Brain* 1947; 70:145–170.
6. Livingston WK: *Pain Mechanisms: A Physiologic Interpretation of Causalgia and its Related States.* New York, MacMillan, 1944.
7. Sunderland S: Pain mechanisms in causalgia. *J Neurol Neurosurg Psychiatry* 1976; 39:471–480.
8. Melzack R: Phantom limb pain: Implications for treatment of pathologic pain. *Anesthesiology* 1971; 35:409–419.
9. Devor M: Nerve pathophysiology and mechanisms of pain in causalgia. *J Auton Nerv Syst* 1983; 7:371–384.
10. Anderson LS, Black RG, Abraham J, et al: Neuronal hyperactivity in experimental trigeminal deafferentation. *J Neurosurg* 1971; 35:444–452.
11. Westrum LE, Black RG, Abraham J, et al: Changes in the synapses of the spinal trigeminal nucleus after ipsilateral rhizotomy. *Brain Res* 1968; 11:706–709.
12. DiGuilio AM: Characterization of enkephalin-like material extracted from sympathetic ganglia. *Neuropharmacology* 1978; 17:989–992.
13. Mays KS, North WC, Schnapp M: Stellate ganglion "blocks" with morphine in sympathetic type pain. *J Neurol Neurosurg Psychiatry* 1981; 44:189–190.

11

Chronic Ear Pain From Myofascial Pain Syndrome

James R. Fricton, D.D.S., M.S.

An 11-year-old boy was referred by his pediatrician to the University of Minnesota's TMJ and Craniofacial Pain Clinic to evaluate a 2-year history of traumatically induced bilateral ear pain. The pain was described as a dull, constant pain occurring daily. Multiple normal ear and hearing examinations and missing 44 days from school due to pain led his otolaryngologist to make the diagnosis of malingering. However, an examination of the craniomandibular structures revealed a diagnosis of myofascial pain with referral to the ear.

DISCUSSION

Myofascial pain syndrome (MPS) is frequently overlooked as a common cause of chronic pain because of the complex pain referral patterns, frequent association with joint dysfunction and other disorders, and multiple behavioral and psychosocial contributing factors.[1-2] However, two studies of pain clinic populations have revealed that MPS is the cause of pain in 55.4% of a chronic head and neck pain population and 85% of a back pain population.[2-3] In addition, a recent epidemiological study of young females (ages 20–40 years) revealed that MPS occurs in nearly 35% of this general population.[4]

The clinical characteristics involve pain referred from trigger points within myofascial structures, either local or distant from the pain. A trigger point is the localized tender area in a firm band of skeletal muscle, tendon, or ligament. These points can occur in any skeletal muscle of the body, although they occur most frequently in the head, neck, shoulders, and lower back. The patterns of referral for each trigger point are consistent among different persons. This area of referral is termed the "zone of reference." In this case, the trigger points were in muscles that can refer pain to the ear, including the masseter, digastric, lateral pterygoid, and sternocleidomastoid (Fig 11–1).

The primary diagnosis of MPS was established according to the following clinical criteria: 1) the presence of trigger points; 2) pain complaints that follow patterns of referral from the trigger points that were consistent with past reports; and 3) reproducible alteration of pain complaints with specific palpation of the responsible "active" trigger points. Active trigger points are hypersensitivity and cause pain.

Palpation was done with sustained, deep, single finger pressure using the spadelike pad of the distal phalanx of the index finger by moving it across the muscle band at the area of tenderness. The resulting alteration in pain occurred immediately or within seconds. In locating a trigger point, the "jump sign" was often elicited. This sign is the patient's behavioral reaction to the tenderness of palpation and may include turning away of the head, wrinkling of the face or forehead, or a verbal response such as "that's it" or "oh, yes."

The development of trigger points can be divided into two basic concepts:

1. Factors that directly traumatize a muscle by direct injury or by repetitive microtrauma from habits that produce muscle tension. The most frequent habits for masticatory MPS include poor postural stability due to malocclusion and oral parafunctional habits.

2. Factors that weaken a muscle and predispose it to the development of trigger points through such factors as nutritional disturbances, structural disharmony, lack of exercise, sleep disturbances, or the presence of other disorders, such as joint problems.

In this case, trauma from playing football resulted in injury to both the tympanic membrane and the adjacent muscles. The inner ear healed, but the muscles continued to be strained by oral habits including clenching, bruxism, pencil chewing, gum chewing, and tongue thrust.

Lack of recognition that myofascial pain can cause ear pain leads to misdiagnosis, inadequate management, and serious psychosocial consequences. If the pain continues and repeated attempts at management fail, the patient is prone to develop a chronic pain syndrome and the complex behavioral and psychosocial problems associated with it. If this occurs, management often requires a more costly team approach to rehabilitation that has less potential for success. Early recognition of this disorder will allow simpler, more effective, and less costly management.

In this case, the pain continued to affect the child's school performance,

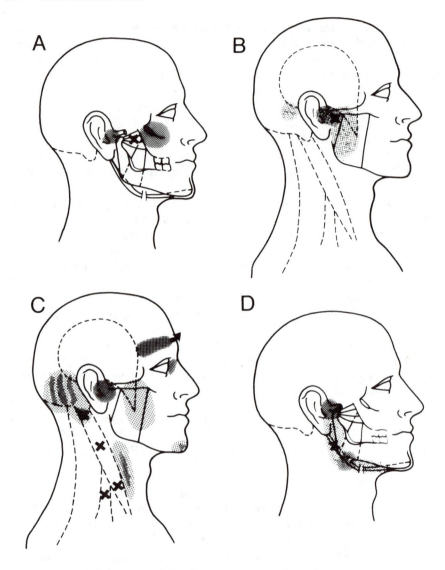

FIG 11–1.
A–D, pain can be referred to the ear from myofascial structures including the masseter, digastric, lateral pterygoid, and sternocleidomastoid. (From Fricton J, Kroening R, Hathaway K: *TMJ and Craniofacial Pain: Diagnosis and Management.* St. Louis, IEA Publishers, 1988. Used by permission.)

which led to low interest, poor grades, and absenteeism. His mother, convinced that the pain was "real," had conflicts with doctors and school administrators, and reinforced the child's pain behaviors. The child was inactive, frequently expressed pain verbally and with facial expressions, and took excessive analgesics. The family was strained with frequent conflicts and feelings of anger and hopelessness.

MANAGEMENT

The final goals for management of myofascial pain is lasting inactivation of the responsible trigger points and restoration of normal resting muscle length with full range of motion. Failure to achieve these goals will lead to minimal or short-term pain relief. The means of achieving pain relief is through passive and active stretching of the involved muscle during counter-stimulation of the trigger point. The means for long-term maintenance of relief is through regular muscle stretching and strengthening exercises, as well as long-term control of contributing factors. A home program of muscle stretching exercises will reduce the activity of any remaining trigger points by physical strain. Strengthening exercises will improve muscle tone and ability to maintain good posture.

Evaluating the present range of motion of muscles is the first step in prescribing a set of exercises. A slightly limited mandibular opening will often indicate the presence of trigger points within the elevator muscles: temporalis, masseter, and medial pterygoid. If the mandibular opening is measured as the interincisal distance, a normal range of opening is generally between 42–60 mm, or approximately three knuckles-width (nondominant hand). A mandibular opening with trigger points in the masseter will be between 30–40 mm (two knuckles). If contracture of masticatory muscles is present, the mandibular opening can be as limited as 10–20 mm. Other causes of diminished mandibular opening must also be considered and should include structural disorders of the temporomandibular joint, such as ankylosis, internal derangements, and gross osteoarthritis. Inactivation of the trigger points with passive and active stretching of the muscles will increase the opening to the normal range as well as decrease the pain. Passive stretching of the muscle during counter-stimulation of the trigger point can be accomplished by placing a properly trimmed and sterile cork or other object between the incisors while the spray and stretch is accomplished. Active stretching by the patient can be accomplished through the exercise demonstrated in Figure 11–2. It must be emphasized that rapid, excessive stretching of the muscle should be avoided to reduce potential injury.

The range of motion for the neck can be determined by the degree of neck flexion, rotation, and lateral flexion. The normal range of motion for neck flexion is 80–90° with the chin touching the chest. The normal rotation of the neck

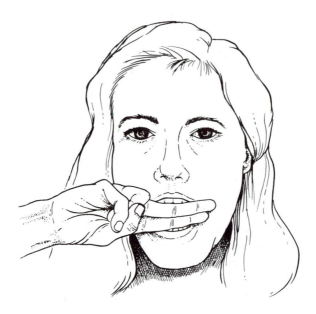

FIG 11–2.
Jaw stretching exercise. This exercise can be performed gradually and gently three times daily for 1 minute each time with optional simultaneous application of heat or ice. Jaw should be stretched slightly beyond the point of tightness and pain. Patient should avoid over-stretching with acutely strained jaws or with acute closed locking from a TMJ internal de-rangement. (From Fricton J, Kroening R, Hathaway K: *TMJ and Craniofacial Pain: Diagnosis and Management*. St. Louis, IEA Publishers, 1988. Used by permission.)

should be a full 90° left and right from the center with the chin pointed directly toward the shoulder or beyond. The normal range of motion for lateral neck flexion is 45° with the ear toward the relaxed shoulder. Any perceived tautness or pain of the muscles with a decrease in range of motion in these movements is often caused by trigger points. However, cervical osteoarthritis, ankylosis, and other joint problems may also cause limitation.

Passive and active stretching of the neck muscles can be accomplished with the exercise demonstrated in Figure 11–3. In this exercise, slow movement with avoidance of crepitation is important in preventing or reducing cervical degen-erative joint disease.

One of the most common causes of failure in managing myofascial pain is due to the lack of recognition and subsequent control of the contributing factors that may perpetuate the trigger points or complicate management. For this reason, control of contributing factors needs to be accomplished with treatment of the muscle. The two most common contributing factors include poor posture and muscle tension-producing habits.

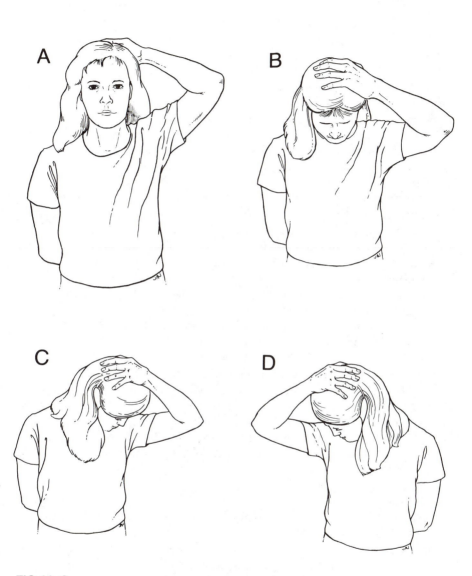

FIG 11–3.
A–D, neck stretching exercise. This exercise can be performed gradually and gently six times daily for 1 minute each time; simultaneous application of heat or ice can be used to reduce pain. Patient should be cautioned to avoid overstretching with an acutely strained neck, severe cervical osteoarthritis with nerve compression, disk disease, or recent surgery in the area. (From Fricton J, Kroening R, Hathaway K: *TMJ and Craniofacial Pain: Diagnosis and Management.* St. Louis, IEA Publishers, 1988. Used by permission).

Poor postural contributing factors, whether structural or behavioral in nature, will perpetuate trigger points if not corrected. In general, a muscle is more predisposed to developing trigger points if it is held in sustained contraction in the normal position or if it is in an abnormally shortened position. A loss of posterior teeth, malocclusion, a class II or class III jaw skeletal discrepancy, a short leg, a small hemipelvis, or an excessive lordosis of the cervical spine can place strain on the masticatory or cervical muscles. Poor posture also occurs due to behavioral factors such as holding a phone to the head with the shoulder, twisting the neck to improve visualization during a task, repetitively holding the head forward while studying for hours at a time, or holding the tongue against the lower teeth. Correcting poor postural habits through education and long-term reinforcement is essential to preventing a reduced trigger point from returning.

An occlusal postural imbalance can be corrected with an occlusal stabilization appliance, also termed a flat plane splint. This appliance should be constructed to cover all teeth in the maxilla or the mandible and should be adjusted to provide as ideal an occlusion as possible with full centric occlusion and centric relation contacts, anterior disclusion, and anterior protrusive and lateral guidance. A stabilization appliance can be adjusted periodically for months while head, neck, and body postural corrections are made that will alter the maxilla-mandible relationship. Postural corrections include placing the tongue on the palate, holding the back straight, positioning the thorax up with the shoulders back, and tilting the pelvis up and back. Once the symptoms have been resolved and the appliance has not required any adjustments for one to two months, permanent stabilization of the occlusion at the original vertical dimension can be accomplished through a coronoplasty (occlusal adjustment). In some situations, orthodontics, restorative dentistry, or fixed and removable prosthodontics may be required to improve structural occlusal problems.

The most common muscle tension-producing oral habits include clenching, bruxism, and gum chewing. In addition to self-report, identification of these habits can be made with examination for tooth wear, tongue and cheek ridging, and masseter hypertrophy.

Reducing these oral habits can be very helpful in managing both masticatory and cervical muscles affected. Teaching control of oral habits is a difficult process because of their relationship with anxiety, stress, and the pace of daily life style. Simply telling a patient not to clench his or her teeth may be helpful with some, but with others, it may result in noncompliance, failure, and frustration. Methods of reducing clenching and bruxism include biofeedback, occlusal adjustment, splints, psychotherapy, autosuggestion, and drug therapy. A comprehensive approach that integrates cognitive, behavioral, and somatic approaches may be most successful. Enhancing cognitive awareness of the habit can be accomplished through sensory cues such as a timer that beeps every half hour or sandpaper placed on telephone receivers, door handles, or faucets to provide a tactile reminder to check the habit. Once aware of the habit, behavioral strategies such as biofeedback and muscle relaxation techniques can be effective in teaching patients what it feels like to hold muscles in a relaxed state. If the patient desires, stress management may also be used to teach how to avoid increasing the habits during stressful life events. It is important to avoid stating that the pain is directly caused by stress, since at best this creates a feeling of impotency in controlling "stress" in patients' lives and thus, the pain, and at worst, will insult patients by implying that the pain is not "real." In addition to cognitive and behavioral approaches, somatic therapy such as a stabilization appliance may be used to reduce the traumatic effects of bruxism by providing more stable, broader muscle contraction patterns to disperse the occlusal forces.

The 11-year-old child with ear pain was given a set of exercises by the physical therapist to stretch the jaw and neck muscles and posture the tongue gently on the palate. This latter exercise helped relax the muscles by stabilizing the jaw and preventing tooth contact. The patient was fitted for a stabilization splint to protect the muscles from further postural and oral habit strain, and to remind him to avoid poor oral habits. Finally, a behavioral therapy program was implemented by the psychologist to change oral habits, to comply with exercise and splint therapies, and to reduce pain behaviors. It was agreed to reduce pain behaviors by not discussing the pain at home and by setting up a time-contingent schedule for reducing analgesic use. Daily attendance at school was begun and coordinated with the patient's pediatrician, school nurse, and school principal. It was agreed by all parties, including the patient, that with the diagnosis and treatment clear, the pain could not be used as a reason to stay home from school. This management program was expected to last 6 months.

In the ensuing 3 months, he used the splint regularly, reduced most poor oral habits, but exercised irregularly. His school attendance was excellent and grades improved dramatically. His ear pain was reduced to mild discomfort that occurred once a week. However, family conflicts continued to occur and the family was referred to family therapy. Although short-term success was achieved, long-term improvement will depend on maintaining exercises, eliminating poor oral habits, and resolving family conflicts.

REFERENCES

1. Travell J, Simons DG: Myofascial pain and dysfunction: The trigger point manual. Baltimore, Williams & Wilkins Co., 1983, pp 63–158.
2. Fricton J, et al: Myofascial pain syndrome of the head and neck. A review of clinical characteristics of 164 patients. *Oral Surg* 1985; 60:615–623.
3. Fishbain DA, Goldberg M, Meagher BR, et al: Male and female chronic pain patients categorized by DSM III. Psychiatric Diagnostic Criteria. *Pain* 1986; 26:181–197.
4. Fricton J: Longitudinal outcome study of TMJ disorders. Progress report to NIDR, grant 1223–DE 07460–03.

12

Jaw Pain From a Temporomandibular Joint Internal Derangement

James R. Fricton, D.D.S., M.S.

A 22-year-old woman presented for a second opinion regarding treatment for a 2-year history of daily right jaw pain with daily right occipital to frontal headaches. An oral surgeon had previously recommended surgery on the right temporomandibular joint (TMJ) after an arthrotomogram had revealed the presence of a TMJ internal derangement. The patient, wanting to avoid surgery, participated in a nonsurgical team management program that consisted of physical therapy, behavioral changes, and a mandibular stabilization splint. There is considerable controversy over the choice of surgical vs. nonsurgical treatment of TMJ internal derangements. Surgical proponents suggest that pain and dysfunction in the TMJ will continue unless the structural defect is corrected. Nonsurgical proponents suggest that pain and dysfunction can be alleviated by promoting the natural remodeling capacity in the joint with physical therapy, splints, and behavioral changes to reduce strain on the joint. The American Dental Association standards for craniomandibular disorders state that conservative reversible treatment should be implemented prior to consideration of surgery.[1] This case illustrated the use of comprehensive conservative care for a late stage TMJ internal derangement.

DISCUSSION

Temporomandibular joint internal derangements (TMJ ID) are characterized by a progressive displacement of the articular disk and interference with normal

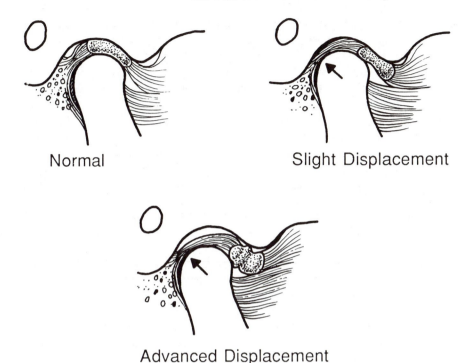

FIG 12–1.
In the late stage TMJ internal derangement, the condyle can become posteriorly displaced (arrow), the disk becomes anteriorly displaced and blocks normal translation of the condyle (C). (From Fricton J, Kroening R, Hathaway K: *TMJ and Craniofacial Pain: Diagnosis and Management.* St. Louis, IEA Publishers, 1988. Used by permission.)

translation of the condyle (Fig 12–1). This dysfunction can result in clicking, locking, jaw pain, headaches, and eventual degenerative changes in the joints.

Temporomandibular joint internal derangements are often associated with TMJ capsulitis and its attendant pain, tenderness, and joint swelling. Rasmussen presented evidence that this progressive displacement goes through five clinical stages, each with specific signs and symptoms that can be helpful in establishing the diagnosis.[2]

The presence and stages of TMJ ID can be confirmed with arthrotomography, but clinical diagnostic criteria can also be highly predictive.[3–4]

Stage I is characterized by reciprocal clicking of the TMJ upon opening and closing. The opening click reflects the condyle moving beneath the posterior band of the disk until it snaps into its normal relationship on the concave surface. The closing click reflects a reversal of this process, with the condyle moving under the posterior band of the disk until it snaps off the disk and onto the posterior attachment. The click occurs at 10–40 mm upon opening, and then from 0–20 mm upon closing. The opening and closing clicks do not occur at the same incisal opening. As the disk becomes further displaced, it begins to interfere with normal translation of the condyle.

Stage II begins when the disk becomes anteriorly and medially lodged relative to the condyle, thereby blocking translation and causing clinical locking. The locking can usually be reversed immediately by the patient and becomes intermittent, depending upon postural stresses placed on the joint-disk apparatus. Repetitive clicking and intermittent locking add to the strain of the posterior, medial, and collateral ligaments and create laxity in them. Patients frequently open with an initial jaw thrust and an anterior translation of the condyle. Occasionally, a patient can also exhibit an excessive opening as a result of ligament laxity and joint hypermobility, eventually resulting in either closed or open locking of the joint.

In *stage III,* an acute, sustained closed-lock occurs. With an *acute closed-lock,* the disk becomes permanently lodged anteriorly and interferes with normal condylar translation. The opening becomes acutely restricted to 20–30 mm, with no joint noise, since only joint rotation can occur. Subsequent to the joint dysfunction, masticatory muscles frequently become tender and painful as a result of the protective splinting of the joint. This may lead the clinician to mistakenly suspect that myofascial pain is the primary diagnosis. However, muscle trismus can result in pain and limited opening in a similar fashion as the acute closed-lock. The TMJ capsule is also usually tender.

After stage II occurs and the locking cannot be disengaged through mobilization, soft tissue remodeling leads to *stage IV.* In this stage, normal daily jaw function forces the soft-tissue disk further anteriorly until the jaw opens almost normally. The posterior attachment and collateral ligaments are allowed time to remodel with deposition of fibrous connective tissue. A single opening click or fine crepitus can occur as a result of irregular interferences in translation. Most of the masticatory muscles continue the protective splinting and cause further pain.

If permitted to continue, soft tissue remodeling progresses to the hard tissue remodeling of *stage V.* Radiographic changes become evident on the condylar head and occasionally on the articular eminences. Disk perforation and bone-to-bone contact will elicit coarse crepitus upon opening and closing. Occasionally, the muscle splinting or capsulitis will subside. If remodeling is successful, patients can progress to a normal opening with minimal pain, but with continued joint noise. In other cases, the bony degenerative changes progress with severe erosion, loss of vertical dimension, joint and muscle pain, and a severely compromised jaw function. In some situations, the degenerative joint disease (DJD) or TMJ capsulitis is accompanied by degeneration of other joints due to a systemic rheumatic disease.

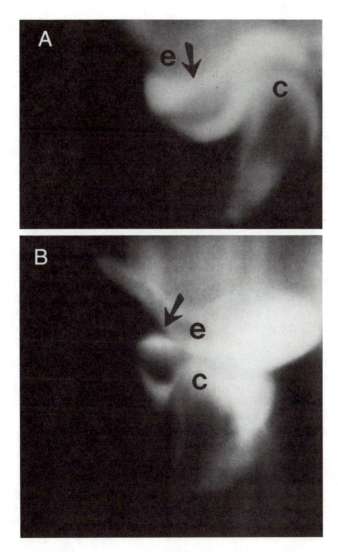

FIG 12–2.
Diagnosis of a TMJ internal derangement can be confirmed by an arthrogram. In A, the disk (arrow) is shown displaced anterior to the condyle *(c)*. In B, translation of the condyle is limited and does not reach the articular eminence *(e)*. (From Fricton J, Kroening R, Hathaway K: *TMJ and Craniofacial Pain: Diagnosis and Management.* St. Louis, IEA Publishers, 1988. Used by permission.)

In this case, the patient had a 1-year history of jaw cracking and difficulty opening the mouth prior to seeking care. She developed jaw pain, headaches, neck stiffness, tinnitus, and an uneven dental occlusion over the next year and consulted her dentist. The patient was referred to an oral surgeon with a diagnosis of a "TMJ" disorder. An arthrotomogram revealed a late stage TMJ ID in the right TMJ (Fig 12–2). At the time of examination, her jaw range of motion (incisal opening) was 43 mm with mild restriction, pain on opening, and jaw deviation to the right. There was no noise in the right TMJ, but a nonreproducible opening click in the left TMJ. Most muscles of mastication and posterior cervical muscles were tender.

MANAGEMENT

Figure 12–3 is a flow chart that can be used to guide clinicians in choosing the appropriate treatment plan for TMJ ID. The management of joint disorders follows similar principles when managing any persistent pain in the head and neck. After a thorough examination, the clinician establishes a problem list consisting of the chief complaints, physical diagnosis, and contributing factors. After discussing the problem list and treatment plan with the patient, the clinician can proceed with management by treating the physical diagnosis and controlling the contributing factors. Improved long-term stability will be unlikely if a comprehensive approach is not used. The general goals of managing joint problems include:

1. Reducing the chief complaints.
2. Improving functioning of the joints involved.
3. Reducing the need for future health care for the problem(s).

The general philosophy of treatment planning is to proceed initially with noninvasive, reversible, conservative modalities such as a splint, in conjunction with physical therapy and, if this proves unsuccessful, consideration of invasive, irreversible treatment such as surgery. Orthodontics, prosthodontics, and orthognathic surgery are considered to be irreversible treatments and not part of the initial management of these disorders.

Treatment of *stage I and II, TMJ internal derangement* will vary depending on the characteristics of reciprocal clicking. Reciprocal clicking can be eliminated by 1–4 mm anterior positioning of the jaw after maximum opening and closing in the forward position. Myofascial pain is also involved in the majority of cases that involve jaw pain, headaches, and neck pain, and may also need to be addressed. The degree of disk displacement can be determined by the amount of jaw opening that occurs prior to clicking. In general, the greater the incisal opening is at the point where the clicking occurs, the further the disk is displaced.

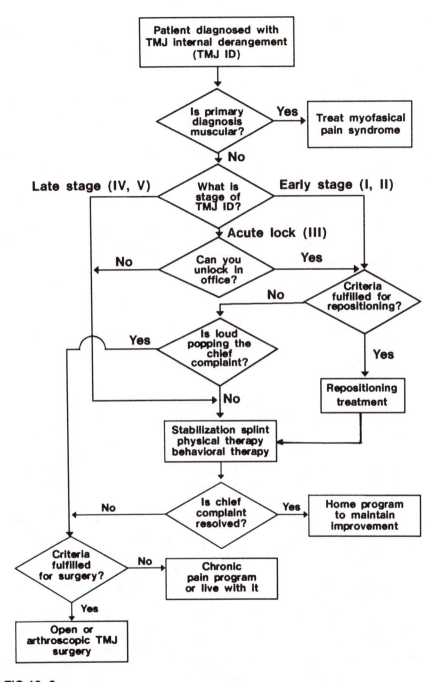

FIG 12–3.
This flow chart illustrates the sequencing of treatment for each stage of a TMJ internal derangement. Conservative care is implemented prior to consideration of surgical care. (From Fricton J, Kroening R, Hathaway K: *TMJ and Craniofacial Pain: Diagnosis and Management.* St. Louis, IEA Publishers, 1988. Used by permission.)

Each of these factors help in deciding the most appropriate treatment. There are three general approaches to treating a Stage I disorder: (1) repositioning splint with exercises and control of contributing factors; (2) stabilization splint with exercises and control of contributing factors; and (3) surgical disk repair with exercises and control of contributing factors.

Patients with asymptomatic reciprocal clicking (Stage I), should be educated about the disorder's potential progression and proper jaw function, asked to avoid oral parafunctional habits, and should be observed for a defined period. Because of the potential for excellent results in the properly chosen symptomatic Stage I or II patient, full time or part time jaw repositioning in conjunction with exercises and control of contributing factors is considered first in treatment planning. The purpose of jaw repositioning is to reposition the condyle into a more functionally favorable relationship with the disk and relieve pressure on retrodiscal tissues. This allows the condyle to translate normally without clicking, and pain and dysfunction are reduced. Although long-term experience with this approach is limited, there are some reports on its short-term efficacy.[5–7] However, past studies have emphasized the importance of patient selection and the difficulty in stabilizing the occlusion after repositioning. Specific criteria have been identified to help predict long-term maintenance of the improvement:

1. Repositioning of 2 mm or less required to eliminate the click.
2. Tomographic evidence of a posteriorly displaced condyle.
3. A shallow articular eminence.
4. The need to change posterior occlusion for other reasons, such as Class II occlusion, loss of teeth, or need for crowns or orthodontics.
5. A normal joint or a joint with the same stage TMJ ID on the opposite side.
6. Minimal behavioral and psychosocial contributing factors.

If a patient fulfills these criteria and repositioning is recommended, he or she should be aware of the probable need for post-repositioning occlusal treatment, particularly with full time use. Since this may be quite extensive and costly, a full discussion of the entire treatment plan is warranted before repositioning begins. If the patient agrees, treatment, including exercises and the control of contributing factors, can proceed.

If repositioning is not a viable option for patients with Stage I ID, a stabilization splint with exercises and control of contributing factors is indicated. Although clicking is usually not eliminated, it may be reduced to a soft click, and pain is usually lessened. Past studies have reported that clicking is the symptom most resistant to treatment with this approach.[8] In these cases, patients should be made aware of this limitation. The major advantage of this approach is that extensive occlusal stabilization procedures are unnecessary, since the maxillomandibular relationship remains unchanged. However, if teeth are missing or malposed, it is important to provide basic occlusal stability by completing a coronoplasty, restorative dentistry, or orthodontics.

If a repositioning or stabilization splint approach does not satisfactorily reduce the patient's clicking or pain from a stage I TMJ ID, an open surgical repair procedure can be recommended. The purpose of this procedure is to surgically remove adhesions and reposition the disk in a harmonious relationship with the condyle by mechanically freeing the disk to allow posterior repositioning. Although technically difficult, these procedures have the advantage of leaving the disk intact and allowing a near normal, condyle-disk functional relationship. However, further research is required to determine the long-term stability of improvement in pain relief, joint function, and prevention of structural joint changes as compared to other approaches.

Acute locking of the MTJ (stage III TMJ ID) occurs when the disk has been abruptly lodged anterior to the condylar head and blocks normal translation of the condyle. This allows rotation of the condyle only upon opening and diminishes the incisal opening to 20–35 mm. Pain and tenderness in and around the joint usually accompanies this condition. The reciprocal click is absent in an acute lock, but mild crepitus may be palpated. The condylar translation cannot be detected with palpation upon opening and the jaw deviates to the affected side. Unless the condition was initiated by trauma, patients usually describe a history of noise and periodic locking on the affected side. Although it is possible to have an asymptomatic joint during this stage, a patient frequently has increased pain from capsulitis and myofascial pain. Therefore, this condition should be treated as early as possible. The treatment options for an acute lock include the following, in order of preference:

1. Immediately unlocking the joint with a joint mobilization technique, with or without sedation. This should be followed by exercises and an immediate repositioning splint.
2. Use physical therapy modalities three times per week with jaw mobilization and a splint for 2–3 weeks.
3. TMJ surgery with a meniscectomy or repair procedure, or arthroscopic surgery.

Initial treatment of an acute lock includes attempting to unlock or reduce the condyle-disk fixation using a manual mobilization technique. This technique is designed to distract the condyle inferiorly and then anteriorly in order to disengage the condyle and allow the disk to shift posteriorly. If much pain, tenderness, and restriction is present in the TMJ or masticatory muscles, the use of I.V. sedation with diazepam (5–10 mg), or another sedative or muscle relaxant with mobilization can be helpful. Once the joint is unlocked, it is critical to keep it unlocked by instructing the patient about range-of-motion exercises, eating a soft diet, anti-inflammatory medication, and inserting a splint to disengage the disk.

If permanent locking persists, stage IV TMJ ID and soft tissue remodeling begins with the disk and associated attachments gradually stretch and change shape. These changes permit an increased range of jaw motion. Pain during this period varies, and treatment depends on the presence or absence of pain complaints and functional problems. The presence of a stage IV ID without symptoms does not warrant intervention. It is possible that degenerative changes may develop in Stage V, but this stage may also be asymptomatic and may not compromise function.

If pain or bothersome dysfunction is present in stage IV, a comprehensive treatment program can be initiated, depending on the degree of myofascial pain, limitation of jaw function, and the presence of contributing factors. This program includes:

1. Stabilization splint.
2. Physical therapy modalities with range-of-motion and postural exercises.
3. Behavioral program to reduce contributing factors.

If significant dysfunction *and* TMJ noise and pain remain after conservative treatments, open or arthroscopic TMJ surgery can be considered. With either a surgical or nonsurgical approach, special consideration should be given to the successful management of contributing factors, and to whether the derangement is the primary cause of symptoms. If so, the potential for successful treatment is improved.

Once stage V TMJ ID begins, the *hard tissue remodeling* occurs with subsequent crepitation in the joint. As with stage IV, pain and dysfunction vary considerably and do not correlate with structrual changes in the joint. However, all factors need to be considered in developing a treatment program. If no pain or dysfunction is present with minor degenerative changes in the joint, patients should be made aware of the condition, but no intervention is warranted. When pain and dysfunction are present with minor degenerative changes, conservative treatment similar to that suggested for stage IV is warranted. If improvement in jaw function is minimal, or condylar degeneration progresses and increases the risk of developing an anterior open bite, TMJ surgery is warranted.

In the 22-year-old woman, an evaluation revealed an additional diagnosis of myofascial pain causing some headaches and neck stiffness. Contributing factors included clenching, jaw thrust, excessive caffeine intake, sleep disturbance, phone bracing with the shoulder, and dental occlusal discrepancy. The conservative management program included an exercise program, behavioral therapy, and a stabilization splint. The exercise program, to be completed 6 times per day, involved jaw and neck stretching, balanced head and shoulder posture exercises, and posturing the tongue gently on the palate. The patient was instructed in a behavioral therapy program by a psychologist in order to change each contributing factor to reduce strain on the joint. Finally, a hard acrylic stabilization splint was inserted over the mandibular teeth and adjusted to protect the muscles and joint by distributing forces over all teeth. The patient was reminded to avoid clenching. This program took place over 6 months, with periodic visits to adjust the splint and monitor compliance. During the first month, the pain was aggravated due to the joint adjusting to the splint and exercises. After this, the symptoms gradually subsided as the patient reduced clenching and other habits, began using a phone headset, and developed good sleeping habits. Compliance with the splint and exercises was good. After 6 months, she had no jaw pain except with excessive chewing, mild headaches once a week, no jaw limitation or joint noise. A follow-up examination 2 years later revealed a normal range of motion (56 mm), no jaw pain, no joint noise, and occasional headaches. The headaches were determined to be due to neck muscular tension.

REFERENCES

1. Griffiths RH: Report of the President's conference on the examination, diagnosis and management of temporomandibular disorders. *J Am Dent Assoc* 1983; 106:75–77.
2. Rasmussen OC: Description of population and progress of symptoms in a longitudinal study of temporomandibular joint anthropathy. *Scand J Dent Res* 1981; 89:196–203.
3. Wilkes CH: Arthrography of the temporomandibular joint in patients with the TMJ pain dysfunction syndrome. *Minn Med* 1978; 61:645–652.
4. Schiffman E, Anderson G, Fricton J, et al: Diagnostic criteria for intra-articular TM disorders. *Community Dent Oral Epidemiol,* in press.
5. Clark G: Treatment of jaw clicking with temporomandibular repositioning: Analysis of 25 cases. *J Cranio Prac* 1986; 2:263–270.
6. Anderson GC, Schulte JK, Goodkin RJ: Comparative study of two treatment methods of internal derangement of the temporomandibular joint. *J Prosthet Dent* 1985; 53:392–396.
7. Maloney F, Howard JA: Internal derangements of the temporomandibular joint III: Anterior repositioning splint therapy. *Aust Dent J* 1986; 31:30–39.
8. Agerberg G, Carlsson GE: Late results of treatment of functional disorders of the masticatory system. *J Oral Rehabil* 1974; 1:309–316.

13

Acute Herpes Zoster, Ophthalmic Division

Theresa Ferrer-Brechner, M.D.

A 46-year-old woman presented with crusty, extremely painful lesions in the ophthalmic division of the trigeminal nerve. The lesions started 5 weeks prior to admission after receiving chemotherapy and radiation therapy for cancer. A diagnosis of acute herpes zoster was made and she was treated with oral steroids, intravenous acyclovir, and intravenous cimetidine without any resolution of the lesions within 5 weeks. The lesions and severe pain persisted, and because of the hyperesthesia and edema, she kept her right eyelid closed (Fig 13–1). Examination revealed highly sensitive and painful encrusted herpetic lesions following the distribution of the right ophthalmic division of the trigeminal nerve.

DISCUSSION

Acute herpes zoster (AHZ) is a neural infection caused by varicella-zoster virus. After a bout of infection during childhood, the virus lies dormant in the dorsal root ganglion for years. It is hypothesized that with a condition of decreased immune response (i.e., aging, chemotherapy, stress), the virus becomes opportunistic and sets an antidromic infection along the course of somatic nerves, characterized by painful cutaneous eruptions along the course of the nerves. Eventually, the viral infection destroys the large somatic fibers, thus inducing a condition of deafferentation pain of postherpetic neuralgia. The incidence of AHZ is said to be approximately 125/1,000,000/year with both sexes equally susceptible.[1] The incidence is increased in patients with lymphoproliferative

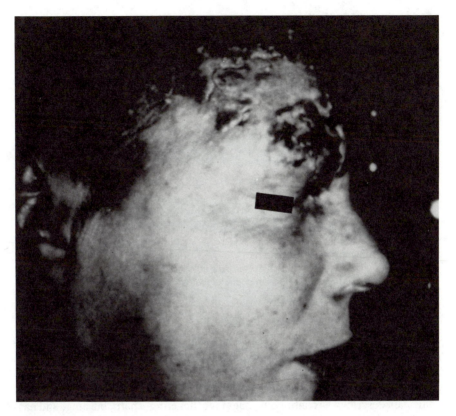

FIG 13–1.
Patient with severe herpes zoster involving the ophthalmic division of the trigeminal nerve, taken fifth week from onset. Zoster lesions have not responded to topical and systemic administration of steroids, cimetidine, and acyclovir.

malignancy, especially in those with severe disease and treated with aggressive chemotherapy and radiation therapy. Older individuals have 5–10/1,000 incidence of AHZ, children 0.5/1,000.[2] The most commonly afflicted areas are the V1 division of the trigeminal nerve and the thoracic areas, T5–10.[3]

Acute herpes zoster usually presents with pain, dysesthesias, or paresthesias along the course of the affected nerves, followed a few days later by cutaneous vesicular eruptions. These lesions usually scab within a week and heal within a month, except in unusually immunocompromised individuals as exemplified by the patient presented here. Viral cultures of the vesicles usually show the presence of the varicella virus. Older patients seem to have more severe pain than younger individuals. Systemic symptoms such as fever, stiff neck, headache, nausea, and regional/diffuse adenopathy can occur in 5% of patients and is not an indication of prognosis.

TABLE 13–1.

Treatment for Acute Herpes Zoster

Antiviral agents
  Iodoxuridine in DMSO
  Cytosine arabinoside (ARA-C)
  Adenosine arabinoside (ARA-A)
  Symmetrel (Amantadine HC1)
  Acyclovir
  Adenosine monophosphate (AMP)
Steroids
  Systemic administration
  Intralesional injection
  Oral administration
  Epidural injection
Repetitive nerve blocks
  Sympathetic block
  Somatic nerve block
Symptomatic treatments
  Topical application of Burrow's solution or calamine lotion
  Narcotic and nonnarcotic analgesics
  Topical aspirin

The greatest problem with AHZ is the development of postherpetic neuralgia (PHN), which is an aftermath of the irreversible destruction of the large somatic fibers by the varicella viruses, thus inducing a condition of ''anesthesia dolorosa,'' pain in an area of numbness. The result is a condition of chronic neuropathic pain described as continuous, nagging, flickering, sharp, burning, and nagging. The treatment of PHN is extremely difficult once destruction of the somatic nerves is complete, probably due to retrograde destruction of afferent fibers that can occur with peripheral deafferentation.[5] Therefore, early treatment of acute herpes zoster is important to prevent the complete destruction of somatic nerves as seen with PHN. The treatments are variable and aimed primarily at the early resolution of the lesions. Studies that look at the prevention of PHN are lacking.

Severe and recalcitrant AHZ is common in patients with depressed immune response, e.g., in elderly patients and cancer patients receiving chemotherapy. These groups of patients develop recalcitrant lesions beyond the normal course of the disease and have a higher incidence of developing postherpetic neuralgia.[6] Because of these risks, these patients need to be treated aggressively with modalities that can acutely decrease pain, shorten the life span of the disease, and decrease the incidence of postherpetic neuralgia.

Various treatments have been advocated for AHZ (Table 13–1). When treating AHZ, the goals are to decrease the pain as rapidly as possible, decrease the time for resolution of lesions, and decrease the incidence of postherpetic neuralgia. However, despite the variety of treatments proposed, none of the treatments have been shown to significantly achieve all of the above goals in a well controlled study. Antiviral treatments, such as acyclovir, have been administered both topically and intravenously, in an attempt to reduce the course of the disease in both normal and immunocompromised patients with AHZ, but results have not been statistically significant.[7] Although there is some evidence that antiviral agents may reduce the severity of AHZ and possibly reduce the incidence of postherpetic neuralgia, further studies are necessary to confirm this effect in more controlled studies.

Steroids, such as ACTH, cortisone, prednisone, triamcinolone, and prednisolone have been used for the treatment of AHZ. Double blind studies with systemic triamcinolone reduced the pain of AHZ in individuals over 60 years, but did not influence the pain in individuals below 60 years of age.[8] Intralesional injection of steroids has been anecdotally reported to decrease pain and incidence of PHN, but controls are lacking.[9] Epidural steroids with or without anesthetics have been demonstrated to decrease or arrest pain in 100 patients.[10]

Neural blocking with local anesthetics injected into sympathetic ganglion can dramatically relieve the patient's pain. When done repeatedly, it has been claimed to decrease healing time, reduce duration of pain, and possibly reduces

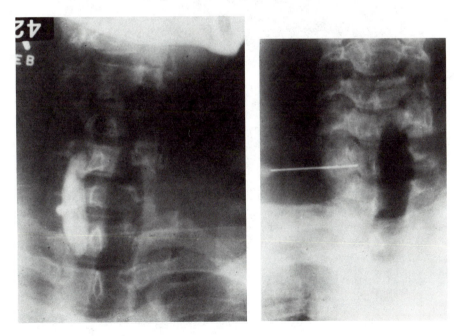

FIG 13–2.
Needle placement for upper and middle cervical sympathetic ganglion block and spread of 10 cc solution of 0.5% lidocaine with 40 mg Depomedrol.

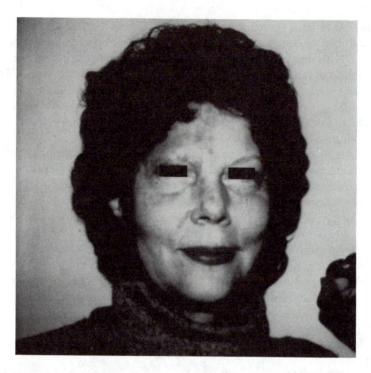

FIG 13–3.
Appearance of the same patient in Figure 13–1 after four upper and middle cervical ganglion blocks, showing total disappearance of herpes zoster crusty lesions and ability of the patient to wear a wig, signifying decreased hyperesthesia.

the incidence of PHN.[11] In a large series of 483 patients, Calding reported that repeated sympathetic block reduced pain, healing time, and PHN, but the study was not controlled.[12]

In this particular patient, institution of steroids and antiviral agents during the first 4 weeks failed to produce any change in the severity of her lesions and pain. A series of upper and middle cervical ganglion blocks were done two times a week for 3 weeks, according to our protocol (Fig 13–2). By the fourth block, her lesions were 90% resolved, she was able to open her eyes, and also wear a wig (Fig 13–3).

As mentioned, the use of sympathetic blocks can be a useful technique for recalcitrant and severe herpes zoster. The best time to start is around 3–4 weeks from onset, when it becomes obvious that the natural course of the disease is prolonged and/or traditionally less invasive approaches have not altered the course of the disease. Sympathetic nerve blocks with local anesthetics have been implied to decrease significantly the occurrence of postherpetic neuralgia.[13]

A recent study in Japan has shown that the severity of acute herpes zoster lesions is correlated with maximum antibody titers to varicella virus and not necessarily to the age of the patients. Those patients with high antibody titers also required longer duration of treatments with sympathetic nerve blocks.[14] In these series, daily blocks were done until the patient's pain visual analogue scale was decreased 1–2 on a scale of 10. An average of 19 blocks on outpatients and 135 blocks on inpatients were recorded, which is a much higher number than that practiced in the U.S.A.

In summary, AHZ can be a debilitating type of pain problem associated with varicella virus-induced vesicular eruptions along the course of a somatic nerve. Treatment should be aimed toward immediate pain control, shortening the course of the disease, and prevention of the dreaded postherpetic neuralgia.

REFERENCES

1. Ragozzino MW, Melton LS III, Kurland LT, et al: Population-based study of herpes zoster and its sequelae. *Medicine* 1982; 61:310–316.
2. Brown GR: Herpes Zoster: Correlation of age, sex, distribution, neuralgia, and associated disorders. *South Med J* 1976; 69:576–578.
3. Hope-Simpson RE: The nature of herpes zoster: A long term study and a new hypothesis. *Proc Roy Soc Med* 1965; 56:9–20.
4. Watson CP, Evans RJ, Watt VR, et al: Postherpetic neuralgia. 208 cases. *Pain* 1988; 35:289–297.
5. Noordenbos W: *Pain.* Elsevier, Amsterdam, 1959, p 182.
6. Molin L: Aspects of the natural history of herpes zoster: A follow-up investigation of outpatient material. *Acta Derm Venereol (Stockh)* 1969; 49:569–583.
7. Whitley RJ, Chien LT, Dalin R, et al: Cancer and the collaborative group. Adenosine arabinoside therapy of herpes zoster in the immunocompromised. NIAID Collaborative Antiviral Study. *N Engl J Med* 1976; 294:1192–1199.
8. Eaglestein WH, Katz R, Brown JA: The effects of early corticosteroid therapy on the skin eruption and pain of herpes zoster. *JAMA* 1970; 211:1681–1683.
9. Epstein Z: Herpes zoster and post zoster neuralgia. Intralesional triamcenalone therapy. *Calif Med* 1971; 115:6–10.
10. Schreuder M: Pain relief in herpes zoster. *S Afr Med J* 1983; 63:820–821.
11. Calding A: The effect of regional sympathetic blockade in the treatment of herpes zoster. *Acta Anaesthesiol Scand* 1969; 13:133–141.
12. Calding A: Treatment of pain: Organization of a pain clinic. Treatment of acute herpes zoster. *Proc Roy Soc Med* 1973; 66:541–543.
13. Dan K, Higa K, Noda B: Nerve block for herpetic pain, in HL Field, R Dubner, R Cervero (eds): *Advances in Pain Research and Therapy, vol 9.* New York, Raven Press, 1985, pp 831–838.
14. Higa K, Dan K, Manabe H, et al: Influencing the duration of treatment of acute herpetic pain with sympathetic block: Importance of severity of herpes zoster assessed by maximum antibody titers to varicella zoster virus in otherwise healthy patients. *Pain* 1988; 23:147–157.

14

Postherpetic Neuralgia, Head and Neck

Steven B. Graff-Radford, D.D.S.

A 75-year-old woman had a continuous, right-sided, frontal pain that had been present for 4 years. The pain was described as a throbbing, burning, aching sensation and it was reported to follow a herpes zoster infection of the right V1 nerve distribution. The herpes zoster infection lasted for 2 weeks, of which the patient was hospitalized for 10 days, and received acyclovir in doses of 500 mg three times daily. Additional treatments included the use of prednisone orally and topically. Once discharged, the patient received treatments of carbamazepine (Tegretol), phenytoin (Dilantin), various narcotic medications, and a transcutaneous electrical nerve stimulation (TENS) unit. She reported that none of these treatments were effective. At the time of presentation, the patient was taking either acetaminophen (Tylenol) and codeine, or Darvocet 3–4 times per day, and between 10–20 mg of diazepam (Valium) at bedtime. Physical examination revealed an area of scarring secondary to herpes zoster infection in the right V1 distribution. When compared to the left side, both with light touch and pinprick, a decreased reactivity to pinprick and an increased reactivity to light touch were revealed. The rest of the examination was within normal limits. The rest of the physical examination included a myofascial evaluation, temporomandibular joint evaluation, and cervical spine evaluation, all of which were within normal limits. A diagnosis of postherpetic neuralgia was made based on the history of continuous unilateral burning and throbbing pain secondary to the clearing of an infection of herpes zoster.

DISCUSSION

It has been estimated that the incidence of herpes zoster is approximately 125/ 100,000/year in the general population. There is no specific affliction with regard to sex or race, but often it will follow a period of immunosuppression such as in lymphoproliferative malignancies or after chemotherapy, radiation therapy, or AIDS. With age, the incidence of herpes zoster progresses, with the rate in children being between .5/1,000 to 10/1,000 in octogenarians.

Postherpetic neuralgia is a pain syndrome characterized by a constant burning and aching pain, often superimposed with sharp, shooting electriclike pains or formications. The pain is required to be present without the existence of herpes zoster lesions, which usually last 4–6 weeks. It is estimated that between 10–20% of all people with herpes zoster will develop postherpetic neuralgia.

The skin in the painful area usually manifests some scarring and often pigmentary changes. There is usually hyperesthesia and hypalgesia in the painful area. These changes are usually limited to the dermatomes affected by the varicella-zoster virus. The most frequent site for the distribution of herpes zoster is the thoracic dermatomes, followed by the cranial and cervical dermatomes, and then by lumbar, sacral, and generalized dissemination. As with herpes zoster, the incidence of postherpetic neuralgia is age related, with approximately 70% of patients with postherpetic neuralgia being over the age of 60.

Diagnosis of this affliction is not a difficult one, but the treatments are somewhat more perplexing and often multiple treatments result in no benefit.

TREATMENTS

The treatment of postherpetic neuralgia may be divided into preventive treatments and those aimed at the problem once it has been established. The preventive treatments include the use of antiviral medications during the acute zoster infection, or the use of sympathetic blockade within the first 6 months of the disease process. There is little, if any, evidence that substantiates the prevention of postherpetic neuralgia through antiviral treatment, steroid administration, or sympathetic neural blockade. Various studies have suggested that approximately 80% of patients can be prevented from developing postherpetic neuralgia if sympathetic blockade is carried out early. These studies, unfortunately, do not answer whether the 20% that go on to have postherpetic neuralgia are the same 20% that would have been afflicted with this problem despite treatment.

Antidepressants

Two double blind studies support the use of antidepressants, particularly amitriptyline, in the treatment of postherpetic neuralgia. A double-blind crossover study by Watson in 1982 suggested that a median dose of 75 mg per day reduced the pain far more effectively than placebo. This relief was not dependent on depression. In summary, tricyclic antidepressants are the most effective treatment available at present for postherpetic neuralgia.

Phenothiazines have been suggested for the treatment of chronic pain and in 5 case studies, Taub reported the combination of amitriptyline and fluphenazine to be very effective. In an ongoing double blind study being conducted by the author, approximately 68% pain reduction has been obtained with a combination of amitriptyline and fluphenazine vs. 38% pain reduction with amitriptyline alone. This study, although not completed, suggests that fluphenazine in low doses, between 1–3 mg, may be effective in potentiating the well-known effects of amitriptyline.

Steroids

Steroids have been reported in a small series to be effective when injected locally in the region of the affected dermatomes. Unfortunately no double blind study has been conducted. Epidural steroids were also reported to be effective, but once again, no control was used in the study.

Various other medications have been tried. These include carbamazepine, which has shown little success, and baclofen, also with little success, Valproic acid has been combined with amitriptyline, but not in a double-blind fashion, and oral vitamin E and vitamin B_{12} administration has been suggested without any rigorous trial.

Topical Applications

Recently, the use of a substance P depleting chemical, capsaicin, applied to the affected dermatome 5 times per day for the first week and 3–4 times per day for subsequent weeks, has been reported to be effective in approximately 50% of patients. In an uncontrolled study by the author, 13 patients were treated with capsaicin without benefit. Additional topical therapies have included aspirin, either dissolved in chloroform, or aspirin dissolved in Vaseline Intensive Care cream. Both of these studies have reported favorable results. Unfortunately, neither have been scientifically controlled.

Surgical Therapy

No effective surgical approach has been found for postherpetic neuralgia, although cordotomy, rhizotomy, and sympathectomy have been attempted. Virtually all surgical approaches have worked on occasional patients, but in general, they are not effective. The most effective of these surgical approaches appears to be a dorsal root entry zone lesion described by Friedman and Nashold, with 10 of 17 patients benefiting from this approach.

Stimulation-Produced Analgesia

The use of acupuncture of TENS to produce central inhibition has been described in numerous uncontrolled studies. Many of these claim significant efficacy. A well-done single blind study showed that acupuncture was of little value in postherpetic neuralgia. Again, the use of TENS in general is not too encouraging, although there are reports of dramatic improvements in certain patients.

Interpleural Catheterization

In a study of 5 patients with postherpetic neuralgia who received placement of an intrapleural catheter and daily infusions of lidocaine into the interpleural space, approximately 50% of the patients became pain free during the infusion. One of these patients continued in a pain-free state following the infusion. The other patients returned to their baseline pain following removal of the catheter after 10 days. Further evaluation of this technique is required prior to any definitive comments.

RECOMMENDED MANAGEMENT OF POSTHERPETIC NEURALGIA

If the patient is seen within 6 months of initiation of postherpetic neuralgia, it is suggested that he or she undergo at least one diagnostic sympathetic nerve block. Should this block be successful, a series of up to three blocks should follow. Again, if these are successful, a maximum of six blocks should be entertained. The evaluation of these patients should include assessment of pain reduction through visual analog scales or other such pain evaluation tools, as well as an evaluation of the patient's functional ability. Should there be no response after the first block, the initiation of amitriptyline should begin. Because of the age and poor medical health of these patients, very low doses of amitriptyline should be initiated. It is suggested that 10 mg be the starting dose, and that the patient be titrated with increments of 10 mg every 3–4 days. All medications should be taken at bedtime. Should there be a problem with morning drowsiness and the inability to function early in the morning, this dose may be split between the dinner hour and bedtime. The average dose of amitriptyline is anywhere between 75–150 mg per day. The use of fluphenazine may be initiated if the effects of amitriptyline are not sufficient. It is important to reserve the use of fluphenazine because of the potential side effects of tardive dyskinesia. In an ongoing study, during which approximately 43 patients have been treated with a combination of amitriptyline or amitriptyline and fluphenazine, there has been no case in which tardive dyskinesia has resulted.

In addition to the use of amitriptyline, it is suggested that a trial of topical capsaicin should be initiated. One of the biggest problems with this form of treatment is the burning sensation that results from this cream, and it has been suggested by Watson that if combined with topical lidocaine, patients are able to tolerate the burning better.

BIBLIOGRAPHY

Bernstein JE, Vickers DR, Dahl MV, et al: Treatment of chronic postherpetic neuralgia with topical capsaicin. *J Am Acad Dermatol* 1987; 17:93–96.

Loeser JD: Herpes zoster and postherpetic neuralgia: Review article. *Pain* 1986; 25:149–154.

Max MB, Schafer SC, Culnane M, et al: Amitriptyline, but not Lorazepam, relieves postherpetic neuralgia. *Neurology* 1988; 38:1427–1432.

Tenicela R, Lovasik D, Eaglstein W: Treatment of herpes zoster with sympathetic blocks. *Clin J Pain* 1985; 1:63–67.

Watson PN, Evans RJ: Treatment of postherpetic neuralgia. *Clin Neuropharmacol* 1986; 9:533–541.

15

Physical Therapy Evaluation and Treatment of Auricular Pain

Josette Fast, P.T.

A 46-year-old woman complained of a 17-year history of auricular and retroauricular pain of insidious onset. Previous diagnoses for this patient included temporomandibular joint (TMJ) dysfunction, C2 radiculopathy, and cervical dysfunction. Treatment for these diagnoses did not benefit the patient, however. Previous treatment consisted of trigger point injections, transcutaneous electrical nerve stimulation, ultrasound, hot packs, electrogalvanic stimulation, and cervical traction. The patient's main pain complaint (P1) was that of a constant and exquisitely tender area located behind the left ear on the mastoid process. She rated P1 as a 10:10 on a visual analogue scale (VAS). Another primary area of complaint was the patient's constant left auricular pain. She described it as a needle piercing her ear drum (P2). She felt these two pains were related. Secondary areas of discomfort were that of constant neck tightness (P3) and left shoulder ache (P4). According to the patient, palpation of P1, hugging other people with the left side of her head and neck, an action she now avoided, and stress aggravated P1. Palpation of P1 was the only aggravating factor in regards to P2. Chewing or talking were considered to have no effect on her pains. Moist heat eased P1 and nothing eased P2. Rest did not change the patient's pain, but P1 and P2 would, occasionally, awaken the patient from sleep. The patient usually slept prone, with her head rotated left and her left arm in flexion and abduction. She awakened in the morning with an increase of P4. P1 and P2 began insidiously 17 years prior to coming to the pain clinic. Her pain intensity had remained the same since the onset, but frequency had progressed to that of a constant status. P3 and P4 also began insidiously and had been present for 2 years.

The patient had been in a high stress job during the last 8 years. Fifty percent of her work hours were spent on the phone. She held the phone between her left shoulder and ear. During childhood, she was involved in minor accidents without incurring injuries to the head or neck regions.

PERTINENT EXAMINATION FINDINGS

Posture

The patient presented with abnormal posture congruent and her aberrant and extensive telephone use: 1) elevated left shoulder; 2) forward head; 3) neck on right side bending on shoulders with compensation of head on left side bending on neck.

Active Range of Motion

The temporomandibular joint was full and painless; the left shoulder was full and painless; the cervical spine showed essentially full range of motion with P3 present during all movements. Of note the patient rotated her head to the right during flexion and extension. Upon further testing, the patient had 2 cm more right rotation of C1–C2 than she did to the left. Repeated motion tests ruled out the possibility of disc derangement.

Palpation Findings

1. Cervical joints—left apophyseal joints of O–C1 and C1–C2 were stiff but painless, while the remaining left apophyseal joints were sore but not stiff. Right apophyseal joint of C1–C2 was painful but not stiff. The remaining right apophyseal joints were unremarkable.

2. Soft tissue—the left cervical paraspinals, levator scapula, and upper trapezius were tight and sore. There were latent trigger points of the sterno-cleidomastoid (SCM) muscles bilaterally.

Comparable Signs

Comparable signs are those found during the physical examination that reproduce a patient's pain and that, which repeated at a later time, will again elicit the same pain. The only comparable sign found for P1 was with light palpation of the P1 area (left mastoid process). No comparable signs were found for P2 and P4, but P3 was present with all active cervical motions.

ASSESSMENT

The initial assessment could only be vague in terms of P1 and P2, considering the comparable signs and lack thereof. P1 and P2 seemed secondary to musculoskeletal pathology due to behavior of symptoms. However, no structure was identified upon the physical examination. P3 seemed secondary to cervical joint and soft tissue dysfunction, and faulty posture and body mechanics. Though P4 was not elicited, P4 seemed secondary to abnormal body mechanics during sleep.

TREATMENT

Treatment was planned to focus, initially, on the cervical, postural, and body mechanics problems identified, doubting if P1 or P2 would somehow be affected.

With such an extended history of pain, one may be curious about the psychological profile of this patient. Evaluation findings from our clinic psychologist revealed the patient to be somewhat depressed but no other major factors were present with which to contend or modify during treatment.

Sessions 1 and 2

To establish the patient's sense of responsibility toward her own rehabilitation and to eliminate perpetuating factors involved in P3 and P4, the patient was instructed in posture, body mechanics, and in relaxation and postural exercises. At the end of the second session the apophyseal joints of the patient's upper cervical spine were mobilized, which had no effect on P1 or P2.*

At this time, review of the initial examination findings and the noneffectiveness of cervical joint mobilization began to reveal a possible cause for P1 and P2. Keeping in mind the actions of the left SCM muscle and where it inserts, consider the following:

1. The patient's history of holding the phone between her left ear and shoulder maintained the SCM in a shortened position.
2. The patient's sleeping posture and the fact that P1 and P2 could

---

* *Mobilization is a gentle, rhythmical oscillation of one joint surface on another to decrease pain and/or increase mobility and is within the control of the patient, as opposed to chiropractic manipulation.*[1]

awaken her from sleep, possibly indicates that if the SCM was dysfunctional, it was being stretched in this position and aggravated the pain.

3. The patient's postural deviations are congruent with a dysfunction of the left SCM.
4. Cervical flexion and extension were done with right rotation, which had to be secondary to a soft tissue structure since joint mobilization did not change this quality of movement.
5. Light palpation of the P1 area provoked P1, indicating that if the pain was secondary to a soft tissue structure, it had to be a superficial structure, which the SCM is.
6. P1 was provoked locally over the mastoid process, which is where the SCM inserts.
7. The patient felt P2 was related to P1.
8. Active trigger points of the SCM are known to refer pain to the ear and behind it.[2]

The above factors seemed to incriminate the left SCM as a most likely cause for P1 and P2. The following treatment sessions focused on this muscle.

Session 3

The left SCM was sprayed and stretched with a vapocoolant as prescribed by Travell and Simons.[2] There was an immediate and significant decrease in sensitivity of the P1 area as determined by palpation. The patient did not pull away with palpation as she had done prior to the spray and stretch. The patient was instructed to do a stretching exercise of the SCM as part of her home program.

Session 4

The gains made in session 3 carried over to the next treatment session as palpation of P1 did not cause the patient to pull away as she had done during the initial evaluation. The patient reported she felt as if something was "breaking up." Spray and stretch was repeated and the patient reported a further decrease in the pain intensity of P1.

Session 5

The patient stated P1 was of the same intensity as at the end of the previous session, but her neck felt stiff. Active cervical range of motion was full but slow, secondary to an increase in P3. The patient's cervical spine was mobilized, after which her active cervical movements were normal and painfree. Spray and stretch was repeated as done previously, with the patient reporting a 75% decrease in pain intensity.

Session 6

The patient came to session 6 stating she was not experiencing the sharp piercing into her ear, but rather a mild discomfort at the entrance to the external auditory meatus. This was indicative of P2 resolving. The treatment of session 5 was rendered.

Session 7

The intensity of P1 was significantly less, P2 was completely resolved, and the patient was able to wake in the morning without her usual P4. The same treatment as was rendered in session 5 was administered. At the end of the treatment, the patient was given a hug on her left side, which she had been avoiding. This was no longer a functional deficit, as she was able to tolerate this without provocation of P1.

Session 8

The patient was reassessed and discharged. Subjectively, P1 was no longer constant and now rarely occurred. It presented as only a momentary jab, which the patient rated a 1.5:10 on the VAS. P2, P3 and P4 were resolved. Functionally, the patient was able to tolerate ipsilateral hugs.

Objectively, the patient's posture and palpation findings were within normal limits. Interestingly, no deflection of the head and neck during flexion and extension was now noted. Measurement of C1–C2 rotation to the right and left were equal.

DISCUSSION

The patient presented in this case study seems to have had pain secondary to dysfunction of the left SCM. The dysfunction may have initially been instigated by her benign childhood accidents, and later facilitated and perpetuated by years of improper posture, body mechanics, and stress. Once attention was paid to these factors, the patient was able to make significant gains in diminishing the intensity and location of her pains, and in improving function.

REFERENCES

1. Maitland G: *Vertebral Manipulation.* London, Butterworths, 1986.
2. Travell JG, Simons D: *Myofascial Pain and Dysfunction—The Trigger Point Manual.* Baltimore, Williams and Wilkins, 1983.

16

Whiplash Injury

Avrom Gart, M.D.

A 26-year-old man, the seat-belted driver of his automobile, was stopped at a red light and suddenly rear-ended. He did not experience any direct head trauma or loss of consciousness and walked away from the accident in a panic state. The following morning he awoke in severe pain and could hardly move his neck. He then presented to his family physician, who immediately performed cervical x-rays, which showed no evidence of any fracture or dislocation. The patient was then reassured and a careful history and physical exam were carried out. The exam was significant for tender scalene and sternocleidomastoid muscles, as well as tight and painful posterior cervical paravertebral and suboccipital muscles, bilaterally. Range of motion of the cervical spine was markedly restricted. The neurological exam was completely within normal limits. At this point, the patient was fitted with a soft cervical collar and instructed to wear it at all times over the next 72 hours, during which time he was to rest at home. Anti-inflammatory muscle relaxants and analgesic medication were prescribed on a time-contingent basis. Upon his return visit, the patient complained of a persistent suboccipital headache, as well as continued neck pain and stiffness. The patient was then started on a physical therapy program consisting of moist heat and gentle massage and, gradually, over the next week, his symptoms began improving. He was instructed to wear the cervical collar only while sleeping. He was advised to return to work. Home cervical isometric and stretching exercises were begun, and after 2 weeks, he no longer complained of headaches. His neck pain and stiffness gradually improved over the next 2 months. At that point, physical therapy was discontinued and the patient was discharged.

DISCUSSION

Whiplash is a word used to describe the group of symptoms resulting from an acceleration-deceleration force applied to the cervical spine. These injuries are most often a result of automobile accidents, but also can occur from falls and other types of sudden body impact. It is implied that there has not been any direct head trauma, and that the medical findings are solely attributable to the abrupt movement of the head and neck upon the torso.

Mechanism of Injury

When a stationary motor vehicle is struck from the rear, the occupant's torso is thrust forward by an accelerating seat back. This causes the unrestrained head and neck to bend backward relative to the body until the occiput strikes either the headrest or the thoracic spine. Following this so-called hyperextension phase, the head and neck then rebound into flexion as the car stops or hits another vehicle in front of it. Hence, the descriptive title "whiplash" finds its way into the medical jargon.

In the initial phase of hyperextension, the anterior cervical musculature and soft tissue structures act to limit the degree of neck motion. Unfortunately, the occupants of a motor vehicle involved in a rear-end collison are usually caught off guard, and by the time the anterior musculature is activated via the stretch reflex, the majority of the hyperextension phase has already been completed.[1] There also may be additional forces limiting hyperextension if the head happens to be rotated to one side during the moment of impact.

Pathology and Associated Clinical Symptoms

The onset of cervical symptoms usually manifests within 24 hours of the accident. This depends upon the amount of muscle tearing and hemorrhage, trauma to capillaries and nerve fibers, and the subsequent rate of formation of soft tissue edema. Damage to bony elements and soft tissue structures may be observed to vary from minor sprains to vertebral fractures, resulting in a neurologic deficit. It is the severity of these injuries and symptoms that helps classify each case into three clinical categories: mild, moderate, and severe.

Approximately 95% of whiplash injuries can be classified as mild. Tearing of muscle fibers in the scalenes, sternocleidomastoids, and longissimus colli muscles is most common. This results in progressive pain and stiffness of the neck, with associated occipital headache caused by a combination of muscle spasm and irritation of the greater or lesser occipital nerves.

Pain is often found to radiate down the arm in a nondermatomal pattern. The most likely explanation is from myofascial pain referral, which usually improves with muscle healing and progressive exercises. Paresthesia along the ulnar aspect of the hand is also a relatively frequent complaint, usually due to spasm of the scalene muscles compressing the lower trunk of the brachial plexus, thus causing a thoracic outlet syndrome. Neurodiagnostic testing can be quite helpful in distinguishing neurogenic from muscular pain symptoms.

Injuries that are classified as moderate in severity occur in approximately 3% of cases. More extensive damage takes place to the anterior cervical muscles, with intense soreness and difficulty in swallowing. Tearing of the anterior longitudinal ligament of the lower neck can cause pharyngeal edema or retropharyngeal hematoma formation with subsequent symptoms of dysphagia shortly after the accident. Derangement of the lower cervical disc may occur with possible nerve root impingement and radicular symptoms. Temporomandibular joint pain is not uncommon and can be caused by either muscle spasm in the masseter and pterygoid muscle complex, or by intra-articular joint dysfunction itself.[2] The forces involved in this type of injury are often sufficient to cause a cerebral concussion with associated symptoms of hyperirritability, insomnia, retro-orbital headache, fatigue, and decreased concentration and memory.[3] Autonomic nervous system dysfunction manifested by cold hands, excessive sweating, vertigo, nystagmus, and occasionally Horner's syndrome can result from traction on the cervical sympathetic chain.[4] Tinnitus and blurred vision are frequently encountered and are either caused by damage to the inner ear or eye itself, or by injury to the vertebral artery.

Injuries of a severe nature are rare and only occur in less than 1% of patients. Neurological deficit occurs and either affects the upper limbs alone, or in the most extreme case, quadriplegia can result. Intrinsic damage is found in the lower cervical cord with or without vertebral body involvement. Stretching, stenosis, or occlusion of the vertebral arteries can cause vertigo, ataxia, or ischemic damage to the brain stem and occipital lobes. Cerebral concussion occurs at this degree of acceleration, with its previously mentioned symptoms.

MANAGEMENT

A detailed history and thorough physical examination is the first step in the management of whiplash injuries. Initial x-ray studies of the cervical spine are usually not of great value unless, of course, a fracture or dislocation is sustained. It is, however, important to perform x-rays, both to reassure the patient and for medicolegal aspects of the injury.

Patients who sustain severe neurologic damage will require both emergency and long-term inpatient care in a multidisciplinary rehabilitation facility. Injuries of moderate severity may require short-term hospitalization and neurologic observation and testing. As soon as symptoms become less acute, the patient can be managed on an outpatient basis, similar to treating a mild injury.

In the initial phase of injury, medication is definitely indicated. Usually a combination of analgesic, anti-inflammatory, and muscle relaxant medications can be prescribed. Careful use of tranquilizers is effective in lessening anxiety and can be substituted for muscle relaxants in appropriate cases. It is important to prescribe medication on a time contingent basis, rather than having patients take a pill on an as-needed basis. "Pill taking" has been shown to be a pain reinforcing behavior that, if left to the patient's control, can often perpetuate symptoms.

A properly fitted cervical collar is used to stabilize the head and neck in a specific position, which is determined by the history and clinical examination. The goal in aligning the head and neck is to decrease nerve root irritation and also to allow the injured cervical muscles and ligaments some degree of relaxation, which helps relieve pain. This is accomplished by having the head held in a slightly flexed position that separates the facets and opens the foramina.

The duration for wearing the collar varies among patients. However, it is usually felt that initially, the collar should be worn both during the day and at night while sleeping. After approximately 1 week, the patient should wear the collar only during the night to help prevent the neck from moving into unwanted positions. In most cases, the collar can be discarded after 4 weeks.

During the initial period of recovery, patients are advised to remain home from work and to rest. Physical therapy is also not advised at this time because, in most cases, the anxiety involved in traveling to and from treatments usually nullifies their effectiveness.

Once the acute phase has passed, initiation of physical therapy in the form of heat, massage, and eventually exercise, is begun. Both heat and massage enhance circulation, help in the removal of accumulated fluids, and promote a state of general relaxation. The object of exercise is to elongate the soft tissue musculature to a normal range, minimize the periarticular fibrous contracture of the zygapophyseal joints and, by muscular action, increase circulation to the deep neck tissues.[5] Isometric and stretching exercises improve both tone and flexibility, which in turn help correct posture and neck function. Alternative treatment with acupuncture and electrotherapy have also been found to be successful in many patients.

RECOVERY

The rate of recovery is based upon the severity of the injury and the patient's physiological makeup. It is the responsibility of the physician to determine the length of treatment and return the patient to the work environment as soon as possible.

REFERENCES

1. Tennyson SA, King AI: A biodynamic model of the human spinal column. Society of Automotive Engineers Paper 760771, Society of Automotive Engineers Proceedings SP-412, Mathematical Modeling Biodynamic Response to Impact 31–44, 1976.
2. Weinberg S, Lapointe H: Cervical extension-flexion injury (whiplash) and internal derangement of the temporomandibular joint. *J Oral Maxillofac Surg* 1987; 45:653–656.
3. Rubin W: Whiplash with vestibular involvement. *Arch Otolaryngol Head Neck Surg* 1973; 97:85–86.
4. Khurana R, Nirankari V: Bilateral sympathetic dysfunction in post-traumatic headaches. *Headache* 1986; 26:183–188.
5. Cailliet R: *Neck and Arm Pain*. Philadelphia, FA Davis Co, 1979, pp 60–85.

PART II

Upper Extremity Pain

17

Reflex Sympathetic Dystrophy of Upper Extremities

Lido Chen, M.D.

The patient is a 54-year-old woman who sustained a crush injury to her right hand 1 year earlier and underwent three operations consisting of a local orthopedic procedure, a contracture release, and a nerve graft. She describes her pain as "pins and needles with burning," which started immediately following the injury. The pain usually starts from the local area over the dorsum of her right hand between her thumb and index finger and spreads proximally to her entire upper extremity. She has not been able to wear any clothes with long sleeves due to the extreme sensitivity of her skin to light touch. She also noticed right upper extremity swelling, occurring intermittently without regard to the position. The pain is not relieved by rest; however, it can be exacerbated by exercise. Prior to her presentation to our pain management center, she had been treated with occupational therapy and transcutaneous electrical nerve stimulation (TENS). Her past medical history is otherwise unremarkable. Her current medication consists of only acetaminophen (Tylenol) with codeine for pain. Physical examination reveals decreasing sensation to pinprick over the dorsal sensory distribution of the radial nerve and hyperesthesia over the diffuse forearm and hand. A moderate decrease in joint motion of her wrist and hand is noted, as well as soft tissue swelling throughout the entire right upper extremity. The skin is dry and shiny. There is no change in hair or nail growth.

DISCUSSION

The diagnosis of reflex sympathetic dystrophy (RSD) requires a high index of suspicion for this disease complex in patients with neuropathic pain. Since its clinical manifestation can vary widely among individuals, the clinical diagnosis is usually based on the triad of the character of pain, vasomotor disturbances, and trophic changes. The picture of pain is consistent with any other neuropathic pain, which is characterized by burning, hyperpathia, and hyperesthesia with spontaneous activity. Patients often complain of vasomotor and/or sudomotor disturbances, which indicates sympathetic dysfunction. The change in skin color and temperature, edema, increases or decreases in hair and nail growth, sweating, etc., are also signs of sympathetic hypo- or hyperactivity. When RSD has progressed into the subacute and chronic stages, trophic changes over the affected extremity will become obvious, including changes in skin turgor, compliance of the soft tissue, and stiffness of the joints with muscle wasting. The above three criteria for a diagnosis of RSD can represent dysesthetic neurogenic pain, which may not be sympathetic-dependent, therefore, the response to the sympathetic block is advocated by some clinicians as an essential criteria for the diagnosis of RSD. For any case where the diagnosis of RSD is uncertain, a sympathetic block should be undertaken to help direct treatment.

Other adjuncts can be used to help in establishing the diagnosis and in documenting objective evidence of RSD. These include plain x-ray film, three phase bone scans (TPBS), psychogalvanic responses, and thermography. Evidence of periarticular osteopenia (Sudeck's atrophy) on x-ray is most commonly utilized by orthopedic surgeons as an aid to diagnose RSD. Unfortunately, this radiologic finding is not specific. The duration of disuse must be disproportional to the degree of osteopenia. Radiologists use TPBS to facilitate or exclude an early diagnosis in patients who have less specific signs and symptoms. Psychogalvanic reflexes such as skin conductance responses, skin potential responses, and thermography are also valuable in measuring sympathetic dysfunction.

Our patient had typical neurogenic pain with evidence of vasomotor disturbances. She was suspected to have ''possible RSD'' and underwent a diagnostic right cervicothoracic ganglion block. This block resulted in complete relief of pain, consistent with a local anesthetic (no placebo) effect. She was, therefore, recommended to continue with a series of therapeutic sympathetic blocks, as well as physical and occupational therapy.

PATHOPHYSIOLOGY

The initiating event of RSD is usually minor or major local tissue damage, secondary to any kind of trauma or disease. Fractures of the forearm have been shown by Drucker to be the most common event for RSD.[3] The degree of tissue damage may not correlate with the degree of pain.

There are different theories in the literature for the pathophysiology of RSD. The "artificial synapse" of injury by Doupe (1944), emphasizes the peripheral arm of the reflex circuit. This theory proposes the formation of "artificial synapse" between somatic afferent and sympathetic efferent fibers at the site of injury. Due to the tonicity of impulses from sympathetic efferent fibers, antidromic as well as orthodromic conductions in the sensory fibers occur at the artificial synapse, resulting in pain and changes in the threshold to sensory stimulation peripherally. The theory of the "vicious cycle of reflexes" by Livingston in 1944, emphasizes the importance of a central response in the mechanism of pain. Despite the presence of an irritative focus in the periphery, changes in the central regulating mechanism occur in the spinal cord and/or at high levels. Spontaneous neuronal hyperactivity of the internuncial pool in the dorsal horn of the spinal cord and high levels can perpetuate the pain. A proposed "cerebral biasing mechanism" by Melzack in 1971 also explains pain as a loss of an inhibitory projection system in the brain stem. There are numerous other proposed theories for RSD, including hypersensitivity of somatic afferent nerves to catecholamines secreted at peripheral sympathetic terminals and possible abnormal membrane properties of nerve regeneration after injury. There may be individual variation in the neurophysiology of the mechanism of RSD, since the clinical manifestation can be broad and varied. The combination of different theories may need to be involved at times to illustrate one particular case.

Our patient had a documented injury that initiated the pain and did not complain of any pain associated with emotional or psychological stress. It is most likely that she has a peripheral mechanism for her pain; however, this does not exclude other possibilities, such as central components contributory to her pain. Her complete resolution of pain with the stellate ganglion block favors the likelihood that peripheral mechanisms caused her pain.

Classification of RSD is made according to Drucker's staging and denervation hyperesthesia syndrome, identifying sensory change (pain), vasomotor disturbances (skin temperature, edema, sweating), sudomotor changes (hair and nail growth), and musculoskeletal changes (muscle power and radiological findings). Acute, subacute, and chronic stages represent the progress of the disease. The details of these stages are included in Table 17–1). The duration of each stage may differ from case to case relating to the severity of the injury.

STAGING

The acute stage, which is also called the denervation phase, is the first stage of RSD. The clinical signs of RSD at this stage are of acute sympathetic denervation. Pain is usually moderate in severity and localized to the area of injury. The

TABLE 17–1.

Classification or Staging of RSD

Changes	Stages		
	Acute	Subacute	Chronic
Sensory change	Burning pain Hyperesthesia	Burning and hyperesthesia Increase in intensity and persistence Increase by emotional and psychic stimulation	Decrease in burning and hyperesthesia
Vasomotor change			
Cutaneous blood flow	Increased	Decreased	No change
Skin temperature	Increased	Decreased	No change
Skin color and turgor	Glossy, smooth, dry, ruborous	Glossy, gray, cyanotic	Smooth, tight
Subcutaneous edema	Spongy, soft	Brawny	Brawny
Sudomotor change			
Hair growth	Increased	Decreased	Decreased or normal
Nail growth	Increased	Decreased	Decreased or normal
Musculoskeletal change	Bony rarefaction in subchondral spongiosa	Bone rarefaction in shaft and epiphyses	Sudeck's atrophy Pericapsular fibrosis Muscle wasting

subacute stage, also called the hypersensitivity phase, is the second stage of RSD. Pain at this stage results from increases in sympathetic activity and hypersensitivity to catecholamines, resulting in pain that has become more intense and persistent, and can be aggravated by emotional or psychic stimulation. The chronic stage, also called the reinnervation phase, is the last stage of the disease, marked by trophic changes. There may be a decrease or no change in sympathetic activity at the stage.

There are transitional periods from stage to stage, during which clinical classification can be difficult. The variation in clinical manifestations of RSD may also make it impossible to specifically indicate the stage of the disease in some patients. This classification is meant to aid in directing and predicting the outcome of the treatment. Our specific patient has burning pain with evidence of vasomotor changes, indicating the denervation stage.

TREATMENT

The treatment of RSD involves a broad spectrum approach, aimed at decreasing the pain and maintaining or resuming the function of the affected extremity. The treatment plan is tailored to each individuals needs, and usually contains multiple modalities such as serial sympathetic blocks, physical therapy, sympathectomy, psychotherapy, stimulation techniques, and trials of different medications.

Sympathetic blocks are advocated as the first choice of treatment for RSD. The purpose of the blocks is to break the cycle of pain and change the cutaneous pain threshold by interrupting the sympathetic outflow. This modality alone can provide complete relief of pain if it is initiated very early in the disease, before the involvement of the musculoskeletal system. However, it is more commonly utilized with other modalities, especially physical therapy. Measurement of the psychogalvanic reflex response, thermography, and cutaneous pain thresholds have successfully documented the improvement in RSD after a sympathetic block.

The efficacy of sympathetic blocks varies from 50%–90%. This difference is most likely due to a combination of using different criteria for diagnosis, a failure to classify patients into different stages for success rates, and possible incompleteness of the sympathetic block. RSD in the acute stage will have an overall response rate of 80%–90%, compared to a 40%–50% response rate in the chronic stage. Therefore, the aggressiveness of performing sympathetic blocks is determined at first by the stage of RSD; the earlier it is, the more aggressive the treatment should be, and the better the result will be. Patients with chronic RSD should be considered for surgical sympathectomy as early as possible if failure in progress with sympathetic blocks is encountered. There is a lack of a consistent protocol in the literature regarding the approach and number of sympathetic blocks performed. Different approaches can be used to achieve the sympathetic block: central blocks via epidural or subarachnoid routes, ganglionic blocks (cervicothoracic ganglion for face, neck, and upper extremity; lumbar sympathetic ganglion for lower extremity), and peripheral block (intravenous Bier blocks), can all achieve a sympathectomy using local anesthetics or other medications, including reserpine, guanethidine, bretylium, or calcium channel blockers. The selection of approach of the sympathetic block and the number of blocks should be individualized. The main goal is to achieve as complete a sympathectomy as possible with each sympathetic block, and to minimize the number of blocks as much as possible. Therefore, monitoring the completeness of the sympathetic block should be routine. The easiest and simplest method to monitor a sympathetic block is by measuring the subsequent degree of temperature rise and observing the vasodilatation. A complete sympathetic block is difficult to achieve in the upper extremity because the contribution to sympathetic fibers can be from as low as the T5 level. Cervicothoracic stellate ganglion blocks can be accomplished with 5–20 mL of local anesthetic solution, generally starting with a lower volume, and increasing as indicated and tolerated.

The increasing duration of pain relief with sympathetic blocks outlasts the duration of local anesthetic, and the intensity of pain should gradually decrease as the sympathetic blocks are carried out.

Whenever the patient's pain relief has reached a plateau with the sympathetic blocks, the blocks are discontinued. The frequency of blocks may vary from a continuous technique with a catheter, to timely intermittent outpatient injections. If a patient obtains complete relief of pain from the local anesthetic blocks, yet fails to respond favorably to duration of pain relief (and placebo effect is ruled out), a neurolytic block can be considered. However, neurolytic blocks to the upper extremity can be technically difficult to perform safely and are not commonly accepted by most anesthesiologists. Physical therapy appointments, if indicated, should be arranged immediately after the sympathetic block so that the patient suffers minimal amount of pain and has a maximal tolerance to the therapy. This is necessary in order to achieve the best effect from both modalities.

Physical therapy is an energetic program and is indicated in the vast majority of cases. It provides temporary pain modulation, a decrease in edema, and an increase in musculoskeletal function by various methods, including heat or cold treatments, hydrotherapy, massage, pressure dressing, active and passive range of motion, and stretching and strengthening exercises. Initially, these exercises can temporarily intensify the pain. Patients should all be discharged with a home exercise program to maintain the degree of pain relief and the functional level of the affected limb achieved during therapy.

Surgical sympathectomy can help 90% of the patients who do not obtain sympathetic relief from an adequate trial of blocks. It can be performed for both upper and lower limbs safely without any serious side effects.

Electrostimulation technique can be used to increase the relief of pain. Transcutaneous electrical nerve stimulation (TENS) has provided good success in the acute stage of RSD, and should be tried in conjunction with physical therapy. TENS has also been documented to be very effective as the first choice of treatment in pediatric patients. Dorsal columns stimulation can be provided for patients with the chronic stage of RSD refractory to other modalities.

Psychotherapy, such as hypnosis and biofeedback, has been shown to decrease sympathetic activity. Behavioral treatment can also help a patient understand his or her own responsibility in the course of RSD, especially when RSD has entered the chronic stage and the chronic pain syndrome has intervened. All of these can be instituted for patients with RSD to help alleviate the pain.

Medical treatment, such as trial of α-blockers, β-blockers, or calcium-channel blockers are reported in the literature with variable success rates. Systemic cortisone treatments are also advocated; however, not all of these reports have been double blind controlled studies to date, and no uniform protocols are available regarding the dosage of drug or the duration of treatment.

REFERENCES

1. Kozin F: The reflex sympathetic dystrophy syndrome. *Am J Med* 1976; 60:321–338.
2. Sunderland S: Pain mechanisms in causalgia. *J Neurol Neurosurg Psychiatry* 1976; 39:471–480.
3. Drucker WR: Pathogenesis of post-traumatic sympathetic dystrophy. *Am J Surg* 1959; 97:454–465.
4. Carroll Weller, *Adv Neurol* 1974; 4:485–590.
5. Procacci P: Cutaneous pain threshold changes after sympathetic block in reflex dystrophies. *Pain* 1975; 1:167–195.
6. Payne R: Neuropathic pain syndromes, with special reference to causalgia and reflex sympathetic dystrophy. *Clin J Pain* 1986; 2:59–73.

18

Carpal Tunnel Syndrome

Chang-Zern Hong, M.D.

A 42-year-old woman, who had been working in a post office as a mail distributor for 10 years, presented with a 2-month history of nocturnal pain, numbness, and tingling of the thumb, the second, and third fingers of the right hand. The pain spread into her right forearm and sometimes even to her right shoulder. The symptoms in the right hand also occurred in the daytime while at work. In the last several days, similar symptoms had occurred in her left hand. She denied any history of acute injury to her right upper extremity or her neck. She also denied any other significant medical problems. On examination, the abnormal findings included positive Tinel's sign on the right hand, and positive Phalen signs on both sides. The opposition strength of the right thumb was slightly reduced (4/5). There was a slightly decreased pinprick sensation over the right index and middle fingers. No obvious muscle atrophy was noticed. A nerve conduction study and electromyogram (EMG) were performed on the upper extremities. The distal sensory latencies were prolonged in the bilateral median nerves. The distal motor latency was prolonged in the right median nerve, but was normal in the left median nerve. The median motor conduction velocity of the forearm segment was normal on both sides. The conduction study done on the ulner nerves bilaterally was normal for both motor and sensory fibers. The EMG findings were also normal. These findings suggested that the patient had bilateral carpal tunnel syndrome. Other laboratory values including complete blood cell count, and levels of blood glucose, serum electrolytes, rheumatoid factors, ANA, and uric acid, were all within normal limits. She was treated conservatively. Treatment consisted of use of a cock-up splint at night, and oral, anti-inflammatory medication. The patient was to avoid using both hands for heavy work. The pain and tingling were rapidly reduced. A follow-up nerve conduction study showed significant improvement. Two months later, she returned to work to a different job (with less hand activities involved.)

TABLE 18–1.

Etiological Factors of Carpal Tunnel Syndrome (CTS)

Acute CTS
 Trauma
  Fractures or dislocation of wrist bone
  Sprain of wrist
  Hematoma
  Cut wounds
  Contusion
 Acute inflammation
  Insect sting
  Acute synovitis
  Acute infection
 Vascular disorders
  Thrombosis of median nerve
  Aneurysm of median nerve
Chronic CTS
 Local lesion affecting the median nerve
  Tenosynovitis—nonspecific, traumatic
  Tumor—osteoma, lipomas, lipofibromas, hamartomas, hemangiomas
  Ganglia
  Infections
  Familial CTS—thickening of flexor retinaculum
 Systemic diseases
  Diabetes mellitus
  Rheumatoid disease
  Lupus erythematosus
  Gout
  Amyloidosis
  Tuberculosis
  Pregnancy, postmenopausal state, contraceptive pill
  Lymphatic leukemia
 Idiopathic CTS

DISCUSSION

The carpal tunnel syndrome (CTS), is a compression neuropathy of the medial nerve at the wrist. The carpal tunnel is a narrow canal formed by the carpal tone and the transverse carpal ligament (flexor retinaculum).[1–2] The median nerve passes through the carpal tunnel along with the tendons of the long flexors of the fingers. After entering the tunnel, the nerve divides into lateral and medial branches. The lateral branch gives off a muscular branch to the thenar mass, and the first lumbrical and cutaneous branches to the thumb and index finger. The medial branch divides into a muscular branch to the second lumbrical, and cutaneous branches to the adjacent sides of the index and middle fingers and adjacent sides of the middle and ring fingers.

The possible causes of CTS are listed in Table 18–1. The most common causes are those with nonspecific tenosynovitis due to vocational stress.[3-4] Repetitive hand activities involving pinch or grasp during wrist flexion may be a contributing factor in CTS.[5]

Table 18–2 summarizes the pathogenesis, clinical findings, and electrodiagnosis at different stages of CTS. The diagnosis of CTS depends on clinical symptoms and signs, and should be confirmed by electrodiagnostic study.[6-8] Due to the high incidence of bilaterality, in CTS, a bilateral nerve conduction study is required, even if the patient has only unilateral symptoms.[9] Peripheral neuropathy or cervical radiculopathy should also be ruled out.[10] The electrodiagnostic test may also have prognostic value.

The effects of acute peripheral nerve compression can be classified into three grades.[11] When the duration of compression is less than 30 minutes with a compression pressure up to 300 mm Hg, the nerve conduction block is probably due to ischemia, and is completely reversible (grade 1). If the compression pressure is increased, or if the duration of compression is prolonged, or both, acute demyelinating block (grade 2), or even wallerian degeneration (grade 3), may occur. In an electrodiagnostic test, selective involvement of only motor fibers with relatively normal sensory can be a frequent finding in acute CTS.[7]

TABLE 18–2.

Pathogenesis and Clinical Manifestation of Carpal Tunnel Syndrome (CTS)

Stage	Pathology	Symptoms/Signs	Electrodiagnosis
Acute CTS			
Grade 1	No histological lesion	Transient paresthesia, pain, and weakness	Reversible conduction block, normal EMG
Grade 2	Local demyelination	Paresthesia, pain, and weakness	Conduction block, slow conduction, normal EMG
Grade 3	Wallerian degeneration	Paralysis and sensory loss	Conduction block, slow conduction, EMG: acute denervation
Chronic CTS			
Stage 1	Intrafunicular anoxia	Paresthesia, pain; positive Tinel and Phalen signs	Slow conduction
Stage 2	Intrafunicular edema	Paresthesia, pain, weakness, and sensory impairment	Conduction block, slow conduction, normal EMG
Stage 3	Funicular fibrosis; axonal degeneration	Paralysis and sensory loss; thenar muscle atrophy	Conduction block, slow conduction, EMG: chronic denervation

The pathogenesis of CTS due to chronic compression to the median nerve has been discussed in detail by Sunderland.[2, 12] The initial lesion is an intrafunicular anoxia caused by obstruction to the venous return from the funiculi of the median nerve as the result of increased pressure in the carpal tunnel. The large myelinated fibers are usually affected earlier than the small fibers. Not all funiculi or all fibers are affected to the same degree at the same time. Therefore, the clinical symptoms in the initial stage are usually mild and variable. Nocturnal paresthesias, including painful numbness and tingling of the affected hand over the area supplied by the median nerve (thumb, index and middle fingers, and radial half of the ring finger), are the common early symptoms. Usually no definite sensory impairment or motor weakness of the affected hand can be identified in neurological examination. The Phalen sign and Tinel's sign are valuable to detect the early stage of CTS. The Phalen wrist flexion test is the maneuver used to increase the compression force to the median nerve by maximal flexion of the wrist for one minute continuously.[6] The median nerve slides proximally and is forced against the proximal edge of the flexor retinaculum. Tinel's sign is the development of a tingling sensation over the area supplied by the injured nerve when this nerve is percussed firmly over or distal to the site of the injury. At this early stage, the nerve conduction study shows increased distal latency of the median nerve (i.e., increase of conduction time in the distal segment across the carpal tunnel). Electromyographic (EMG) study on the thenar muscles usually shows normal findings since no axonal degeneration occurs at this time.

The secondary stage includes the development of intrafunicular edema due to impaired capillary circulation with leakage of protein into the surrounding tissue. The edema finally causes enlargement of the median nerve at the margin of the flexor retinaculum. A demyelinative lesion of the median nerve becomes severe and more extensive, and finally, axonal degeneration occurs in some fibers. Clinically, pain and paresthesia become progressively more severe. Mild weakness in thumb opposition may occur. The sensory impairment in the thumb, index, and third fingers, and radial half of the ring finger is usually remarkable. Tinel's sign is positive. Nerve conduction study usually shows remarkably prolonged distal latency in the median nerve, and reduced amplitude of the evoked potential upon stimulation above (but not below) the carpal tunnel due to conduction block. Electromyogram study may still be within normal limits, or may show mild denervation in the thenar muscles if the muscle weakness is marked.

In the third stage, the deforming force interrupts the blood supply and also contributes direct mechanical force to the median nerve. The final outcome is the fibrous connective tissue replacement of the contents of the funiculi with severe axonal degeneration. Few regeneration axons are successful in penetrating this tissue, with most terminating when they reach the fibrosed segment by contributing to the swelling of the median nerve at that site. At this stage, the pain or paresthesias may not be as severe as in the earlier stages. However, the motor weakness and sensory loss (anesthesia) may become very obvious. Thenar muscle atrophy is usually prominent. Nerve conduction study of the median nerve shows reduced amplitude of the evoked compound muscle or nerve potential, not only from the proximal stimulation above the carpal tunnel, but also from the distal stimulation below the carpal tunnel, due to severe axonal degeneration. The motor and sensory distal latencies may be quite prolonged. Electromyogram study usually shows severe chronic denervation (large polyphasic motor unit potentials and reduced recruitment).

MANAGEMENT

The appropriate treatment of CTS depends on the cause and the severity of the disease. Mild cases of CTS usually respond to conservative treatment satisfactorily. However, if a progressive lesion causing compression is identified, even in the early stage, surgical intervention is usually required. Surgical decompression should be considered in the advanced cases of CTS, or in the mild cases that do not respond to conservative management. For a progressive compression neuropathy, the earlier the decompression surgery is performed, the better the prognosis. An electrodiagnostic test (EMG and nerve conduction study) is usually helpful to determine if surgery is required.

The conservative management of CTS includes the following treatment programs:[2, 3, 6]

1. Rest of the wrist and hand:
   a. Avoid overloading or repetitive activities of the affected hand.
   b. Use of cock-up wrist splint at night (to avoid overflexion of wrist during sleeping), or when doing "relatively heavy" activities.
2. Anti-inflammatory agents, local or systemic:
   a. Nonsteroidal anti-inflammatory drugs (oral).
   b. Steroid hormone (oral or local injection).
3. Agents to relieve the pressure in the carpal tunnel: diuretics (systemic) and hyaluronidase (local) have been tried in the past, but are not often used today.
4. Physical therapy:
   a. Heat—hot pack or ultrasound to improve local circulation and to reduce pain.
   b. Hydrotherapy to relieve the pain and to make exercise more comfortable. Stretching of flexor tendons since tensed flexor tendons may cause increased pressure of median nerve compression.[5] Strengthening exercise of the intrinsic and extrinsic muscles of the hand.

5. Occupational therapy: Therapeutic exercise with functional activities, energy saving techniques, training for daily living activities if needed, and prevocational programs.
6. Vocational rehabilitation: Change of occupation may be required to avoid recurrence.

REFERENCES

1. Cailliet R: Hand Pain and Impairment. Philadelphia, FA Davis Co, 1971.
2. Sunderland S: The carpal tunnel syndrome, in *Nerves and Nerve Injury*. New York, Churchill Livingstone, 1978, pp 711–727.
3. Phalen GS: The carpal tunnel syndrome. Seventeen years' experience in diagnosis and treatment of six hundred fifty-four hands. *J Bone Joint Surg* 1966; 48:211–228.
4. Phalen GS: The carpal tunnel syndrome. Clinical evaluation of 598 hands. *Clin Orthop* 1972; 83:29–40.
5. Smith EM, Sonstegard DA, Anderson WH: Carpal tunnel syndrome: Contribution of flexor tendons. *Arch Phys Med Rehabil* 1977; 58:379–385.
6. Gordon C, Bowyer BL, Johnson EW: Electrodiagnostic characteristics of acute carpal tunnel syndrome. *Arch Phys Med Rehabil* 1987; 68:545–548.
7. Johnson EW: Carpal tunnel syndrome, in Johnson EW (ed): *Practical Electromyography,* ed 2. Baltimore, Williams & Wilkins, 1988, pp 187–205.
8. Stevens JC: The electrodiagnosis of carpal tunnel syndrome. *Muscle Nerve* 1987; 10:99–113.
9. Bendler EM, Greenspun B, Yu J, et al: The bilaterality of carpal tunnel syndrome. *Arch Phys Med Rehabil* 1977; 58:362–364.
10. Yu J, Bendler EM, Mentari A: Neurological disorders associated with carpal tunnel syndrome. *Electromyogr Clin Neurophysiol* 1979; 19:27–32.
11. Gilliatt RW: Acute compression block, in Sumner AJ (ed): *The Physiology of Peripheral Nerve Disease*. Philadelphia, WB Saunders, 1980, pp 287–315.
12. Sunderland S: The nerve lesion in the carpal tunnel syndrome. *J Neurol Neurosurg Psychiatry* 1976; 39:615–626.

19

Thoracic Outlet Syndrome

Avrom Gart, M.D.

A 42-year-old moderately obese woman presented with right-sided neck, scapular, and arm pain, accompanied by paresthesias in the fourth and fifth digits of the right hand. She stated that her right arm often felt cold, especially while doing overhead work. Physical examination revealed decreased sensation to light touch and pinprick in the right upper extremity corresponding to the eighth cervical and first thoracic dermatomes. Hyperabduction of the right arm obliterated the radial pulse. Initial diagnostic testing included normal cervical spine radiographs. However, nerve conduction studies indicated a prolonged right ulnar F-wave and somatosensory-evoked response. Following a poor response to a course of physical therapy, surgical exploration of the thoracic outlet via the supraclavicular approach was performed, which revealed a cervical band that compressed both the subclavian artery and lower trunk of the brachial plexus. This structure was resected, and subsequently the patient's symptoms improved. Physical examinations and repeat nerve conduction studies were found to be normal.

DISCUSSION

The term "thoracic outlet syndrome" refers to a group of physical signs and symptoms whose actual etiology, in many cases, remains unclear. It is generally agreed upon, however, that entrapment of the neurovascular bundle at some point along its anatomical pathway through the cervicobrachial region contributes to the cause of this painful condition. Anatomical variation does exist, especially in the attachments of both the scalenus anterior and medius muscles to the first rib, which may compromise the course of the nerves and vessels traveling through this region on their way into the arm. Specifically, the lower trunk of the brachial plexus and the subclavian artery are those structures most often at risk. A cervical rib usually associated with the seventh cervical transverse process has been found to be the etiologic factor in some situations. Others contest that the costoclavicular space, which is bounded by the inner third of the clavicle and subclavius, the first rib, and the superior border of the scapula, is the site of neurovascular compression.

SIGNS AND SYMPTOMS

A patient's presentation and complaints will usually reflect the severity and duration of the lesion involved, although this will seldom help locate its anatomical site. Symptoms of dull, aching pain are often described and localized to the supraclavicular fossa, anterior shoulder, neck, and arm. Sensory disturbances corresponding to the lower trunk of the brachial plexus (eighth cervical and first thoracic dermatomes) usually precede a demonstrable motor deficit and are felt along the medial border of the arm, forearm, hand, and into the fourth and fifth digits. As the lesion progresses, objective sensory findings become apparent and are followed by intrinsic muscle weakness manifested by grip strength loss, along with atrophy of the thenar eminence. Vascular compromise of the subclavian artery may cause ischemic pain with repetitive arm usage, or signs of Raynaud's phenomenon. Obstruction of venous return leads to peripheral edema and stiffness.

PROVOCATIVE TESTING

The following physical maneuvers have been designed to reproduce the patient's symptoms or diminish the radial pulse. However, it should be noted that they are often positive in normal individuals.

Adson's Test.—Symptoms caused by the so-called scalenus anticus syndrome, cervical rib or band, or abnormal first rib may be found by radial pulse obliteration using this maneuver. In this test, the patient is seated, with the arms resting comfortably on the thighs. The examiner palpates the radial pulse while the patient deeply inspires with the head extended and rotated to the affected side. Diminution or obliteration of the radial pulse during the test is considered positive.

Shoulder Hyperabduction Test.—The examiner palpates the radial pulse while the shoulder is slowly hyperabducted with the elbow flexed. If the pulse is obliterated with greater ease compared to normal subjects, the test may be considered positive.

Shoulder Bracing Test.—Bracing the shoulder backward in an exaggerated military position approximates the first rib and clavicle. In the cases of costoclavicular space narrowing, reproduction of symptoms or obliteration of the radial pulse is considered a positive test.

CLINICAL INVESTIGATION

Radiological Assessment.—Standard cervical spine radiographs will detect an obvious cervical rib, abnormal first rib, clavicle, or other bony anomaly. Apical lordotic views are necessary to rule out a Pancoast tumor invading the brachial plexus.

Arterial Studies.—Subclavian artery compression may be seen during arteriography with arm or head positions that reproduce the patient's symptoms. Simple blood pressure measurements in both arms may be widely asymmetrical. A bruit of the subclavian artery may be detected using Doppler ultrasonography.

Venous Studies.—Comparison of the venous pressure in both arms may be performed using phlebography. Venography or flow studies using isotopic tracers injected into the distal arm may demonstrate venous compression.

Nerve Conduction Studies.—Peripheral entrapment syndromes should routinely be ruled out using standard studies across the elbow and wrist. Brachial plexus lesions must be investigated by stimulation in the supraclavicular fossa at Erb's point. Recently, ulnar F-wave studies and somatosensory-evoked responses, in both anatomical and provocative arm positions, have been found to be useful.[1-3]

DIFFERENTIAL DIAGNOSIS

Lesions involving the lower cervical spinal cord such as a spinal tumor, syringomyelia, motor neuron disease, arachnoiditis, or cervical disc disease.
Pancoast tumor involving the brachial plexus.
Brachial plexopathy.
Ulnar nerve entrapment at the elbow or wrist.
Carpal tunnel syndrome.

MANAGEMENT

Conservative Treatment

Significant improvement in symptoms can be expected in the majority of cases with a regular physical therapy and home exercise program. Daily stretching, strengthening, and postural exercises for the neck and shoulder muscles help to relieve tension on the neurovascular elements in the thoracic outlet. A sling or figure eight harness can be used in an attempt to relieve acute symptoms in special cases. Those patients exhibiting a definitive clinical neurologic deficit or vascular compromise may warrant surgical intervention.

Surgical Treatment

Since both symptoms and causes of the thoracic outlet syndrome are unique to each patient, a thorough clinical investigation is necessary. There are two common surgical exposures that are currently used, each with their own benefits and risks. The first and most popular approach is via the supraclavicular region. The anterior scalene muscle is easily resected, which then allows exploration of the brachial plexus, removal of any cervical rib or band, or resection of the first rib.[4] Complications, although very rare, include infection, injury to the brachial plexus, phrenic nerve paralysis, or thoracic duct injury. The second approach, posterior thoracoplasty via the transaxillary route, has been used for resection of the first rib in some cases.[5] Neurologic symptoms usually respond better than do vascular symptoms with this approach. Complications include pneumothorax, infection, pleural effusion, brachial plexus injury, or damage to the ulnar, intercostal, or long thoracic nerves, and breast thrombophlebitis.

In cases of neurovascular compression caused by the clavicle, resection of the clavicle, including the periosteum, is performed. This exposure, however, may result in unwanted disfigurement or a delayed plexus stretch injury and is, therefore, used less frequently.

Those patients whose symptoms are caused by compression from the pectoralis minor require direct transection of the tendon.

CONCLUSION

The signs and symptoms of thoracic outlet syndrome must be viewed with caution as they mimic the common complaints associated with a variety of other conditions. Careful history and physical examination, along with a complete diagnostic evaluation, is necessary in order to reach an accurate clinical diagnosis. Surgical treatment should only be considered in those patients who fail to respond to a thorough course of conservative management.

REFERENCES

1. Wulff CH, Gilliatt DM: F Waves in Cervical Rib Patients. *Muscle Nerve* 1979; 2:452–457.
2. Glover JL, Worth RM, Bendick PJ, et al: Evoked responses in the diagnosis of thoracic outlet syndrome. *Surgery* 1981; 89:86–93.
3. Chodoroff G, Lee DW, Honet JC: Dynamic approach in the diagnosis of thoracic outlet syndrome using somatosensory evoked responses. *Arch Phys Med Rehab* 1985; 66:3–6.
4. Hempel GK, Rusher AH Jr, Wheeler CG, et al: Supraclavicular resection of the first rib for thoracic outlet syndrome. *Am J Surg* 1981; 141:213–216.
5. Johnson C: Treatment of thoracic outlet syndrome by removal of first rib and related entrapments through posterolateral approach. *J Thorac Cardiovasc Surg* 1974; 68:536–545.

20

Polymyalgia Rheumatica With Giant Cell Arteritis

I. Jon Russell, M.D., Ph.D.

A 67-year-old white woman developed an aching pain in her shoulders, neck, back, and hips with 3 hours of morning stiffness. All of her joints exhibited normal range of motion, there was no synovitis, and no soft tissue tenderness. She was mildly anemic (Hb, 12.6 g/dL) and had an elevated sedimentation rate (ESR, 54 mm/hr). Treatment with naproxen 250 mg twice daily provided some relief. Three months later she developed a severe headache associated with jaw claudication. Her temporal arteries were thickened and very tender. A biopsy on the right revealed narrowing of the lumen with granulomatous inflammation of the vessel wall. She was treated with 60 mg/day of prednisone and felt completely well by the second day of therapy. Her ESR and Hb normalized within 1 month. She was able to taper the dosage of the prednisone and discontinue it after 18 months without recurrence of her symptoms.

DISCUSSION

As health care has improved over the past 100 years, the proportion of individuals over the age of 65 years has increased substantially. It is not surprising, therefore, that a group of diseases fairly unique to those over the age of 50 might become more apparent.

The patient described above had three infectious illnesses (diphtheria, rheumatic fever, and Bright's disease) as a child, but survived all of them to live a long and healthy life. It wasn't until age 67 years that she developed a vague syndrome of severe, disabling, musculoskeletal pain, which a series of physicians variously diagnosed as degenerative joint disease, psychogenic rheumatism, and fibrositis syndrome over a period of several months.

A little osteoarthritis might be expected at her age, since the frequency of that disorder increases progressively with age, but that was not the cause of her severe pain. Psychogenic rheumatism is defined as a psychiatric disorder in which the patients have selected the musculoskeletal system as the somatic manifestation of their distress. That diagnosis was incorrect because she was psychiatrically normal. Finally, fibrositis syndrome was not the correct diagnosis because she did not exhibit the typical pattern of tender points which characterize that syndrome. Even if a sufficient number of tender points had been symptomatic to make the diagnosis of fibrositis syndrome, an elevated sedimentation rate should have prompted her physicians to seek an associated inflammatory process.

The course of her disease was altered by the onset of severe headaches that persisted for 2 months before she again sought medical attention. At that point, an astute medical resident obtained a history of jaw claudication, noted the tenderness of the temporal arteries, and felt their induration. On that basis, he made the presumptive diagnoses of *polymyalgia rheumatica* with *giant cell (temporal) arteritis*.

The clinical model of polymyalgia rheumatica has traditionally been based on a triad of *shoulder and pelvic girdle pain* in an individual *over the age of 50* years with a *sedimentation rate >50 mm/hr*. An increased specificity of those findings is obtained when they have been present for more than 2 weeks, are not associated with muscle weakness, and are relieved within 2 days after initiating low dose corticosteroids.[1]

A large collaborative British study evaluated the clinical features of 236 patients with unequivocal polymyalgia rheumatica and compared them to 253 patients with conditions that mimic that disorder. They found that the most valuable criteria for differentiation were *bilateral shoulder pain or stiffness,* an *ESR >50 mm/hr,* a duration of *morning stiffness >1 hr,* an *age of 65 years* or more, plus *constitutional symptoms* like depression or weight loss for at least 2 weeks' duration. It was also observed that a *rapid change in the ESR* during a course of 10 mg/day prednisone therapy was valuable in supporting the diagnosis.[2]

The constitutional symptoms are often present for weeks to months before the diagnosis is made. They include fever, headache, visual disturbances, malaise, and anemia. It seems that no list of diagnostic criteria is unassailable. For example, there are cases reported in which the onset occurred in the decade before age 50 years and patients with an otherwise typical clinical picture have been reported to have an ESR <49 mm/hr.[3-4]

The apparent relationship between polymyalgia rheumatica and giant cell arteritis is not a constant one, since only 10%–20% of patients with polymyalgia rheumatica have giant cell arteritis, and 30% of patients with giant cell arteritis have polymyalgia rheumatica. The presence of giant cell arteritis in this patient was suspected because of her jaw claudication and severe headache. The temporal arteries were thickened and tender to palpation, further supporting that possibility. It should be recognized that patients with advanced atherosclerosis can exhibit palpably firm temporal arteries. Occasionally, a much younger patient with severe headaches can have very tender temporal arteries without any histologic abnormality in the vessel.

The diagnosis of giant cell arteritis is confirmed by finding granulomatous lesions in the arterial wall that narrow the vascular lumen. Thus, a decision must be made regarding who should have a temporal artery biopsy. Not every patient with polymyalgia rheumatica will progress to giant cell arteritis, so not every patient with polymyalgia rheumatica needs to have a temporal artery biopsy. Patients who exhibit symptoms suggestive of ischemia, such as visual changes or jaw claudication, should have a temporal artery biopsy performed. Another relative indication for biopsy is failure of the symptoms of polymyalgia rheumatica to resolve completely with low dose corticosteroid therapy. Once the diagnosis of giant cell arteritis is made histologically, 60 mg/day of corticosteroid is indicated.

The prevalence of giant cell arteritis in the general population seems to depend on ethnic distribution and average age. It appears to be more common among people of Scandinavian descent, but less common in blacks and Hispanics. In Denmark, the annual incidence in the general population was 22/100,000, which rose to 77/100,000 for individuals over the age of 50 years.[5] Women had an incidence rate 4–5 times higher than was seen in men. By contrast, a study in Shelby County, Tennessee, disclosed only a 0.35/100,000 annual incidence in the overall population, increasing to 1.58/100,000 for those over age 50 years. The incidence was 7 times greater for whites than blacks and 7 times greater in females than males.[6] Approximately 1.5% of random autopsies show evidence of giant cell arteritis in either the temporal artery or aorta.

The visual symptoms associated with giant cell arteritis are particularly important because the disease can ultimately cause irreversible blindness. Although the onset of blindness can be quite sudden, it is usually preceded by visual symptoms like ptosis, diplopia, blurring, or TIA-like episodes. Once vision is lost in one eye, progression to the contralateral eye is almost inevitable within days to weeks unless treatment intervenes.

Typical laboratory abnormalities in polymyalgia rheumatica and giant cell arteritis include an elevation in the sedimentation rate, a mild to moderate anemia, a normal or elevated peripheral leukocyte count, a normal or elevated platelet count, mild abnormalities in liver function tests, and, occasionally, synovial fluid inflammation.[7]

One of the problems associated with the diagnosis of polymyalgia rheumatica is the difficulty in distinguishing it from rheumatoid arthritis.[8] Patients with polymyalgia rheumatica can exhibit a symmetric synovitis involving the large joints that can even cause bony erosions. Usually, the rheumatoid factor will be negative in polymyalgia as it is in seronegative rheumatoid arthritis. On the other hand, completely healthy individuals can develop rheumatoid factor positivity with age. The coexistence of rheumatoid factor with the pain pattern of polymyalgia rheumatica certainly could mimic seropositive rheumatoid arthritis.

Recent studies with histocompatibility antigens have indicated a substantially higher frequency of HLA DR-4 antigen positivity in seropositive rheumatoid arthritis than seronegative rheumatoid arthritis.[9] There was also a higher frequency of HLA Leu 2 + Leu 7 + lymphocyte subsets in rheumatoid arthritis as compared to polymyalgia rheumatica or normal controls. These tests are not readily available to the clinical practitioner, but they do suggest that those populations are different.

The cause of giant cell arteritis and/or polymyalgia rheumatica is not known. It is suspected that an inflammatory process is initiated in a genetically susceptible individual by an infection or actinic injury to the vessel wall, which then becomes self-perpetuating, unless interrupted by immunosuppressive therapy.

MANAGEMENT

Since the initial manifestations of polymyalgia rheumatica are often nonspecific, they may resemble anything from a flulike illness to a malignancy. As a result, the diagnosis can be delayed inappropriately, or the workup can involve the use of unnecessary diagnostic studies. A high index of suspicion for this disorder in elderly individuals is the best defense against missing the diagnosis.

Patients over the age of 50 years who complain of musculoskeletal pain or have vague constitutional symptoms should be examined carefully and have an ESR drawn. In the presence of musculoskeletal symptoms typical for polymyalgia, but no evidence for ischemia to suggest giant cell arteritis, treatment should be initiated with 10–15 mg of prednisone daily in a single morning dose. That therapy should be continued for 12 months or longer with gradual tapering of the dosage. Monthly monitoring of the patient's symptoms and the sedimentation rate provide sensitive measures on which to base decisions regarding changes in therapy.

Failure of the symptoms to resolve under these conditions should raise suspicion of an occult malignancy or of giant cell arteritis. When giant cell arteritis is clinically suspected, one or both of the temporal arteries should be biopsied to establish the diagnosis histologically. The pathologist should view at least one section every millimeter to avoid missing intermittent, localized lesions. Occasionally, the opposite temporal artery will also need to be examined because the first biopsy is negative.

Patients with a typical clinical pattern for giant cell arteritis should begin therapy with 60 mg of prednisone daily to avoid progressive ischemic injury. If a temporal artery biopsy has not already been done, it should be performed within 1–3 days of initiating therapy, so the histologic changes are not obscured by treatment.

The prognosis of treated polymyalgia rheumatica and/or giant cell arteritis is very good. Corticosteroid therapy may need to be continued for several years, but gradual decreases in dosage after the first month are possible in most cases. Factors that contribute to an increased mortality are the requirement for a maintenance dosage >10 mg of prednisone per day and progression of the disease to visual loss.[9] The survival curves for men with giant cell arteritis are not much different than the curves for the general population. On the other hand, it appears that women with giant cell arteritis have a measurably decreased survival rate as a consequence of this disease.[10]

Long-term treatment with corticosteroid can lead to drug-induced complications, including thinning of the skin, osteopenia, infection, and atherosclerosis. For that reason, the dosage should be tapered to below 10 mg/day as soon as possible, while maintaining control of the disease activity.

REFERENCES

1. Hunder GG, Disney TF, Ward LE: Polymyalgia rheumatica. *Mayo Clin Proc* 1969; 44:849–875.
2. Bird HA, Esselinckx W, Dixon A, St. J. Mowat AG, Wood PHN: An evaluation of criteria for polymyalgia rheumatica. *Ann Rheum Dis* 1979; 29:980–986.
3. Dailey MP, McCarty DJ: Polymyalgia rheumatica begins at 40. *Arch Intern Med* 1979; 139:743–744.
4. Chuang TY, Hunder GG, Ilstrup DM, et al: Polymyalgia rheumatica: A ten year epidemiologic and clinical study. *Ann Intern Med* 1982; 97:672–680.
5. Boesen P, Sorensen SF: Giant cell arteritis, temporal arteritis and polymyalgia rheumatica in a Danish county: A prospective investigation, 1982–1985. *Arthritis Rheum* 1987; 30:294–299.
6. Smith CA, Fidler WJ, Pinals RS: The epidemiology of giant cell arteritis: Report of a ten year study in Shelby County, Tennessee. *Arthritis Rheum* 1983; 26:1214–1219.
7. Healey LA: Polymyalgia rheumatica and the American Rheumatism Association criteria for rheumatoid arthritis. *Arthritis Rheum* 1983; 26:1417–1418.
8. Doloug JH, Forre O, Kass E, et al: HLA antigens in rheumatoid arthritis: Association between HLADRW4 positivity and IGM rheumatoid factor production. *Arthritis Rheum* 1980; 23:309–313.
9. Gram E: Survival in temporal arteritis. *Trans Ophthalmol Soc UK* 1980; 100:108–110.
10. Gram E, Holland A, Avery A, et al: Prognosis in giant cell arteritis. *Br Med J [Clin Res]* 1981; 282:269–271.

PART III

Chest Pain

21

Post-thoracotomy Pain Syndrome

Lido Chen, M.D.

The patient is a 35-year-old man who underwent right thoracotomy for removal of a right upper lobe lesion 3 months before being seen in the pain management center. He relates that his pain has never disappeared completely following the upper lobectomy. This pain is described as an intermittent shooting sensation radiating from back to front, and is accompanied by a continuous, dull aching over the area of the right scapula and flank regions. Physical examination reveals that the shooting pain is along the T6 distribution and the dull aching pain is mainly over the right infrascapular region. There is a negative Tinel's sign over the scar. His past medical history is not significant for any other major diseases.

DISCUSSION

Post-thoracotomy pain syndrome (PTS) is the term commonly used to describe pain that develops following thoracotomy, without regard to the primary etiology. Clinicians tend to relate this syndrome to pleurisy or intercostal neuralgia. However, the cause of pain in PTS often goes beyond these entities.

In the clinical evaluation of PTS, one should at first exclude visceral pain. Many of the structures inside the chest cavity, including the heart, pericardium, lungs, trachea, bronchi, esophagus, and thymus are innervated by visceral branches of the thoracic sympathetic trunks and vagal parasympathetic nerves. It is well known that chest pain can result from pathology in these structures. Common examples are angina pectoris and pulmonary embolism. The treatment for these processes is obviously entirely different from the persistent somatic pain of PTS, and is aimed at correcting the underlying pathology.

Once a visceral etiology has been excluded, the pain is then more likely to have a somatic origin. This somatic pain originates from musculoskeletal structures composing the chest cavity itself (ribs, external oblique muscle, internal oblique muscle, parietal pleura, etc.), or the surrounding muscles used to support the chest wall (pectoralis major and minor, latissimus dorsi, teres major and minor, paraverteral muscles, etc.). Somatic pain originating from intrinsic structures of the chest cavity often presents clinically as intercostal neuralgia, and is commonly secondary to pleurisy (or pleuritis), nerve entrapment syndrome, neuroma, rib trauma and costochondritis, etc. Somatic pain originating from structures extrinsic to the chest cavity often has a myofascial component secondary to intraoperative positioning, incision, pressure from a retractor to the involved muscles, etc. It is also possible that a combination of the two exist simultaneously in one patient.

In addition to the above physiological reasons for the pain, PTS can exist in patients with "chronic pain syndrome," indicating no clear-cut physical findings, yet patients can display an inability to cope with the activities of daily living. A complete and thorough psychological evaluation is therefore helpful in determining the etiology of pain and directing the appropriate treatment.

Our patient was felt clinically to have somatic pain including intercostal neuralgia and myofascial pain involving the lattissimus dorsi and paravertebral muscles.

DIFFERENTIAL DIAGNOSIS

The first step in approaching a patient with PTS is to distinguish between visceral and somatic etiologies using the history and characteristics of the pain. Visceral pain is usually associated with a sensation of pressure or tightness, and is poorly localized. It can radiate to the neck, shoulder, or arm. The presence of other cardiac or pulmonary disorders should also alert the clinician to the possibility of a visceral etiology.

Somatic pain, from either intercostal neuralgia or myofascial pain, after thoracotomy is usually associated with an increase or change in pain with respiration. Intercostal neuralgia is a well-localized sharp pain radiating from back to front along the distribution of the intercostal nerve over the affected dermatome. Intercostal neuralgia can also be associated with changes in cutaneous sensation such as burning, paresthesia, hyperesthesia, or dysesthesia. Localized tenderness, with or without a positive Tinel's sign, is suggestive of local pathology such as neuroma, nerve entrapment, costochondritis, or rib trauma. Therefore, a detailed examination of the scar and painful area should be performed. If intercostal neuralgia is not associated with any change in cutaneous sensation, or if no local pathology is suspected, a chest x-ray should be examined for any evidence of pleurisy.

Myofascial pain from thoracotomy can involve numerous muscles, both anteriorly and posteriorly. It usually manifests as a dull aching with individual patterns of referred pain that do not follow the distribution of the intercostal nerves. Specific trigger points may exist; however, they are not an absolute finding.

TREATMENT

The treatments for PTS are directed at the underlying causes of pain. When intercostal neuralgia is suspected, diagnostic intercostal nerve blocks with local anesthetics should be performed, including, minimally, one dermatome above and one dermatome below the pathology. These should be performed on at least two occasions. Temporary relief of the pain is expected, and if not obtained, the patient needs to be reevaluated for other sources of pain. It is rare when repeated local anesthetic blocks alleviate the pain permanently. Commonly, more aggressive treatment is required for permanent relief, such as intercostal neurectomy, ganglionectomy, rhizotomy by neurosurgeon, cryoneurolysis, or neurolytic block, depending on the availability of these services and the tolerance of the patient. Intercostal neurectomy or rhizotomy carry the possibility of pain recurrence; however, these procedures are better tolerated by the patient than is ganglionectomy, especially when other multiple medical problems exist. Intraoperative cryoneurolysis has been documented to decrease the demand for immediate postoperative analgesia and to enhance the value of physiotherapy. However, relief from persistent intercostal neuralgia following thoracotomy remains debatable. Difficulty in accurate placement of the cryoprobe via the percutaneous approach may have contributed to the less than satisfactory success rate with this treatment modality. Neurolytic block can also be performed using phenol; however, the possibilities of postblock neuritis and spreading of neurolytic solution proximally have limited its clinical usage.

It is worth mentioning that scar-related pain secondary to nerve entrapment or neuroma may give a clinical picture of intercostal neuralgia. Therefore, scan injection with local anesthetics and steroids should be undertaken before doing a diagnostic intercostal nerve block whenever there is suspicion of scar-related pain problems. If there is localized tenderness that suggests possible rib trauma or costochondritis, trigger point injection can be performed.

If the PTS is thought to be myofascial in origin, physical therapy and other adjuncts such as trigger point injection, transcutaneous nerve stimulation, and muscle strengthening exercises should be arranged on an individual basis. Nonsteroidal anti-inflammatory drugs can be administered. The patient with chronic pain syndrome may also benefit from psychotherapy, behavioral modification, and biofeedback.

Out patient was treated initially with intercostal nerve blocks at T5, T6, and T7 with incomplete resolution of pain. Physical therapy was begun and his pain gradually responded. During this phase of therapy, he received a total of four intercostal nerve blocks to facilitate the physical therapy. He did not require more aggressive therapeutic measures and currently has only minimal pain.

BIBLIOGRAPHY

Conacher ID: Percutaneous cryotherapy for post thoracotomy neuralgia. *Pain* 1986; 25:229–238.

Glynn CJ, Floyd JW: Cryoanalgesia in the management of pain after thoracotomy. *Thorax* 1980; 35:325–327.

Katz J: Cryoanalgesia for post thoracotomy pain. *Lancet* 1980; 1:512–513.

Netter F: *The Ciba Collection of Medical Illustrations,* Vol 1. 1983, pp 76–78.

22

Acute Herpes Zoster Involving the Chest Wall

Steven D. Waldman, M.D.

A 48-year-old woman was referred to the pain management center for evaluation and treatment of intractable pain secondary to acute herpes zoster. The pain had failed to respond to simple analgesics, nonsteroidal anti-inflammatory agents, and narcotic analgesics. The patient was unable to provide self-care activities because any movement or contact with the rash exacerbated her pain. Severe sleep disturbance was present. The patient's past medical history was significant for breast malignancy.

DEFINITION

Herpes zoster is an infectious disease that is caused by the DNA virus herpesvirus varicella. This virus is the causative agent of both chicken pox (varicella), and shingles (herpes zoster). Primary infection in the nonimmune host manifests itself clinically as the childhood disease chicken pox. It is postulated that, during the course of primary infection with herpesvirus varicella, the virus migrates to the dorsal root or cranial ganglia. The virus then remains dormant in the ganglia producing no clinically evident disease. In some individuals the virus may reactivate then travel along peripheral or cranial sensory pathways to the nerve endings, producing the pain and skin lesions characteristic of shingles. The reason that reactivation occurs in only some individuals is not fully understood, but it is theorized that a decrease in cell-mediated immunity allows the virus to multiply in the ganglia and spread to the corresponding sensory nerves, thus producing clinical disease. Patients who are suffering from malignancies (particularly lymphoma), patients who are receiving immunosuppressive therapy (chemotherapy, steroids, radiation), and patients suffering from chronic diseases who are generally debilitated, are much more likely to develop acute herpes zoster than the healthy population. These patients all have in common a decreased cell-mediated immune response, which may be the reason for their propensity to develop shingles. This may also explain why the incidence of shingles increases dramatically in patients over 60 years of age and is relatively uncommon under the age of 20 years.

SIGNS AND SYMPTOMS

As viral reactivation occurs, ganglionitis and peripheral neuritis causes pain that is generally localized to the segmental distribution of the posterior spinal or cranial ganglia affected. Approximately 53% of cases involve the thoracic dermatomes, 20% the cervical region, 17% the trigeminal, and 11% the lumbosacral. Rarely, the virus may attack the geniculate ganglion, resulting in facial paralysis, hearing loss, vesicles in the ear, and pain. This combination of symptoms is called the Ramsay Hunt syndrome. Herpetic pain may be accompanied by flulike symptoms and generally progresses from a dull aching sensation to unilateral, segmental, bandlike dysesthesias and hyperpathia. Since the pain of herpes zoster usually precedes the eruption of skin lesions by 5–7 days, erroneous diagnosis of other painful conditions such as myocardial infarction, cholecystitis, appendicitis, and glaucoma may be made. Some pain specialists feel that in some immunocompetent hosts, when reactivation of the virus occurs, a rapid immune response may attenuate the natural course of the disease and the rash may not appear. This segmental pain without rash is called zoster sine herpete and is by necessity a diagnosis of exclusion.

In most patients, however, clinical diagnosis of shingles is readily made when the rash appears. Like chicken pox, the rash of herpes zoster appears in crops of macular lesions that progress to papules and then to vesicles. At this point, should the diagnosis of herpes zoster be in doubt, it can be confirmed by isolation of the virus from vesicular fluid (differentiating it from localized herpes simplex infection), or by Tzanck smear of the base of the vesicle, which will reveal multinucleated giant cells and eosinophilic intranuclear inclusions. As the disease progresses, the vesicles coalesce and crusting occurs. The area affected by the disease can be extremely painful and the pain tends to be exacerbated by any movement or contact with clothing, sheets, etc. As healing takes place, the crusts fall away leaving pink scars in the distribution of the rash, which gradually become hypopigmented and atrophic. As a general rule, the quicker all the vesicles in a given patient appear, the quicker the rash will heal. The clinical severity of the skin lesions of herpes zoster varies widely from patient to patient;

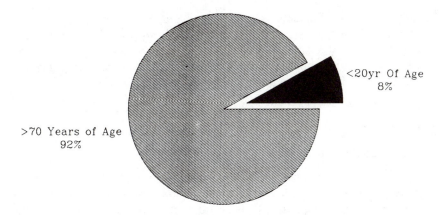

FIG 22–1.
Postherpetic neuralgia. Pain one year after acute attack.

however, the severity of skin lesions and scarring tends to increase with age, as does the duration of pain (Figure 22–1). In most patients, the hyperesthesia and pain generally resolve as the skin lesions heal. Unfortunately, pain may persist beyond lesion healing. This most common and feared complication of herpes zoster is called postherpetic neuralgia. Again, the elderly suffer this dreaded complication of pain and dysesthesia at a higher rate than the general population suffering from acute herpes zoster (Figure 22–2). The symptoms of postherpetic neuralgia can vary from a mild self-limited problem to a debilitating, constantly

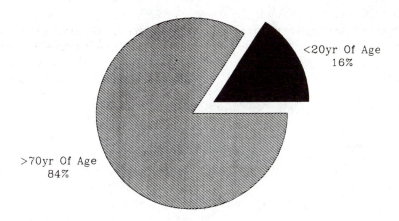

FIG 22–2.
Postherpetic neuralgia. Pain beyond lesion healing.

burning pain that is exacerbated by light touch, movement, anxiety, and/or temperature change. This unremitting pain may be so severe that it often completely devastates the patient's life and can lead to suicide. It is the desire to avoid this disastrous sequela to a usually benign self-limited disease that dictates all therapeutic efforts for the patient suffering from acute herpes zoster.

TREATMENT

Basic Considerations

The therapeutic challenge of the patient presenting with acute herpes zoster is twofold: 1) the relief of acute pain and symptoms, and 2) the prevention of complications, including postherpetic neuralgia. It is the consensus of most pain specialists that the earlier in the natural course of the disease treatment is initiated, the less likely the patient will develop postherpetic neuralgia. Furthermore, since the older patient is at highest risk of developing postherpetic neuralgia, early and aggressive treatment of this group of patients is mandatory.

Careful initial evaluation, including a thorough history and physical exam, is indicated to rule out occult malignancy or systemic disease that may be responsible for the patient's immunocompromised state and to allow early recognition of changes in clinical status that may presage the development of complications, including myelitis or dissemination of the disease.

Treatment Options

There are as many therapeutic approaches to the treatment of acute herpes zoster as there are clinicians treating the disease. Inherent problems in assessing the efficacy of a specific treatment centers around the fact that the disease has many different clinical expressions, and that the natural history of the disease, as well as the incidence of complications, including postherpetic neuralgia, cannot be reliably predicted in any single patient. Most studies looking at the efficacy of a proposed treatment have failed to take these problems into account and, therefore, only the most general conclusions may be reached.

Nerve Blocks

Sympathetic neural blockade appears to be the treatment of choice to relieve the symptoms of acute herpes zoster as well as to prevent the occurrence of postherpetic neuralgia. Sympathetic nerve block appears to achieve these goals by blocking the profound sympathetic stimulation that is a result of the viral inflammation of the nerve and ganglion. If untreated, this sympathetic hyperactivity can cause ischemia secondary to decreased blood flow of the intraneural capillary bed. If this ischemia is allowed to persist, endoneural edema forms, increasing endoneural pressure and causing a further reduction of endoneural blood flow with irreversible nerve damage. This damage appears to preferentially destroy large myelinated nerve fibers (which are metabolically more active), and spares small fibers. Noordenbos was first to report this phenomenon and correlate it with the pain symptomatology of herpes zoster. He postulated that large neural fibers modulate or inhibit entry of pain impulses into the central nervous system, while small fibers enhance entry of pain impulses into the central nervous system. Therefore, enhanced transmission of painful stimuli, as well as misinterpretation by the central nervous system of the non-noxious stimuli of the small fibers as pain would result if large fibers were preferentially destroyed. Interestingly, Noordenbos' theory of "fiber dissociation" predated Melzack and Wall's Gate Control Theory by 6 years. His theory may also explain the clinical finding of Winnie and others that sympathetic neural blockade is more efficacious when utilized early in the course of the disease by presumably interrupting the neural ischemia before irreversible large fiber changes occur.

For patients with acute herpes zoster involving the trigeminal, geniculate, cervical, and high thoracic regions (Fig 22–3), blockade of the stellate ganglion

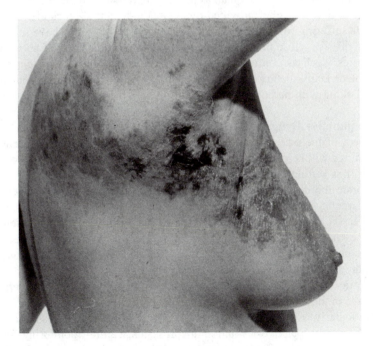

FIG 22–3.
Photograph of acute herpes zoster involving the chest wall.

with local anesthetic on a daily basis should be implemented immediately. For patients with acute herpes zoster involving the thoracic, lumbar, and sacral regions, daily epidural neural blockade with local anesthetic should be implemented immediately. As vesicular crusting occurs, the addition of steroids to the local anesthetic may decrease neural scarring and further decrease the incidence of postherpetic neuralgia. These sympathetic blocks should be continued aggressively until the patient is pain free and should be reimplemented at any return of pain. Failure to utilize sympathetic neural blockade immediately and aggressively, especially in the elderly, may sentence the patient to a lifetime of suffering.

Drug Therapy

Narcotic Analgesics.—Narcotic analgesics may be useful to relieve the aching pain that is often present during the acute stages of herpes zoster as sympathetic nerve blocks are being implemented. They are less effective in the relief of neuritic pain that is often present. Careful administration of potent, long-acting narcotic analgesics, such as oral morphine elixir or methadone on a time-contingent rather than on an as needed approach, may represent a beneficial adjunct to the pain relief provided by sympathetic neural blockade. Since many patients suffering from acute herpes zoster are elderly or may have severe multisystem disease, close monitoring for the potential side effects of potent narcotic analgesics, such as confusion or dizziness that may cause a patient to fall, is warranted. Daily dietary fiber supplementation and milk of magnesia should be started along with narcotic analgesics to prevent the side effect of constipation.

Adjunctive Drugs.—Antidepressants may be useful adjuncts in the initial treatment of the patient suffering from acute herpes zoster. On an acute basis, these drugs will help alleviate the significant sleep disturbance that is commonly seen in this setting. In addition, the antidepressants may be valuable in helping ameliorate the neuritic component of the pain that is not as effectively treated with narcotic analgesics. After several weeks of treatment, the antidepressants may exert a mood-elevating effect that may be desirable in some patients. Care must be taken to observe closely for central nervous system side effects in this patient population. These drugs may cause urinary retention and constipation that may be mistakenly attributed to herpes zoster myelitis.

Anticonvulsants may also be of value as an adjunct to sympathetic neural blockade in the management of pain secondary to acute herpes zoster. They may be particularly useful in relieving persistent paresthetic or dysesthetic pain. As with the narcotic analgesics and antidepressants, careful monitoring for central nervous system side effects is mandatory. If carbamazepine is used, rigid monitoring for hematologic parameters, especially in patients receiving chemotherapy or radiation therapy, is indicated. Phenytoin should not be used in patients with lymphoma, as the drug may induce a pseudolymphoma-like state that is difficult to distinguish from the actual disease.

Minor tranquilizers, such as diazepam and the like, have a limited place in the adjunctive therapy of pain of acute herpes zoster. Although anxiety is often present in this setting, these drugs may actually increase pain perception. In addition, the addiction potential and central nervous system side effects limit their usefulness. Anxiety may be treated pharmacologically with hydroxazine, or perhaps more appropriately with behavioral interventions such as monitored relaxation training and hypnosis.

Antiviral Agents.—A limited number of antiviral agents, including adenine arabinoside, acyclovir, interferon, and possibly adenosine monophosphate, have been shown to shorten the course of acute herpes zoster. Of these drugs, acyclovir and adenosine monophosphate appear to have the least side effects. To date, there has been no convincing evidence that the drugs prevent the occurrence of postherpetic neuralgia. They are probably useful in attentuating the disease in immunosuppressed patients. Careful monitoring for side effects is mandatory with the use of these relatively toxic drugs.

In the past, corticosteroids have been advocated as an adjunct in the treatment of acute herpes zoster. Proponents of this approach cite more rapid healing and a decreased incidence of postherpetic neuralgia. Other studies have been unable to confirm these findings. Local infiltration of affected skin areas with corticosteroid, with or without local anesthetic, may be of value as an adjunct to sympathetic neural blockade in decreasing localized areas of pain not amenable to other treatment modalities. Some authors feel that corticosteroids may increase the risk of dissemination in immunosuppressed patients if used prior to vesicular crusting. Our experience has not confirmed this.

ADJUNCTIVE TREATMENTS

Local application of ice packs to the lesions of acute herpes zoster may provide relief in some patients. Application of heat will increase pain in most patients, presumably due to increased conduction of small fibers, but heat is beneficial in an occasional patient, and may be worth a try if application of cold is ineffective. Transcutaneous nerve stimulation and vibration may also be effective in a limited number of patients. The favorable risk to benefit ratio of all of the above modalities makes them a reasonable alternative for patients who cannot or will not undergo sympathetic neural blockade.

Topical application of aluminum sulfate as a tepid soak provides an excellent drying of the crusting and weeping lesions of acute herpes zoster, and most patients find these soaks quite soothing. Zinc oxide ointment may also be used for protection, especially during the healing phase when temperature sensitivity is a problem. Disposable diapers can be used as an absorbent padding to protect healing lesions from contact with clothing and sheets.

COMPLICATIONS

In most patients, acute herpes zoster is a self-limited disease. However, in the elderly and the immunosuppressed, complications may occur. Cutaneous and visceral dissemination may range from a mild rash resembling chicken pox to a life-threatening, overwhelming infection in those already suffering from severe multisystem disease. Myelitis may cause bowel, bladder, and lower extremity paresis. Ocular complications from trigeminal nerve involvement range from severe photophobia to keratitis with loss of sight. As mentioned above, postherpetic neuralgia occurs more frequently and with greater severity in these elderly and immunosuppressed patients.

CONCLUSION

In view of the devastating effects of inadequately treated acute herpes zoster on patients, their family, and society in terms of cost and lost productivity, it is incumbent for all health care professionals to initiate immediate and aggressive treatment in the form of sympathetic neural blockade, coupled with adjunctive treatments.

BIBLIOGRAPHY

Mayne GE, Brown M, Arnold P, et al: Pain of herpes zoster and postherpetic neuralgia, in Raj P (ed): *Practical Management of Pain*. Chicago, Year Book Medical Publishers, 1986; pp 345–361.

Lilley JP, Su WP, Wang JK: Sensory and sympathetic nerve blocks for postherpetic neuralgia. *Reg Anaesth* 1986; 11:165–167.

Lobato RD, Madrid JL: Clinical and physiopathological mechanisms of postherpetic pain. *Clin J Pain* 1986; 2:253–257.

Reuler JB, Chang M: Herpes zoster: Epidemiology, clinical features and management. *South Med J* 1984; 77:1149–1156.

Winnie AP: Acute herpes zoster, in Dannemiller Pain Management Review Course Proceedings. San Antonio, Dannemiller Foundation, 1988, pp 2c–30c.

Rosner HL, Yerby JT, Brand L: Herpes zoster—Can we change the outcome? *J Pain Sympt Mgmt* 1986; 1:168–170.

23

Fibrositis (Fibromyalgia) Syndrome Associated With Rheumatoid Arthritis and Tuberculosis

I. Jon Russell, M.D., Ph.D.

In September, 1970, a 49-year-old Latin American female nonsmoker presented with a 3-month history of right upper chest discomfort and intermittent productive cough. She also complained of arthralgias, but no synovitis or soft tissue tenderness was found. Her antinuclear antibody (ANA), rheumatoid factor (RF), and erythrocyte sedimentation rate (ESR) were normal, but she had a positive PPD and an obstructive defect on pulmonary function testing. A reticular/nodular infiltrate was seen on her chest x-ray. Diagnoses included bronchiectasis, positive PPD, arthralgias. Courses of erythromycin and penicillin were prescribed. In February of 1978 she presented with morning stiffness and joint pain despite 3900 mg of aspirin/day. Synovitis was found at the proximal interphalangeal (PIP), and metacarpophalangeal (MCP) joints, wrists, elbows, and knees. Her ANA was still negative, RF was positive (1:5120), and ESR was 80 mm/hr. Her chest x-ray showed fibrosis; hand x-rays were unremarkable. Diagnoses included rheumatoid arthritis (RA), rheumatoid lung, positive PPD. NSAIDs and physical therapy were prescribed. In July of 1978 her symptoms changed. The musculoskeletal pain was more severe. Morning stiffness lasted more than 4 hours. She exhibited marked tenderness at multiple soft tissue sites typical of fibrositis, but had no articular synovitis. The ESR was 80–100 mm/hr. Hyperglycemia (up to 300 mg/dL) required insulin. Control delayed-type hypersensitivity skin tests and PPD were negative, indicating anergy. After eight unsuccessful attempts, one sputum sample was fluorochrome and culture positive for *Mycobacterium tuberculosis*. Diagnoses: included fibrositis/fibromyalgia syndrome (FS), active tu-

berculosis, inactive RA, adult onset diabetes mellitus (AODM). Isoniazid, etham-
butol, and rifampin were prescribed. In November of 1979, after several pain-free
months, she again developed joint pain and morning stiffness lasting more than 2
hours. She had definite synovitis in many joints, but the previous soft tissue tenderness to palpation was gone. Hand x-rays showed erosions at the MCP joints, ESR
was 50 mm/hr., and PPD again was positive. Diagnoses included RA, AODM,
treated tuberculosis, resolved FS. Hydroxychloroquine and myochrysine were prescribed.

DISCUSSION

It seems apparent from this patient's course that the clinical problem changed
once or twice along the way. It can be viewed as having four phases. In the
first phase, she presented repeatedly over a 2-year period because of her respiratory symptoms, but was noted to also have arthralgias of unknown etiology.
Careful examination by several physicians during that time failed to disclose any
synovitis.

In the second phase, her joint symptoms progressed until they met 7 of the
11 established criteria for classical rheumatoid arthritis.[1] Namely, she had morning stiffness, pain on joint motion, swelling in at least one joint, swelling in at
least one other joint, symmetry of the joint swelling, a positive RF, and a synovial
effusion with more than 2,000 white cells per cubic millimeter, all persisting
for approximately 3 months and documented by her physician.

She then entered a 1-year long third phase characterized by active FS associated with active tuberculosis and no apparent arthritis. She complained bit-
terly of unbearable pain in her neck, back, chest, shoulders, arms, and legs.
The diagnosis of fibrositis was based on tenderness to palpation at sites around
the body.[2] The tender point index (TPI) has been used to quantify the severity
of tenderness at each of 18 sites, as shown in Table 23–1. Normal persons rarely
exhibit a TPI >4, while this patient had a TPI of 18.

Traditionally, this patient would have been given diagnosis of *secondary*
fibrositis syndrome because she had a high titer rheumatoid factor and an elevated
sedimentation rate, suggesting an association with rheumatoid arthritis.[4] Current
terminology would label it ''fibrositis/fibromyalgia syndrome associated with
tuberculosis and rheumatoid arthritis.''

This patient had a dramatic response to a soft tissue injection of corticosteroid, which raised the possibility that her symptoms might benefit from low-
dose oral corticosteroid therapy. In addition, as the lung disease progressed, it
became increasingly important that active tuberculosis be excluded as a pertinent
clinical diagnosis. That possibility was investigated by repeating the PPD and
culturing the sputum. The finding of active tuberculosis was not surprising,
considering the abnormal chest x-ray and the endemic nature of that disease. On

TABLE 23–1.
Tender Point Index (TPI)*

A. Points of Tenderness in Fibrositis/Fibromyalgia Syndrome

Number	Tender Point
1, 2	Occiput: at the suboccipital muscle insertions
3, 4	Low cervical: at the anterior aspects of the intertransverse spaces at C5–7
5, 6	Trapezius: at the midpoint of the upper border
7, 8	Supraspinatus: at origins, above the scapula spine near the medial border
9, 10	2nd rib: at the second costochondral junctions, just lateral to the junctions on upper surfaces
11, 12	Lateral epicondyle: 2 cm distal to the epicondyles
13, 14	Gluteal: in upper outer quadrants of buttocks in anterior fold of muscle
15, 16	Greater trochanter: posterior to the trochanteric prominence
17, 18	Knees: at the medial fat pad proximal to the joint line

B. Severity Scale and Tender Point Index (TPI)

Severity	Patient Response to Pressure (4 kg)
0	No reported tenderness
1+	Tenderness reported verbally, but la Belle indeference, no physical response
2+	Tenderness reported plus an objective physical response (wince, withdrawal)
3+	Tenderness emphatically reported plus an exaggerated, dramatic physical response (wince, jerk, withdrawal)
4+	Untouchable area. The anticipated pain is so bad that the patient refuses to allow the expected palpation

*TPI = Sum of Individual Severities at 18 points.

the other hand, that diagnosis was not seriously considered until she became anergic, because her physicians had been so convinced that her pulmonary problem was rheumatoid lung.

A course of treatment for the tuberculosis seemed to initiate the fourth phase of this patient's illness, characterized by resolution of the FS, reconstitution of her delayed-type hypersensitivity reaction to tuberculin antigen, and the return of active rheumatoid arthritis.

These findings suggest the following hypothetical scenario. The patient was exposed to *Mycobacterium tuberculosis* in the distant past and was probably genetically predisposed to develop rheumatoid arthritis. The combination of the two collaborated to cause a fairly rapid progression of bronchiolitis, as can occur with rheumatoid arthritis patients who smoke. Then, for reasons unknown, the patient's immune response became sufficiently compromised that the tuberculosis underwent a transition from quiescent to active disease.

In the face of active tuberculosis, her cell-mediated immunity was sufficiently suppressed that she no longer exhibited the cell-mediated synovitis of rheumatoid arthritis or delay-type hypersensitivity. Her high titer rheumatoid factor could have resulted either from the chronic tuberculosis process or from the seropositive rheumatoid arthritis. The high ESR seen during the third phase of her disease was most likely due to the tuberculous infection. It can also be elevated in patients with rheumatoid arthritis, but that would be unusual at a time when the arthritis was so quiescent.[5]

There is no apparent explanation for her development of diabetes mellitus during this phase of her disease, except that diabetes is very common in middle-aged Hispanic individuals. There was also considerable physiologic stress from the tuberculous infection, which might unmask a latent tendency to diabetes.

Finally, as her tuberculosis was treated with antibiotics, it would appear that her immune system was reconstituted sufficiently to allow articular inflammation. As a result, she exhibited a recurrence of her polyarticular synovitis.

There is little or no information in the literature to help the clinician understand the so-called "secondary fibrositis syndrome." Primary fibrositis syndrome has now been studied extensively, and there is a growing awareness of its frequency, its diagnostic characteristics, and its management. There is even evidence for immunologic and metabolic contributors to its pathogenesis.[6, 7] In contrast, secondary fibrositis has been almost ignored since the time of Dr. Philip Hench, who used the term "fibrositis" to describe aching stiffness associated with many inflammatory disorders.[8]

Conventional wisdom says that fibrositis seen in association with other diseases is caused by the underlying condition. There is only circumstantial evidence to support that hypothesis. "Associated with" doesn't assume a pathogenic mechanism, so it is a more correct designation than "secondary." On the other hand, the term "secondary fibrositis" is entrenched and is easier to say than "fibrositis associated with rheumatoid arthritis," so the traditional terminology may be here to stay.

Table 23–2 shows a list of conditions commonly associated with FS. It is adapted from Beetham's 1979 review[4] in which he itemized 31 disorders under four major headings: rheumatic diseases, chronic infections, malignant diseases, and endocrine disorders. The frequency with which fibrositis is associated with these disorders is quite variable. The table also shows a profile of relatively inexpensive tests that can be used to screen for associated disorders in patients who first meet the diagnostic criteria for FS.

A retrospective review of all new patients examined in the rheumatology practice at the University of Texas at San Antonio from 1980–1982 disclosed that 17.5% were given the diagnosis of fibrositis syndrome. Two-thirds of those patients (N = 49) had primary FS, while one-third (26) had FS associated with another medical condition, based on Beetham's nomenclature. The most common associated disorders were rheumatoid arthritis (N = 8), systemic lupus erythematosus (N = 8), and hypothyroidism (N = 6). Somewhat less frequent was tuberculosis (N = 2). The remainder was composed of miscellaneous rheumatic conditions.

A study by Dr. Fred Wolfe showed a somewhat different distribution of primary and secondary FS.[9] Fibrositis associated with rheumatoid arthritis was substantially more common than primary FS in his practice. Those differences are not likely due to differences in criteria for the diagnosis of FS because a three-center study showed that the characteristics of FS in San Antonio were not different from those of patients in Wichita or Los Angeles.[10] A more important factor may have been the aggressiveness with which the diagnosis of FS was sought in patients with rheumatoid arthritis. It is likely that FS occurring in association with other disorders is underreported.

Dr. Wolfe also made the observation that patients with rheumatoid arthritis who have associated fibrositis syndrome seem to experience the most severe pain and have the most dramatic complaints about their disease.[11] That observation was indirectly supported by the results of a multicenter rheumatoid arthritis study,[12] which showed that two groups of patients could be identified by canonical analysis. One group had a lot of synovitis without much pain, while the second group had less synovitis, but much more pain.

The clinical features of FS associated with other disorders are essentially those of primary FS . There will be a history of diffuse musculoskeletal pain, and localized tenderness will be present in discrete sites around the body at the so-called tender points. A graphic description of fibrositis pain likens it to the simultaneous sensation of the soreness from yesterday's excessive exertion coupled with a bad sunburn.

The fibrositic symptoms in patients with rheumatoid arthritis seem to have

TABLE 23–2.

Medical Illnesses Associated with Fibrositis Syndrome and Tests That are Useful in Screening for Them

	Tests
Rheumatic disease	
SLE	ANA + ESR
RA (rheumatoid arthritis)	RF + ESR
Polymyositis	CPK
Chronic infections	
TB	PPD + ESR
Chronic syphilis	VDR
SBE (subacute bacterial endocarditis)	Culture + ESR
Endocrine disorders	
Hypothyroidism	T_4 + TSH

Adapted from Beetham WP Jr: *Med Clin North Am* 1979; 63:433.

no clear temporal relationship to the activity of the arthritic disease. When FS occurs with systemic lupus erythematosus, the symptoms tend to be most prominent early in the course of the lupus, often before it can be diagnosed. Interestingly, the FS symptoms tend to recur when the lupus is entering remission. Hypothyroidism is often noted among patients with FS, but a pathologic relationship has not been established. If hypothyroidism were the cause of the FS symptoms, one would expect them to remit with thyroid replacement to the euthyroid state. In the author's experience, only a partial remission of the FS symptoms occurs with thyroid replacement therapy.

An interesting hypothesis to explain the association of musculoskeletal pain with insomnia relates to the regulation of structural protein synthesis.[13] If one function of deep, slow-wave (stage 3 and 4 non-REM) sleep is to repair musculoskeletal tissues injured in the process of normal daily activity and if that stage of sleep is persistently lacking, the failure to maintain those tissues adequately might manifest itself in the form of somatic discomfort.

Any theory that proposes to unify the rather disconnected features of FS must now also explain the rather surprising findings of immunoglobulin deposits in the skin, abnormalities in T-cell subpopulations,[14] and a decrease in natural killer cell activity.[15] One such theory is based on a deficiency of serotonin.[16] It is appealing because serotonin functions as a chemical neurotransmitter for the regulation of deep sleep and central perception of pain. A deficiency of serotonin within the internuncial space would theoretically result in nonrestorative sleep and an exaggerated perception of somatic stimuli. Indeed, recent findings indicate a lower than normal level of serotonin in the sera of FS patients, which is associated with an increased number of platelet membrane receptors for serotonin. There is still much to be learned about this hypothesis.

Some physicians believe that FS patients develop their symptoms due to intolerable ambient stress or because they allow an inappropriate somatic response to stressful stimuli. In fact, one study[17] demonstrated greater frequencies of depression and anxiety in patients with fibrositis syndrome than in rheumatoid arthritis, but other authors[18, 19] have failed to confirm those findings.

The serotonin-related hypothesis gains support from the observed clinical benefit with two different tricyclic drugs (amitriptyline, cyclobenzaprine), and with one benzodiazepine (alprazolam).[16] The tricyclic antidepressants increase internuncial serotonin by blocking the re-uptake of secreted serotonin. The mechanisms responsible for the effects of alprazolam are not known, but it has been reported to inhibit the function of platelets, which store serotonin.

MANAGEMENT

Until there is a more complete understanding of the physiologic processes involved in FS, it appears that a multidimensional therapeutic program is best. Such a program should involve patient education, medication for fibrositis, medication for any associated condition, physical therapy, injection therapy, and regular follow-up.

Patients with FS experience a considerable amount of pain and are understandably frustrated by their inability to sleep normally. The tendency among physicians not well informed about this disorder is to aggressively search for some occult process like a malignancy. Uncertainty on the part of the physician increases the concern of the patient for her own welfare. For example, chest pain in a fibrositis patient is more likely to emanate from the chest wall than from ischemic myocardium. Repeated admissions to the CCU, or a technically impressive demonstration of normal coronary arteries by angiography are inappropriately aggressive measures for such patients and could be avoided by an astute examination.

Fibrositis patients should be informed regarding the soft tissue nature of their disorder, which distinguishes it from arthritis. In doing so, phrases such as "not deforming like arthritis," and "a benign condition," are obviously inappropriate for a patient who has rheumatoid arthritis associated with the FS. Another phrase, "You will just have to live with it," is not very encouraging or supportive. An important message to get across is that the physician is regularly updated about the condition, that he/she is sympathetic with the patient's problem, and will do everything consistent with good medical practice to help. These reassurances may be of value in helping the patient better adapt to troublesome somatic symptoms.

Fibrositis patients should be given an analgesic medication. Most clinicians believe that nonsteroidal anti-inflammatory drugs reduce the severity of the somatic pain. The propionic acid derivatives (ibuprofen, 800 mg three times daily; naproxen, 500 mg twice daily; ketoprofen, 75 mg three times daily) have been most useful. It appears from two clinical studies[20, 21] that naproxen or ibuprofen exert synergistic affects when administered with a sedative hypnotic drug (amitriptyline, 10–50 mg at bedtime, or alprazolam, 0.5–1.5 mg at bedtime, respectively).

Of course, attention should be given to specific treatment of any condition associated with FS. It is beyond the scope of this chapter to discuss in detail the treatment of connective tissue diseases, chronic infections, malignancies, and endocrine disorders, but the treatments routinely utilized to manage those syndromes should be undertaken where applicable.

Physical therapy can be very helpful, but the expense incurred by regular sessions with a therapist tend to be prohibitive. For that reason, it is suggested that a short course of physical therapy be given as a form of patient education, rather than seeing it as definitive and complete therapy. In the author's practice, a therapeutic program was designed and officially dubbed the "fibrositis protocol.'' That allows the physician to order what is needed on a routine basis with a minimum of effort. The same thing could be accomplished by printing up physical therapy orders for FS that become the prescription for the therapist.

The ''fibrositis protocol'' includes heat administered by hydrocollator packs to the back, neck, and shoulders for 30 minutes, followed by deep sedative massage for about 10 minutes. The massage is painful at first, but becomes progressively less uncomfortable with time, as the therapist kneads connective tissues more deeply. The physical therapy program is continued on a two- or three-session per week basis for 3 weeks. The patient will then be instructed to use a hot bath or shower at home, or even to use an inexpensive infrared lamp about 24 in. above the skin, as substitutes for the professional heat device. The massage can, of course, be provided at home by a spouse.

Each therapy session involves some education by the therapist regarding posture principles, body mechanics, and a gradually progressive aerobic isotonic exercise program, in which the ultimate goal is to regularly walk at least 1 mile per day. It is difficult to know exactly how much long-term benefit there is to this program, since it has not been formally tested in a controlled study. Some support for it is derived from a study by Dr. McCain, who demonstrated significantly more benefit from an aerobic exercise program than from stretching exercises.[22] Interestingly, it has been shown[23] that vigorous exercise (running 6 miles/day) will prevent experimental interference with deep sleep and thus, might be of value in correcting the sleep abnormality.

Injection of an anesthetic agent and/or corticosteroids into the area of a tender point can be symptomatically helpful but should be resorted to only occasionally.

The author uses injection to ''break the cycle'' when other more conservative therapies fall short. Triamcinolone (Aristospan) is diluted to 5 mg/mL in 1% lidocaine for injection around one of the following structures: the greater occipital nerve near its foramen, the biceps tendon, a costochrondral junction, a trochanteric bursae, a pes anserine bursae, rarely a lateral epicondyle at the elbow, and even less frequently, a tender point in a muscle. The amount of suspension injected at each of these sites will vary depending on the size of the soft tissue structure. The clinician should be aware that a large volume of injected fluid dissects tissue planes and can induce its own unique sequelae, including hematoma formation. Therefore, a strategically placed depot of medication may be more effective than a large volume splayed around blindly in the soft tissue.

The author has used local injection more as a tide-over intervention or diagnostic test than as definitive therapy. For example, complete relief from disabling chest pain achieved by an injection in the area of costochondral junction can do a lot toward relieving a patient's anxiety about heart disease. It is recommended that soft tissue sites not be repeatedly injected. There is evidence[24] that primary fibrositis syndrome is not benefited by oral corticosteroid therapy.

Besides, repeated soft tissue injections are likely to depress the pituitary adrenal axis, risking additional side effects and adrenal insufficiency.

Finally, a most important aspect of treating fibrositis syndrome is a psychophysiological one regarding the relationship of a patient and physician. A realistic view of the state of the art in 1990 is that we know very little about how to manage FS.

Dr. T.F. Main[25] quips that, "The sufferer who frustrates a keen therapist by failing to improve is always in danger of meeting primitive human behavior disguised as treatment." Physicians treating a chronic condition of unknown etiology can become frustrated when the patient does not respond favorably to honest efforts in her behalf. On the other hand, one would not expect patients with diabetes mellitus to improve if they were given iron in place of insulin. Our ignorance regarding the ideal treatment for FS might understandably lead to therapeutic failures, but we need to realize that it isn't necessarily the patient's fault. The physician's task is to provide patients with the best therapies available, in an environment of hopeful optimism. The physician and patient must both realize and discuss the fact that therapeutic options are still limited and imperfect.

The physician must resist his/her natural inclination to make some change in therapy if the current regimen has not been dramatically effective. Rather, it seems that persistence with therapy and tincture of time are useful allies. Dr. Wayne Katon (personal communication) recommends that the physician tabulate the frequency of visits the patient has made to any health care provider within the last 12 months, and schedule appointments for the patient slightly more frequently than that. This tends to reassure the patient that the physician is there to help, and that the patient will not be rejected because of a less than optimal outcome.

Some rheumatologists have developed expertise in caring for fibrositis syndrome. Some clinical psychologists or psychiatrists have skills, like Jacobsonian relaxation therapy, which aid in the patient's adaptation to musculoskeletal pain. Selective referral for such assistance may be useful adjuncts to other interventions by the primary care physician.

REFERENCES

1. Ropes MW, Bennett GA, Caleb S, et al: Revision of diagnostic criteria for rheumatoid arthritis. *Bull Rheum Dis* 1958; 9:175–176.
2. Wolfe F, Smythe HA, Yunus MB, et al: Criteria for fibromyalgia. *Arthritis Rheum* 1989; 32:S47.
3. Russell IJ, Vipraio GA, Morgan WW, et al: Is there a metabolic basis for the fibrositis syndrome? *Am J Med* 1986; 81:50.
4. Beetham WP Jr: Diagnosis and management of fibrositis syndrome and psychogenic rheumatism. *Med Clin North Am* 1979; 63:433.

5. Pinals RS, et al: Preliminary criteria for clinical remission in rheumatoid arthritis. *Arthritis Rheum* 1981; 24:1308–1315.
6. Russell IJ, Vipraio GA, Michalek J, et al: Abnormal T cell subpopulations in fibrositis syndrome. *Arthritis Rheum* 1988; 31:S98.
7. Russell IJ, Bowden CL, Michalek J, et al: Imipramine receptor density on platelets of patients with fibrositis syndrome: Correlation with disease severity and response to therapy. *Arthritis Rheum* 1988; 30:S63.
8. Hench PS: Differentiation between "psychogenic rheumatism" and true rheumatic disease. *Postgrad Med,* 1946, p 460.
9. Wolfe F, Cathey MA: Prevalence of primary and secondary fibrositis. *J Rheumatol* 1983; 10:965–968.
10. Wolfe F, Hawley DJ, Cathey MA, et al: Fibrositis: Symptom frequency and criteria for diagnosis. An evaluation of 291 rheumatic disease patients and 58 normal individuals. *J Rheumatol* 1985; 12:1159–1163.
11. Wolfe F, Cathey MA, Kleinheksel SM: Fibrositis (fibromyalgia) in rheumatoid arthritis. *J Rheumatol* 1984; 11:814–818.
12. Bombardier C, Ware J, Russell IJ, et al: Auranofin therapy and quality of life in patients with rheumatoid arthritis: Results of a multicenter trial. *Am J Med* 1986; 81:565.
13. Adam K: Sleep as a restorative process and a theory to explain why. *Prog Brain Res* 1980; 53:289–305.
14. Caro XJ, Wolfe F, Johnston WH, et al: A controlled and blinded study of immunoreactant deposition at the dermal-epidermal junction of patients with primary fibrositis syndrome. *J Rheumatol* 1986; 13:1086.
15. Russell IJ, Vipraio GA, Tovar Z, et al: Abnormal natural killer cell activity in fibrositis syndrome is responsive in vitro to IL-2. *Arthritis Rheum* 1988; 31:S24.
16. Russell IJ: Neurohormonal aspects of fibromyalgia syndrome. *Rheumatic Dis Clin North Am* 1989; 15:149–168.
17. Hudson JI, Hudson MS, Pliner LF, et al: Fibromyalgia and major affective disorder: A controlled phenomenology and family history study. *Am J Psychiatry* 1985; 142:441–446.
18. Clark S, Campbell SM, Forehand ME, et al: Clinical characteristics of fibrositis: II. A "blinded," controlled study using standard psychological tests. *Arthritis Rheum* 1985; 28:132–137.
19. Ahles TA, Yunus MB, Riley SD, et al: Psychological factors associated with primary fibromyalgia syndrome. *Arthritis Rheum* 1984; 27:1101–1106.
20. Goldenberg DL, Felson DT, Dinerman H: A randomized, controlled trial of amitriptyline and naproxen in the treatment of patients with fibromyalgia. *Arthritis Rheum* 1986; 29:1371.
21. Russell IJ, Fletcher EM, Michalek JE, et al: Efficacy and safety of ibuprofen and alprazolam in the treatment of primary fibromyalgia/fibrositis syndrome: A double-blind, placebo-controlled study. Unpublished data, 1989.
22. McCain GA: Role of physical fitness training in the fibrositis/fibromyalgia syndrome. *Am J Med* 1986; 81:73–77.
23. Moldofsky H. Scarisbrick P: Induction of neurasthenic musculoskeletal pain syndrome by selective sleep stage deprivation. *Psychosomatic Med* 1976; 38:35–44.

24. Clark S, Tindall E, Bennett RM: A double blind crossover trial of prednisone versus placebo in the treatment of fibrositis. *J Rheumatol* 1985; 12:980.

25. Main TF: The ailment. *Br J Med Psychol* 1957; 30:129.

PART IV

Abdominal Pain

24

Chronic Relapsing Pancreatitis

Theresa Ferrer-Brechner, M.D.

A 45-year-old white woman, known to have chronic relapsing pancreatitis because of severe epigastric pain, nausea, and vomiting, was admitted to the hospital. This was her third admission in the past month because of recurrent pain, and each episode has been characterized by significant increases in serum amylase levels. She has a positive history of heavy alcohol intake up to 3 months ago. She had lost 20 lb in the past month. Her problem started 5 years before this admission, and she has undergone numerous endoscopic pancreatic drainage and open pancreatic cyst drainage procedures, but her pain episodes have not stopped. She has now been admitted with the possibility of total pancreatectomy if medical treatment fails. Her pain has been poorly controlled with 200 mg meperidine (Demerol) given intramuscularly every 3–4 hours as needed.

DISCUSSION

The management of pain from recurrent acute pancreatitis is controversial and treatment recommendations vary from an accommodation of waiting for the acute episode to "burn out" to the most extreme measure, i.e., total pancreatectomy. In treating acute pancreatitis, there are three goals: (1) to relieve pain; (2) to treat complications; and (3) to preserve pancreatic function as much as possible. One important factor in planning the treatment of recurrent pancreatitis is the question of whether the attacks are produced by alcohol intake.

If the patient has alcohol-induced pancreatitis, it is extremely important to

165

tie the physical treatment of recurrent pancreatitis to an alcohol rehabilitation program. A patient has to agree that the alcohol rehabilitation counselor will establish communications with the pain program and that evidence of sobriety will be monitored.

There are non-alcohol-induced causes of pancreatitis; it can be idiopathic, or drug induced, or result from blunt trauma, obstruction of pancreatobiliary drainage, or sepsis. The non-alcohol induced variety is commonly seen in children.[1] Whatever the cause of acute pancreatitis, the primary aim during an acute episode is to immediately alleviate pain and then make definitive plans to develop a longer-range strategic plan for pain control. This plan should include management of narcotic medications during and between episodes of acute exacerbations, a decision about whether neuroablative procedures are indicated, and the establishment of contingency plans when early signs of acute episodes occur.

Pain management of acute pancreatitis includes modalities that are presently used for acute postoperative pain management: pain-controlled analgesia (PCA),[2] epidural/intrathecal opiate analgesia (EOA), or epidural local anesthetic analgesia (ELAA). The choice of technique is dependent on the sophistication of the physician treating the patient. PCA is a modality in which the intravenous narcotic is self-administered through a programmable infusion device that administers pre-set bolus doses when the patient pushes a button. PCA has a proven advantage over intramuscular administration of narcotics in patients with moderate to severe pain in that effective analgesia can be achieved with a 40% lower 24-hour dose of narcotic and lower incidence of side effects.[3] Various types of computerized infusion devices are now commercially available, offering options of continuous infusion rates at indicated times of day and lockout intervals. PCA is extremely effective in patients who have severe pain with acute pancreatitis, who otherwise are treated with intramuscular injection of narcotics. It affords a more stable plasma narcotic level, provides control to the patient of analgesic requirement, individualizes narcotic requirement, and provides more free time to presently overburdened nursing personnel.

In 10 patients suffering from acute pancreatitis with severe pain who were referred to our service, 9 patients had excellent steady pain relief within 2–3 hours of initiation of PCA. The duration of PCA use was dependent on how long the patient was unable to take oral medications (range, 5 days to 6 weeks). When the patients were taking oral liquids, they were switched to oral analgesics such as oxycodone/aspirin or oxycodone/acetaminophen on a time-contingent basis. The PCA was kept beside the patient for 24 hours and if narcotic requirement decreased at least 50%, PCA was discontinued.

Another method of pain control for severe acute pancreatitis is the use of continuous epidural analgesia, either with an opioid or local anesthetic, or a combination of both. The disadvantage of this technique is that it requires the expertise of anesthesiologists who have pain management experience and nursing personnel who understand proper monitoring of patients with possible delayed respiratory depression. After the epidural catheter is placed at the lower thoracic area (T10–12), intermittent injections of dilute local anesthetic (6–10 ml of 0.125% bupivicaine, 0.5 lidocaine) can be injected to give an immediate segmental analgesia. This can be followed by bolus injections of morphine, 3–5 mg in 5–10 mL normal saline, or by continuous infusion of combined narcotic and local anesthetic solution.[4] The possible occurrence of delayed respiratory depression with epidurally administered opiate, especially in narcotically naive patients, should never be underestimated. Training of nurses regarding hourly monitoring of sedation level and respiratory rate is of utmost importance to detect early development of respiratory depression due to cephalad migration of the opiate to the midbrain 8–10 hours after injection in the lumbar or thoracic region.[5] Other common side effects of epidural opiate analgesia are pruritus, nausea, and urinary retention. All of these side effects have been successfully reversed with the use of the opiate antagonist naloxone in low doses (0.2–0.4 mg given IV).

After the acute episode of pancreatitis is over, the question arises as to whether appropriate definitive treatments for pain control are indicated, besides a total pancreatectomy. Disruption of nerve supply to the pancreas by surgical or chemical approach have been described to produce satisfactory pain control. However, patient selection criteria need to be better defined. Denervation should be considered in patients with frequent recurrent disabling abdominal pain (more than 2 episodes per month) resulting in rapid weight loss; each episode should be documented with increases in pancreatic enzyme levels. In this patient, chemical denervation should be tried before a total pancreatectomy is considered.

Chemical denervation of the nerve supply to the pancreas can be achieved by injection of 50%–70% alcohol into the celiac plexus. The technique of celiac plexus block for pancreatitis has been described previously.[6] Essentially, the needles are placed anterior to the T12–L1 vertebral bodies, with the point of the needle on the right side being higher than the left. After negative aspiration, a small amount of contrast material can be injected to demonstrate spread of the solution. The procedure can be done as a two-step process. The first procedure is done with 40–50 mL of dilute local anesthetic (0.25% bupivicaine or 0.5% lidocaine), prognosticating the effect of the ''permanent'' block with alcohol. During the time that the block is in effect, indices for pain and nausea can be measured semiquantitatively with the use of visual analogue scales. If there is 75% pain relief, the block can be repeated with the use of 50%–70% alcohol. Celiac plexus block has been used to alleviate pain from pancreatic cancer and pancreatitis. Efficacy is well demonstrated with pancreatic cancer, but is more questionable in patients with pancreatitis because of recurrence of pain within 6 months. In a study of 16 patients with disabling pain from pancreatitis, 13 patients had substantial reduction of pain within two weeks of nerve block.[7] Ten of the 16 patients showed significant long-term improvement. Repeat block was done in 5 of the 6 remaining patients with continuing pain. Two patients who did not respond to the block eventually underwent pancreatic resection and subsequently died. This demonstrates that celiac plexus block has a place in the management of recurrent pancreatic pain and should be considered before total pancreatectomy.

The prognosis for pancreatic surgery is affected by several factors. Continued alcohol intake indicated shorter survival time than that in patients with nonalcoholic pancreatitis.[8] This emphasizes the importance of ensuring the maintenance of sobriety in the patient with alcohol-induced pancreatitis. Constant contact with the patient's alcohol rehabilitation counselor is of utmost importance. Operations performed on the basis of gross pathology were effective in relieving pain. Ductal drainage has been found helpful in patients with diffusely dilated ducts and has a lower mortality and preservation of endocrine function.[9]

In this patient, intramuscular meperidine (Demerol) was stopped and patient-controlled analgesia was immediately instituted with meperidine (10 mg bolus dose on demand and 10 mg/hr continuous infusion at night in addition to availability of bolus dose). The patient immediately had a marked decrease in pain (90%–20% on pain visual analogue scale) within two hours of PCA initiation. She was maintained on the PCA until the sixth hospital day, when she was able to take oral medications. At that time, she was switched to oral oxycodone and acetaminophen (Percocet), 2 tablets every 4 hours, around the clock. The PCA device was left at the patient's bedside. The next day, her total PCA use was decreased more than 50% and, thereafter, was discontinued. She was sent home shortly. However, she had recurrent episodes for the next two months. Although the pain was controlled with the PCA during her hospitalizations, the patient's weight dropped from 135 to 98 lb. It was then decided that a trial of celiac

TABLE 24–1.

Reported Techniques for the Management of Pain From Recurrent Pancreatitis

I. Management of acute episodes.
  A. Patient controlled analgesia (PCA).
  B. Epidural opiates.
  C. Epidural local anesthetic.
  D. Suppression of pancreatic secretion (calcitonin).
II. Management of recurrent episodes.
  A. Surgical techniques.
    1. Endoscopic cystenterostomy.
    2. Drainage of pancreatic pseudocysts.
    3. Bypass procedures (bilioenteral, duodenojejunostomy).
    4. Total pancreatectomy.
  B. Anesthetic procedures: celiac plexus block.

plexus block with local anesthetic block be done, which afforded complete pain relief. The block was repeated with 70% alcohol, which provided 8 pain-free months and a 25-lb weight gain. The patient also joined the Alcoholics Anonymous program to maintain sobriety.

REFERENCES

1. Synn AV, Mulvihill SJ, Fonkalsrud EW: Surgical management of pancreatitis in childhood. *J Pediatr Surg* 1987; 22:628–632.
2. Ready LB, et al: Development of an anesthesiology based postoperative pain management service. *Anesthesiology* 1988; 68:100–106.
3. Bennett RL, Batenhorst RL, Bevens BA, et al: Patient controlled analgesia: A new concept of postoperative pain relief. *Ann Surg* 1982; 195:700–705.
4. Cohen SE, Tan S, Albright GA, et al: Epidural fentanyl/bupivicaine mixtures for obstetric analgesia. *Anesthesiology* 1987; 67:403–407.
5. Ready LB: Acute perepidural narcotic therapy, in Brown DL: *Problems in Anesthesia,* vol 2. Philadelphia, JB Lippincott, 1988, pp 327–328.
6. Thompson GE, Moore DC, Bridenbaugh LD, et al: Abdominal pain and alcohol celiac plexus nerve block. *Anesth Analg* 1977; 56:1–5.
7. Bell SN, Cale R, Roberts-Thompson IC: Celiac plexus block for control of pain in chronic pancreatitis. *Br Med J* 1980; 281:161–164.
8. Mannell A, Adson MA, McGrath DC, et al: Surgical management of chronic pancreatitis: Long term results in 141 patients. *Br J Surg* 1988; 75:467–472.
9. Gramer M, Daviace J, Engelhalm I: Endoscopic management of cysts and pseudocysts in chronic pancreatitis: Long term follow up after 7 years of experience. *Gastrointestinal Endoscopy* 1989; 35:1–9.

25

Abdominal Pain Secondary to Central Pain Syndrome

Theresa Ferrer-Brechner, M.D.

A 61-year-old black man presented with severe unremitting abdominal pain of 3 years' duration. Extensive gastrointestinal workup by numerous physicians failed to reveal any upper or lower gastrointestinal tract pathology. Past history revealed that 3 months prior to the onset of abdominal pain, the patient had sustained major head trauma when a piece of steel beam weighing 80 lbs landed on his head. He sustained a depressed skull fracture, and emergent evacuation of subdural hematoma was performed. Postoperatively, the patient was left with aphasia and right hemiparesis, which gradually resolved with 6–9 months' speech and physical therapy rehabilitation. Three months after the head trauma, he developed abdominal pain, characterized by a "bandlike" deep sensation through his entire abdomen. The pain had a continuous, burning quality and the patient observed "jerking" movements of his abdominal musculature. Workup included endoscopies, oral cholecystograms, and repetitive upper GI and lower GI tract series. The patient received multiple medication trials that included fluoperazine (Stelazine), meprobamate, Flexaril, acetaminophen (Tylenol #3), Fiorinal, diazepam (Valium), and clonazepam (Clonopin). All lab values (CBC, SMAC-12 panel, blood lead levels) were normal. An electroencaphalogram (EEG) demonstrated rare right frontal delta waves without evidence of seizure activity. A computed tomographic (CT) scan was negative except for some basal ganglia calcifications and few prominent sulci. When first seen in the pain clinic, the patient appeared physically incapacitated with abdominal pain, and assumed a fetal position during history taking. Abdominal exam was within normal limits, except for palpation-induced spasms of the abdominal wall. Bowel sounds were normal. Neurologic exam revealed a mild cranial VII nerve palsy and stuttered speech. Reflexes were equal on both sides. Minnesota Multiphasic Personality In-

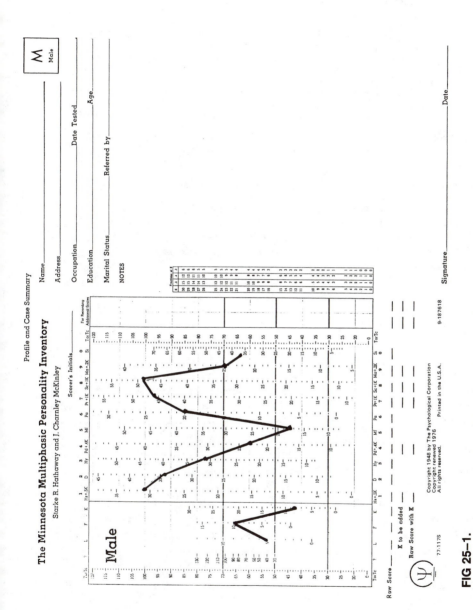

FIG 25–1.
This figure illustrates the patient's Minnesota Multiphasic Personality Inventory (MMPI).

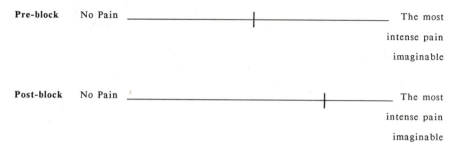

FIG 25–2.
This figure demonstrates there was increase in the patient's subjective pain rating following the differential epidural, even when the sensory block was at the level of T2.

ventory (MMPI) showed a markedly disturbed profile with elevations of several scales above normal interpreted as that of a profile of patients who abruptly lose function and have a high degree of anxiety and depression (Fig 25–1). Neuropsychology testing for cognitive function showed marked impairment in three-dimensional constructional ability, indicating organic brain damage. Differential epidural block was performed indicating no pain relief despite a complete sensory block to a T4 level (Fig. 25–2). A diagnosis of central pain syndrome (CPS) was made.

DISCUSSION

Central pain syndrome (CPS) indicates the occurrence of "spontaneous pain and painful overreaction to objective stimulation resulting from lesions confined to the substance of the central nervous system."[1] Although originally described in patients with thalamic lesions or infarcts, CPS can result from lesions at any level of the central nervous system, from the spinal cord to the cerebral cortex.[2] Traumatic lesions of the parietal cortex with sparing of the thalamus can result in painful peripheral manifestations similar to thalamic pain syndrome.[3] Although pain is usually referred to the hands, face, and feet, this patient had referral to the abdominal wall. Clonic epileptiform muscle jerking, similar to that seen in our patient, has been associated with painful episodes.[4] In patients with total spinal cord transections, complaints of visceral pain has been reported, characterized by cramplike periumbilical painful sensations.

Central pain syndrome results from multiple unique mechanisms, probably working simultaneously, thus giving rise to a wide spectrum of symptoms. These mechanisms can include reorganization of spared sensory fibers, activation of secondary alternative pathways, irritation of central gray masses, loss of inhibitory mechanisms with damage of nociceptive systems, and abnormal firings of central sensory nuclei due to deafferentation.

EVALUATION

The neurological symptoms and pain characteristics seen in CPS patients were recently reviewed.[5] Most of the 27 patients examined neurologically exhibited hypersensitivity to cutaneous stimuli and dysesthesias. The pathognomonic symptom in CPS appears to be sensory abnormality, which affects temperature and possibly pain sensibility. This kind of sensory disturbance is considered a diagnosic criteria for CPS in clinical practice and is the basis for the hypothesis that the crucial factor for the occurrence of CPS is a lesion affecting the spinothalamic system.

Pain characteristics of CPS include: (1) variable onset of pain, starting from first day poststroke to 24–34 months; (2) location varied from superficial or unilateral in 75% (more common in left); (3) the quality of pain most commonly reported were burning, aching, pricking, and lacerating—burning pain was more common in groups with extrathalamic lesions; (4) pain was intensified by joint movements, cold, light touch, and emotional changes; (5) pain did not respond to nonopiate analgesics.

Neurological exams in this group indicated that all patients had some kind of sensory changes in the affected side. Although components varied, decreased sensitivity to innocuous temperature was a common feature in 70%–80% of patients. Abnormal pinprick and cold sensibility was seen in 93%–96% of patients studied. Touch threshold was raised in 85%, and 37% had hypersensitivity to touch, which was more common in thalamic patients. In all patients studied, CSF studies were normal.

MANAGEMENT

Central pain syndrome is one of the most challenging pain problems seen in a chronic pain population. The first step is to establish a definitive diagnosis. In this particular patient, diagnoses was not established for a long period of time because the diagnostic evaluation was primarily focused on the peripheral symptoms of central pain syndrome. Definitive diagnosis was made by a combination of psychometric testing, detailed neurologic exam, cognitive testing for brain damage, and lack of pain relief with a complete sensory and motor block above the area of pain.

Once the diagnosis of CPS is established, treatments for the peripheral symptoms should be discontinued, such as use of narcotic analgesics. Clinical experience and a few systematic studies indicate that analgesics, including opiates, do not relieve CPS.[6] General treatments for CPS have successfully and unsuccessfully been tried, mostly in uncontrolled studies (Table 25–1). The first group of treatments includes a pharmacologic approach. Drugs studied include:

(1) Antidepressant drugs, usually tricyclics (TCA) in mostly uncontrolled studies.[7] It has been theorized that TCAs have specific analgesic effect that occurs at an earlier onset than their analgesic effect.[8] The dose used to induce analgesia was also much lower than that used to successfully treat depression; (2) Antiepileptic drugs have also been reported to alleviate neurogenic pain conditions, such as tic douloureux.[9] In CPS characterized by paroxysmal pain caused by demyelinating diseases, antiepileptic drugs have been helpful. Carbamazepine and phenytoin have been helpful in a small group of patients with poststroke pain syndrome.[10]

In a double-blind crossover study comparing placebo, amitriptyline, and carbamazepine in a small group of patients with CPS suffering from pain but without signs of depression, Leijon and Boivic indicated a statistically significant reduction of pain in comparison to placebo, seen during the second week of treatment. Fewer patients responded to carbamazepine, and the pain relief was not statistically significant in comparison to placebo.[5]

The second group of treatments tried have been neuroablative lesions such as stereotaxic chemical hypophysectomy, and stereotactic mesencephalic tractotomy for thalamic pain.[11–12] Although some efficacy has been found, no comparative studies utilizing less invasive techniques have been done.

The third group of treatments consists of neurostimulatory techniques such as deep brain stimulation and transcutaneous nerve stimulation. Deep brain stimulation, with electrodes placed in the subcortical areas such as the periventricular or thalamic areas, have been shown to induce a descending pain inhibitory system by decreasing actvity in the dorsal horn of the spinal cord. This technique has

TABLE 25–1.

Reported Treatments for CPS

Pharmacologic	Results	Author
Antidepressants		
Amitriptyline	10/15 significant pain relief	Leijon, 1989
Amitriptyline + fluphenazine	100% relief	Taub & Collins, 1974
Hydroxy L-tryptophan	5/7 good results	DeBenedetti, 1981
Tryptophane		King, 1980
Neuroablative		
Peripheral chemical blocks (alcohol/anesthetics)	Poor	
Neurectomies	Poor	White, 1969
Sympathectomies	Short-term relief	Loh, 1981
Chordotomy	Good, but pain recurs	Waltz, 1966
	Poor	White, 1969
Intramedullary tractotomy	Good (only one case)	Drake, 1953

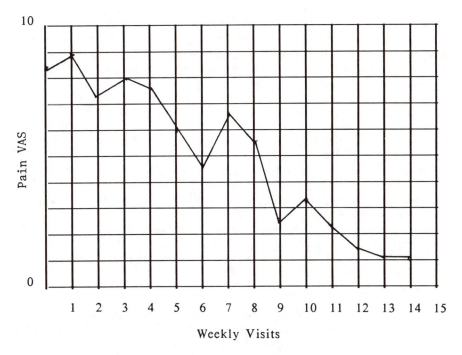

FIG 25–3.
This figure illustrates the patient's weekly visual analogue scale (VAS), showing subjective pain improvement with Sinequan, Tegretol, and TENS (transcutaneous electrical nerve stimulation).

been used for intractable pain, including that due to CPS, when an expert pharmacologic approach has not reduced pain.[13] Thalamic stimulation has also been successful in relieving the painful spasticity associated with CPS.[14]

This particular patient was treated with escalating doses of doxepin, starting with 10 mg/day to 125 mg/day by the third week. Carbamazepine was started in the second week at 150 mg twice daily. In the third week, a trial of peripheral stimulation technique was done. Behavioral management included activities management and education on pacing, coping skills, training, and relaxation.

Pain visual analogue scales (0–10 scale) taken during each visit indicated a gradual decrease in pain ratings from 9 to 2.5 by the eleventh visit, which is in the third month of treatment (Fig 25–3). After 6 weeks, the patient no longer assumed a fetal position and he walked normally to the clinic. His functionality at home improved dramatically.

In summary, CPS should be suspected when there is history of central nervous system trauma or disease in a patient with peripheral pain and negative workup aimed at an area of pain. Definitive diagnosis can be established by doing psychometric testing, cognitive screening, and differential epidural blocks. Treatment includes withdrawal from opiates, and pharmacologic treatments with titration of tricyclics with or without carbamazepine. If these fail, neurostimulatory techniques can be added to the pharmacologic treatment.

REFERENCES

1. Riddoch G: The clinical features of central pain. *Lancet* 1938; 234:1093–1098, 1150–1156, 1205–1209.
2. Dejerine J, Roussy G: La syndrome thalamique. *Revue Neurol (Paris)* 1906; 12:521–532.
3. Fields HL, Adams JE: Pain after cortical injury relieved by stimulation of internal capsule. *Brain* 1974; 97:169–178.
4. Retif J, Brihaye J, Vanderhaegen JJ: Syndrome douloureux 'thalamique' et lesion parietale. *Neurochirurgica (Stuttg)* 1967; 13:375–384.
5. Leijon G, Boivic J: Central post-stroke pain: A controlled trial of amitriptyline and carbamazepine. *Pain* 1989; 36:27–36.
6. Arner S, Mayerson BA: Lack of analgesic effect of opioids on neuropathic and idiopathic forms of pain. *Pain* 1988; 33:11–23.
7. Taub A, Collins WF: Observation on the treatment of denervation dysesthesia with psychotrophic drugs: Postherpetic neuralgia, anesthesia dolorosa, peripheral neuropathy, in Bonica JJ, et al (eds): *Advances in Neurology* vol 4. New York, Raven Press, 1974, pp 309–315.
8. Rascal O, Tran MA, Bonnevialle P, et al: Lack of correlation between plasma levels of amitriptyline and nortriptyline and clinical improvement of chronic pain of peripheral neurologic origin. *Clin Neuropharmacol* 1987; 10:560–564.
9. Thompson T: Carbamazepine therapy in trigeminal neuralgia. *Arch Neurol* 1980; 37:699–703.
10. Agnew DC, Golberg VD: A brief trial of phenytoin therapy for thalamic pain. *Bull LA Neurol Soc* 1976; 41:9–12.
11. Levin AB, Ramirez LF, Katz J: The use of stereotactic chemical hypophysectomy in the treatment of thalamic pain syndrome. *J Neurosurg* 1983; 59:1002–1006.
12. Shieff C, Nashald BS: Sterotactic mesencephalic tractotomy for the relief of thalamic pain. *Br J Neurosurg* 1987; 1:305–310.
13. Hosobuche Y: Subcortical electrical stimulation for control of intractable pain in humans. *J Neurosurg* 1986; 64:533–543.
14. Sigfried J: Effets de la stimulation du noyau du thalamus sur les dyskinesies et al spasticite. *Rev Neurol* 1986; 142:380–383.

26

Chronic Pelvic Pain

Andrea Rapkin, M.D.
Linda Kames, Psy.D.

A 28-year-old divorced nulliparous woman had chronic continuous pelvic pain for 5 years. She described the pain "like cramps only worse, like someone set a fire inside me." She had undergone a laparoscopy, which identified a 5-cm ovarian cyst. Subsequently, an ovarian cystectomy was performed. The cyst was found to be a functional corpus luteum cyst. However, the pain persisted, although neither the patient nor her doctors believed it to be due to the cyst or its removal. Follow-up pelvic exams were all normal. A diagnostic laparoscopy revealed pelvic adhesions more pronounced on the side of the previous cystectomy. At the time of evaluation, the patient had come to the end of her tolerance of the pain. She had requested a hysterectomy out of desperation, but was willing to follow her gynecologist's suggestion that she try the pain management program first.

DISCUSSION

This case illustrates one of the more common presentations of chronic pelvic pain (CPP). Chronic pelvic pain is, by definition, pain that has lasted for more than 6 months. As evidenced by this patient, individuals with chronic pelvic pain are usually exasperated, depressed, and often are no longer able to perform normal activities of living, such as work, exercise, or sexual activity. The patient and her physician, in desperation, may resort to surgical intervention. Often, this results in hysterectomy followed by oophorectomy, loss of childbearing capacity, and need for hormonal replacement. Frequently, the pain will persist.

The etiology of CPP is not always clear. Many conditions are associated with CPP, only some of which are gynecologic. Careful history and pelvic examination must be performed to rule out gastrointestinal, genitourinary, musculoskeletal, or neurologic causes of pain. Laboratory studies such as a complete blood count, erythrocyte sedimentation rate, urine analysis, urine culture, and possibly pelvic ultrasound (if the manual examination is hampered by obesity or pain), are usually performed. If suspected, nongynecologic causes of pain are investigated using appropriate studies (e.g., upper gastrointestinal series, barium enema, and intravenous pyelogram). A diagnostic laparoscopy should follow if the etiology of the pain is still uncertain. Most studies of laparoscopy for chronic pelvic pain reveal that approximately one-third of the patients have endometriosis, one-third have adhesions, and one-third have no obvious pathology.[1]

Pelvic adhesions may result from prior surgery, infection, or inflammation secondary to endometriosis. At the time of laparoscopy, the operator must clarify the diagnosis if adhesions are visualized. Evidence of edema, erythema, or purulent discharge from the fallopian tubes or a tubo-ovarian abscess signifies a subacute infectious process, which is obviously not treated in the same fashion as CPP. In a retrospective review of patients with CPP and those with infertility, we have found that there was no difference in the site, density, or amount of adhesions in those with and without pain.[1] Since many patients with significant pelvic adhesions do not have pain, it is probable that other associated factors are necessary for the induction of pelvic pain. These findings question the role of adhesions as a cause of chronic pelvic pain. Kresch, on the other hand, has implicated pelvic adhesions, particularly those that involve the parietal peritoneum or bowel, as the casue of pelvic pain.[2] A few uncontrolled studies have noted relief of pain after lysis of adhesions.[3] Lysis of adhesions may be performed, when possible, through the laparoscope, though it is not recommended that laparotomy be performed solely for lysis of adhesions, as upward of 70% of the cases in which second look laparoscopy is performed will reveal substantial reformation of adhesions.[4]

Often, laparoscopic evaluation reveals that adhesions are emanating from or adjacent to areas of the peritoneum, which are either pink, red, white, black, or clear and vesiculated. Seventy to ninety percent of these lesions, when subjected to biopsy, will prove to be atypical endometriosis.[5] The flamelike areas of red endometriosis have been overlooked in the past. Unfortunately, these red areas may, in fact, be the most biochemically active. If biopsies of all suspicious areas of peritoneum are performed, the number of cases of chronic pain in which a diagnosis of endometriosis will be made may actually increase by one-third. Endometriosis is initially treated with specific medical or surgical therapy, not through a pain management program.

Regardless of the presence or absence of pathology, most women with CPP have varying degrees of psychological dysfunction, which is often secondary to the chronic pain process. However, the incidence of childhood or adult physical and/or sexual abuse is upward of 50% in patients with chronic pelvic pain.[6]

The pain management clinic approach to CPP, with and without obvious pathology, has been successful in reducing pain by at least 50% in approximately 85% of the cases. This effect has persisted for at least six months.[6] The comprehensive pain management approach to CPP is employed when medical and/or surgical approaches are inappropriate or ineffective, and includes both somatic and psychological therapies. The extensive evaluative component includes a diagnostic nerve block to attempt to assess the locus of pain, a full history and physical examination, and individual and partner psychological interviews. It is expected that the patient undergo a diagnostic laparoscopy before referral to the pain management program, and that the results be incorporated into treatment planning. In addition, a variety of psychological measures are employed, including the Minnesota Multiphasic Personality Inventory (MMPI), Chronic Illness Problem Inventory (CIPI), Beck Depression Inventory (BDI), McGill Pain Questionnaire, UCLA Pelvic Pain Questionnaire, Spielberger State-Trait Anxiety Inventory, and the Dyadic Adjustment Scale.

While each treatment program is individualized according to the woman's needs, the majority of pelvic pain patients follow a structured protocol designed to be completed in 6–8 weeks. Patients receive acupuncture two times a week and psychological therapy once a week. Narcotics and other analgesics are tapered until these can be eliminated. Tricyclic antidepressants are utilized when appropriate. Psychological treatment is based on the type of pain and the patient's psychological status. For intermittent pain, such as dysmenorrhea, stress-inoculation techniques and systematic desensitization are utilized, with menstruation and menstrual-related feelings and activities as the stress and anxiety producing events.[7–8] For chronic continuous pain, general behavioral pain management techniques are applied. All patients receive training in stress management; self-control procedures, such as relaxation and self-hypnosis skills; activity and time management, and anxiety or depression reduction therapy. Crisis intervention, resolution of trauma, and marital and sexual therapy are undertaken when necessary.

At the end of the 8-week program, patients are placed on a follow-up schedule and they continue to be monitored for at least a year. A booster course of acupuncture is administered 6 months post-treatment and, thereafter, at 6-month intervals as needed.

REFERENCES

1. Rapkin AJ: Adhesions and pelvic pain: A retrospective study. *Obstetrics and Gynecology* 1986; 68:13–15.
2. Kresch AJ, Seifer DB, Sachs LB, et al: Laparoscopy in 100 women with chronic pelvic pain. *Obstet Gynecol* 1984; 64:672–674.
3. Goldstein DP, deCholnoky C, Emans SJ, et al: Laparoscopy in the diagnosis and management of pelvic pain in adolescents. *J Reprod Med* 1980; 24:251–256.
4. Adhesion Study Group NICHD: Reduction of postoperative pelvic adhesions with intraperitoneal 32% dextron 70: A prospective, randomized clinical trial. *Fertil Steril* 1983; 40:612–619.
5. Martin DC, Van der Zwagg R: Excisional techniques for endometriosis with the CO_2 laser laparoscope. *J Reprod Med* 1987; 32:753–758.
6. Rapkin AJ, Kames LD: The pain management approach to chronic pelvic pain. *J Reprod Med* 1987; 32:323–327.
7. Meichenbaum D: A self-instructional approach to stress management, in Sarusun I, Spielberger C (eds): *Stress and Anxiety*, vol. 2. New York, Wiley Press, 1975.
8. Wolpe J: *The Practice of Behavior Therapy*, ed 2. New York, Pergamon Press, 1973.

PART V

Back Pain

27

Piriformis Syndrome

Chang-Zern Hong, M.D.

In the last 3 weeks, a 35-year-old male gardener developed right buttock pain with radiation to the lateral aspect of the right lower extremity from the right thigh to the dorsum of the right foot. He also experienced tingling and numbness over the lateral aspect of the right leg and foot. He occasionally felt weakness in the right leg. On examination, the range of motion of the lumbosacral spine was full with no remarkable paraspinal muscle spasm. The straight leg raising test was positive at 70° on the right side with radiation of pain in the sciatic distribution. Tendon reflexes were normal and symmetrical in both lower extremities. Pinprick and touch sensation were decreased over the skin in the area supplied by the peroneal nerve. Muscle strength was reduced (3–4/5) over the peroneal muscles and hamstrings. On palpation, there was a trigger point over the right piriformis muscle with local twitch response and referred pain to the posterior thigh and leg. Tinel's sign was also positive when the sciatic nerve was pressed near the lower margin of the greater sciatic notch. Electromyography (EMG) was performed and revealed chronic partial denervation in the right hamstrings, right peroneal muscles, right tibialis anterior, right extensor hallucis longus, and right extensor digitorum brevis, but negative in the gluteal and paraspinal muscles. A diagnosis of piriformis syndrome was made and the patient was treated conservatively, including physical therapy with ultrasound deep heat therapy, cooling spray and stretch, strengthening exercise, and gentle deep pressure massage. Some improvement was noticed after 2 weeks of physical therapy, but there was still a persistent trigger point over the periformis muscle. A trigger point injection was then given with 0.5% procaine. There was remarkable improvement after the injection. The pain and weakness finally disappeared after 2 months of continuous intensive physical therapy.

DISCUSSION

The true piriformis syndrome is the entrapment of a portion or the whole sciatic nerve by the piriformis muscle, or by the sharp edge of the greater sciatic notch, due to the variation of the course of the sciatic nerve in relation to the piriformis muscle.[1-6] Pace and Nagle, reported 45 cases of "piriformis syndrome" from the patients referred to the Problem Back Service at Rancho Los Amigos Hospital.[7] Their patients did not have the typical sciatic nerve entrapment, as in the true piriformis syndrome, although they believed that muscle spasm and hypertrophy irritated the sciatic nerve. For such a group of patients, it seems more appropriate to use the term "piriformis myofascial syndrome" as described by Simons and Travell.[2] This may be considered as a mild form of piriformis syndrome. Table 27–1 summarizes the clinical pictures of these two syndromes.

TABLE 27–1.

Pathogenesis and Clinical Manifestation of Piriformis Syndrome and Piriformis Myofascial Syndrome

	Piriformis Syndrome	Piriformis Myofascial Syndrome
Pathology	Sciatic nerve entrapment due to variation in pathway of sciatic nerve in relation to piriformis muscle	Trigger point in taut band of piriformis muscle
Incidence	Rare	Not unusual
Symptoms		
Pain and paresthesia	Usually over lateral leg and foot (peroneal nerve distribution)	Usually over posterior thigh and leg, and sole (referred pain pattern)
Weakness	Often (peroneal nerve innervated muscles)	Rare
Signs		
Trigger points	In piriformis muscle	In piriformis muscle
Tinel's sign	Over sciatic nerve, distal to piriformis	Absent
Straight leg raising	Positive	May be positive
Piriformis compression	Pain and weakness on resisted abduction—external rotation of thigh, or passive internal rotation-adduction	Pain and weakness on resisted abduction-external rotation of thigh or passive internal rotation-adduction
EMG	Chronic partial denervation in muscles innervated by peroneal (more) and by tibial (less) nerves	Normal
Treatment	Surgery may be necessary	Surgery usually unnecessary

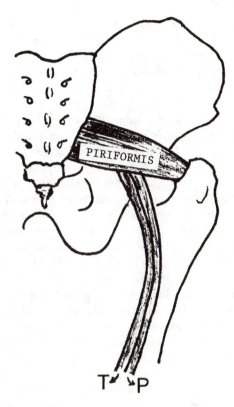

FIG 27–1.
The usual path of the sciatic nerve as the nerve trunk exits the pelvis beneath the piriformis muscle. (T = tibial division and P = peroneal division of the sciatic nerve.)

The piriformis muscle arises from inside the pelvis and runs laterally through the greater sciatic notch to become tendinous and insert on the greater trochanter of the femur. Usually (80–90% of the time), the sciatic nerve leaves the pelvis below the piriformis muscle (Figure 27–1), but the following variations can be found[2, 5]:

- The whole sciatic nerve passes through the muscle (0.8%)
- The peroneal division alone passes through the muscle (7.1%)
- The peroneal division alone passes over the muscle (2.1%)

With such variations, the sciatic nerve, especially the peroneal division, may easily be compressed with the bony edge of the greater sciatic notch, either by passive stretch (adduction, flexion, and internal rotation of the hip), or by active resistive contraction (abduction and external rotation of the hip) of the piriformis muscle. The taught piriformis muscle bands may also entrap the peroneal division of the sciatic nerve or, rarely, the entire nerve as the nerve fibers penetrate the piriformis muscle.[2]

The clinical presentation consists of pain, paresthesia, and weakness of the thigh and leg, as usually seen in sciatica. The symptoms may be triggered or intensified by over activity of the piriformis muscle, trauma to the gluteal area, and prolonged stooping, sitting, squatting, or walking. On physical examination, the trigger point of the piriformis muscles can be detected externally by direct pressure on its lateral and middle portions through the overlying gluteal muscles, or internally by rectal or pelvic examination on the medial, intrapelvic portion of the muscle. The piriformis muscle is tender with referred pain to the posterior aspect of the thigh and leg, and down to the sole.[2] If significant nerve damage occurs, Tinel's sign may be demonstrated with radiation to the lateral aspect of the leg and foot following the pattern of peroneal nerve distribution. With the patient seated, pain and weakness on resisted abduction and external rotation of the thigh are the characteristic findings.[2] The increased piriformis tension makes the leg on the affected side appear shorter and may cause external rotation of that leg when the supine patient is at rest.[2] Straight leg raising may be restricted.

In the case of true piriformis syndrome, there is a variable degree of weakness and atrophy involving the hamstrings and muscles innervated by the peroneal nerve, while muscles innervated by the tibial nerve are less affected.[6] Electromyogram may show evidence of chronic partial denervation in those muscles, but appears normal in the lumbosacral paraspinal muscles and gluteal muscles. Some patients may also have concomitant inferior gluteal nerve entrapment, and thus have weakness, atrophy, and positive EMG findings in the gluteus maximus muscle.[6] Electromyogram findings in the piriformis myofascial syndrome are usually negative. The studies with F-wave, H-reflex, and somatosensory-evoked potentials were found valuable in the diagnosis of piriformis syndrome.[6] Comprehensive evaluation including CAT scan or MRI of the spine is important to rule out lumbosacral radiculopathy, and is usually done before a diagnosis of piriformis syndrome has been considered.

TREATMENT

Surgical treatment with division or section of the piriformis muscle has been recommended for those cases with anatomic variations of the sciatic nerve. However, conservative treatment may be successful. No surgical intervention is required for the piriformis myofascial syndrome.[7] The following consists of a conservative therapeutic approach:

I. Anti-inflammatory medication.

II. Avoid overactivity or overstretching of the piriformis muscle.

III. Physical therapy:

    A. spray and stretch to the piriformis and gluteus maximus muscles[3];

    B. heat therapy to the piriformis muscle;

    C. massage or ischemic compression to the piriformis muscle;

    D. gradual strengthening exercise of the hip muscles;

    E. electrical muscular stimulation of the piriformis muscle to improve contractility or local circulation; and

    F. transcutaneous nerve stimulation of the sciatic nerve to relieve pain.

IV. Trigger point injection to piriformis muscle with 0.5% procaine solution to release the taut band of muscle fibers and to break the vicious cycle.[2-3]

V. Vitamin, nutrition, or hormone supply or others to correct the systemic perpetuating factors of myofascial trigger points.[3] The extra supply of vitamins B and C may be essential for tissue repair around an ischemic area.

REFERENCES

1. Kopell HP: Management of nerve compression lesions of the lower extremity, in Omer GI, Spinner M (eds), *Management of Peripheral Nerve Problems.* Philadelphia, WB Saunders Co, 1980, pp 626–638.
2. Simons DG, Travell JG: Myofascial origins of low back pain: Pelvic and lower extremity muscles. *Postgrad Med* 1983; 73:99–108.
3. Simons DG: Myofascial pain syndrome due to trigger points. *Int Rehab Med Assoc* Nov 1987; Monograph Series No 1.
4. Kopell HP, Thompson WAL: Peripheral entrapment neuropathies of the lower extremity. *N Engl J Med* 1960; 262:56–60.
5. Sunderland S: Sciatic, tibial and common peroneal nerve lesions, in *Nerves and Nerve Injury.* New York, Churchill Livingstone, 1978, pp 967–991.
6. Synek VM: The piriformis syndrome—review and case presentation. *Clin Exp Neurol* 1987; 23:31–37.
7. Pace JB, Nagle D: Piriform syndrome. *West J Med* 1976; 124:435–439.

28

Facet Arthralgia

Theresa Ferrer-Brechner, M.D.

A 55-year-old white woman was referred because of low back pain radiating to the buttocks and back of the leg. Pain was constant but aggravated by prolonged standing, side bending, and twisting movements. The patient had a history of lumbar laminectomy at L4–5 level 2 years prior to referral because of pain and neurological deficit, both of which were resolved after surgery. However, present pain started 8 months later. The pain was described as starting in the left lower back and radiating to the buttocks and back of the leg, stopping at the knee area. Neurological examination was negative for any sensory or motor deficit. Radiologic findings revealed degeneration of the left facet joints at L3–4 and L4–5 levels. Magnetic resonance imaging (MRI) and computed tomography (CT) scan did not reveal any discogenic disease, but confirmed the facet joint arthropathies.

DISCUSSION

The zygoapophyseal joint has recently been implicated as a possible site of intractable low back pain and sciatica. It has been hypothesized to be one of the unrecognized causes for postlaminectomy pain syndrome. In contrast to painful radiculopathy secondary to disc protrusion, the pain usually extends to the buttocks, but rarely below the knee.[1] Radiological examination with MRI scan usually shows degeneration of the facet joints. The innervation of the facet joints are provided by the articular nerve of von Luschka, a branch of the paravertebral somatic nerve as it exits from the intervertebral foramina.[2] The nerve travels along the lateral border of the facet joint that has two branches. One branches off on the upper one-third of the lateral border of the facet joint, and the other continues to the lower one-third of the facet joint. The facet nerve is primarily a sensory nerve and does not have any motor function.

Various methods performed to denervate the facet joint include severing with a scalpel, radiofrequency, injection of neurolytic solution, and recently the use of cryogenic probe.

In 1971, Rees reported his results in severing the posterior rami of the segmental nerves (articular nerve of Luschka), which supplies the lumbar facet articular capsule. He performed the neural interruption by introducing a long scalpel percutaneously, penetrating the lumbar intertranverse ligament, and sweeping the blade in a posterior-inferior fashion. He reported 95–98% success in 2,000 patients.[3]

Shealy destroyed the facet nerve by using percutaneous radiofrequency lesioning to the parafacet area.[1] Electrical stimulation was induced first, confirming proximity of the radiofrequency electrode to the spinal nerve. With controlled lesion temperature monitoring, the patient reported to the surgeon repetitively, regarding the pain intensity and location of the frequency current.

Blocking of peripheral nerves such as the facet nerve can be performed with local anesthetic agents. However, the maximum duration of analgesia can only be 8–10 hours at the most, even with long-acting agents. Injection of neurolytic agents such as phenol or alcohol carries the risk of a paravertebral somatic nerve neurolysis because of its close proximity. In addition, incomplete destruction of the nerve can cause abnormal regeneration and painful neuritis.

Another recent approach to facet arthropathy is use of the percutaneous cryogenic neurolysis of the facet nerve.[4] Animal studies indicate that with freezing to $-20°C$ for 60 seconds, less demyelination, scarring, and inflammatory reduction occur in comparison to crushing thermolysis or cutting of a nerve.[5–7] Freezing has the advantage of normal nerve regeneration with return to normal function and longer duration, in comparison to local anesthetics.[8] In 10 patients with documented facet arthralgia, 9 patients had significant pain relief lasting from 2 weeks to 3 months.[9] The freezing was repeated as often as necessary as an outpatient procedure (Fig 28–1).

TECHNIQUE

The patient is placed in the prone position with a pillow under the iliac crest area. The tips of the spinous processes are identified and a line is drawn running horizontally through them (Fig 28–2). At T12 and L1, a point two inches lateral to the posterior tips of the spinous process is marked. At L2, L3, and L4, points 2-1/2 inches lateral to the posterior tips of the spinous process are marked, and at L5, S1, a point 3 inches lateral to the posterior tip of the spinous process is marked. All these points mark the initial entry of the needle through the skin.

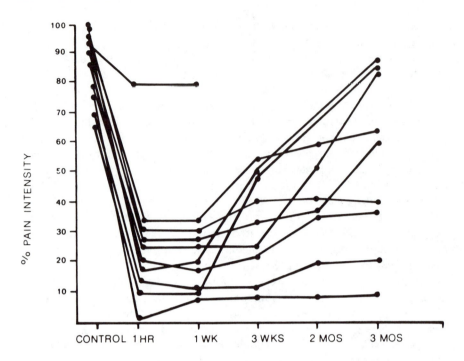

FIG 28–1.
Cross-section of cryoprobe top. (From Brechner T: Percutaneous cryogenic neurolysis of the articular nerve of Luschka. *Reg Anaesth* 6:21. Used by permission.)

The needle is then inserted at an angle perpendicular to the skin. As soon as bony structure is encountered, x-ray is used to confirm the location of the needle. By using these three points, the needle is placed correctly at the course of the facet nerve as described by Fox and Rizzoli.[2] When the needle is properly located, 2 mL of local anesthetic is injected initially for diagnostic purposes. The patient is then examined for any sign of somatic nerve block and changes of pain experience. If pain is relieved both at rest and with pain-provoking movements, and there is absence of sensory block, the block is considered successful.

If the cryoprobe is to be used, a 14-gauge needle with teflon-over-catheter is inserted using the same landmarks. Radiologic confirmation of needle placement is obtained. The needle is withdrawn and the catheter is left in place. The cryoprobe is then introduced through the catheter and x-rays are again taken to confirm proper location.

Some cryoprobes have a stimulating electrode that is capable of delivering direct electrical current that has continuous pulses of 1 msec duration. This electrical stimulation determines the proximity of the cryoprobe electrode tip to

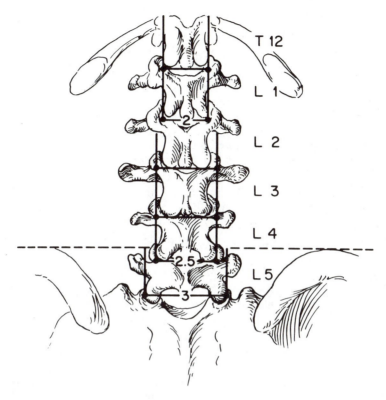

FIG 28–2.
Results of cryogenic facet neurolysis over time. (From Brechner T: Percutaneous cryogenic neurolysis of the articular nerve of Luschka. *Reg Anaesth* 6:22. Used by permission.)

the facet nerve or the spinal nerve root. If the probe is close to the facet nerve, stimulation at 1–2 volts can replicate the characteristic pain of which the patient complained. Severe radicular pain of characteristic dermatomal distribution is provoked by less than 1 volt, and muscle contractions can occur between 1–2 volts when the electrode is in proximity to a spinal nerve. If this occurs, the needle is withdrawn and repositioned until the characteristic reproduction of the original pain is felt by the patient. Following final radiographic and electrical confirmation of proper electrode position, the cryoprobe is activated.

The temperature is monitored by a thermistor probe located at the tip and registered by a meter on the machine. Freezing is performed at −60°C for 60 seconds. It is important to have the probe return to a higher temperature at least 10–20 seconds before removal of the electrode. If one attempts to remove a frozen probe, it tends to adhere to the surrounding tissue and/or the Teflon catheter. The procedure is repeated at two to three levels bilaterally and Band-

Aids are used as dressing. The patients are then returned to the recovery room area and allowed to recover and rest for 2 hours. After this period of time, they are encouraged to become active and perform exercises that would normally produce pain to assist in assessing the success of the procedure.

APPARATUS

The Spembly cryosurgical instrument consists of three components: a delivery system for gaseous nitrous oxide (N_2O), a temperature measuring facility, and a battery operated nerve stimulator. The nitrous oxide delivery system enables N_2O at a pressure of up to 850 psi to be delivered safely to a Joule-Thompson orifice in the tip of the probe. Figure 28–3 shows the cross-section of the probe tip and corresponding differences in pressures. At no time is high pressure gas, contained within the tube, in contact with tissue. The probe contains the freezing probe and electronic stimulator in one unit. The cryoneedle is approximately 15-gauge in diameter, and this includes the coating of polytetrafluoroethylene (PTFE) material for electrical insulation. The entire cryoneedle and connecting cables can be sterilized in a gas autoclave. The probe is connected by 6 feet of flexible tubing to the console unit, which has a gas pressure regulator switch, a nerve stimulator socket, and dials to record gas pressure and probe tip temperature. The refrigerant is N_2O and, at operating pressure of 600 psi, the minimum temperature of $-60°C$ can be achieved rapidly at the tip of the probe.

The presented patient underwent a diagnostic block under fluoroscopy of the facet nerves at L3–4, L4–5, and L5–S1 with 2 cc of 1% at each level. She

DIAGRAM OF CRYOPROBE TIP

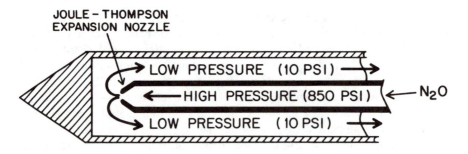

JOULE – THOMPSON EXPANSION NOZZLE

LOW PRESSURE (10 PSI)

HIGH PRESSURE (850 PSI) ← N_2O

LOW PRESSURE (10 PSI)

FIG 28–3.
Landmarks for needle entry aimed toward facet joints of lumbar area. (From Brechner T: Percutaneous cryogenic neurolysis of the articular nerve of Luschka. *Reg Anaesth* 6:20. Used by permission.)

reported 85% pain relief with both the pain visual analog scale and clinical pain estimate (0–10) without sensory loss. Her diary indicated 5 hours of pain relief. She underwent cryoprobe block of the same facet nerves 2 days later as an outpatient, and she obtained pain relief for 2-1/2 months. The procedure was repeated 3 times over the year, the duration being from 2 months to 3-1/2 months between cryogenic blocks. Although pain relief was 75%–80%, the patient was able to resume significant functioning as a volunteer.

REFERENCES

1. Shealy CM: Percutaneous radiofrequency denervation of the spinal facets. *J Neurosurg* 1975; 43:449–451.
2. Fox JL, Rizzoli HV: Identification of radiologic coordinates for the posterior articular nerve of Luschka in the lumbar spine. *Surg Neurol* 1973; 1:343–346.
3. Rees W: Multiple bilateral subcutaneous rhizolysis of segmental nerves in the treatment of the intervertebral disc syndrome. *Ann Gen Pract* 1971; 26:126–127.
4. Carter DC, Lee P, Gill W, et al: The effect of cryosurgery on peripheral nerve function. *J R Coll Surg Edinb* 1972; 17:25–31.
5. Gaster RN, Davidson TM, Rand RW, et al: Comparison of nerve regeneration rates following controlled freezing or crushing. *Arch Surg* 1971; 103:378–383.
6. Poswillo DE: A comparative study of the effects of electrosurgery and cryosurgery in the management of benign oral lesions. *Br J Surg* 1971; 9:1–7.
7. Bagly DH, Beazley RM: Histological changes in peripheral nerves following cryosurgery. *J Sur Res* 1974; 16:231.
8. Lloyd JW, Barnard JDW, Glynn CJ: Cryoanalgesia: A new approach to pain relief. *Lancet* 1976; 10:932–934.
9. Brechner T: Percutaneous cryogenic neurolysis of the articular nerve of Luschka. *Reg Anaesth* 1981; 6:18–22.

29

Acute Nonsurgical Lumbar Disk Protrusion

John Rowlingson, M.D.

A 47-year-old white male hospital administrator had his first episode of low back pain approximately 5 years ago, when he reached awkwardly to catch a falling chair. He developed sharp, nonradiating low back pain which responded to 2 weeks' of treatment that included bed rest, aspirin, and methocarbamol (Robaxin). Thereafter, he was generally symptom-free, except for a few 1-2 day occurrences of mild, activity-related low back pain, until 4 weeks prior to evaluation. Upon this occasion, he developed sharp pain across his lower back at work when stepping off an elevator that had not quite stopped at floor level. Aspirin for 4 days provided mild improvement, and he went on vacation to the beach. The low back pain was exacerbated when the patient did a little jump step over a wave while wading into the ocean. The back pain grew in intensity and was associated with obvious spasm of the paraspinal muscles. The pain level exceeded any that he had experienced previously and was markedly increased with any sitting or with the strain at bowel movement. Because of the persistence of the symptoms in spite of the conservative therapy that had worked before, neurosurgical consultation was sought by the patient. The presence of aching low back pain, radicular pain into his right foot, both accompanied by numbness in his leg, prompted the surgeon to order a CT scan. This revealed a bulging disc at L4–5. The patient was referred to the pain management center for conservative therapy. In addition to the above history, physical examination revealed a decrease in sensation to pinprick in the right L5 dermatome above and below the knee and positive straight leg raising of the right leg beyond 65°. A nonsteroidal anti-inflammatory agent (NSAID) and a muscle relaxant were prescribed for daily use, and the patient was advised to be careful about his activity. This treatment was only moderately successful at decreasing his symptoms over the next week, and he was thus reevaluated when he complained that he "just couldn't get comfortable." His physical exam was as before, and an epidural steroid injection was performed at the L4–5 level. In 3 days he was basically pain free, stopped the muscle relaxants, and started back exercises on a daily basis. Within a month he had gone on a weekend sailing trip and was pleasantly surprised by the amount of bending, pulling, and stretching he was able to do. He stopped his NSAID and continued his back exercise.

DISCUSSION

Eighty-five percent of adults will have low back pain sometime in their lives, and the incidence at any given time in the general population is 20%–25%.[1] As a matter of fact, low back pain is such a common problem one wonders what is wrong with those who do not have it! There is low mortality from spinal disorders, but the morbidity and health care costs are high and impose a significant economic burden on society.[2] The estimated cost on an annual basis is in the $30 billion range. At least equally important is the life disruption of the patients and their families, the problems on the job site, and the image and self-esteem changes in the patient's community. Acute low back pain must be managed effectively because evidence reveals increasing disability secondary to low back pain in spite of ergonomic information, improved diagnostic equipment, and labor-saving mechanical devices.[3]

As in the cited case, the common ages affected are those between 18 and 55 years. Most spinal disorders are activity related, but the patient need not have a physically demanding job. Not all patients will provide the interviewer with the classic history of lifting a heavy object in a "twisted-spine" position that results in sharp, radiating pain into the lower extremity and is ultimately associated with sensorimotor deficits and positive straight-leg raising. Eighty-five percent of herniated discs occur at either L4–5 or L5–S1. It is vital that a careful history be taken by an open-minded physician, since the differential diagnosis for low back pain complaints is vast. It has recently been recognized that a thorough history and physical examination comprise an adequate workup in patients with complaints of localized spine pain and those with pain radiating into the proximal or distal extremity, but *not* associated with any neurologic signs of dysfunction.[2] Furthermore, laboratory studies such as plain x-rays, discograms, and myelograms are contraindicated or at least not common practice (i.e., CT scan, EMG, and laboratory studies for inflammatory disease) at this early stage of the disease.[2] In patients with spinal pain that radiates into the extremity and *is* associated with positive neurological signs, laboratory studies in common practice would include x-rays, CT scan, and/or myelogram.[2] Mooney, writing to expound upon the concept of the disc being a common, chronic, pain-producing structure of the low back, states that a CT scan of the discogram or an MRI is the best test for diagnosing disc disease.[3] There is still a difference of opinion over the significance of physical assessment, functional capacity, and ergonomic-biomechanical data that is being obtained more frequently as part of the thorough workup of the patient with low back pain.

The cited case represents a typical patient because he had postural low back pain in the distant past, and another episode shortly preceding the onset of pain associated with radicular signs and symptoms. Cailliet notes that the five most common structures for producing pain from the lower back are the posterior longitudinal ligament, the deep paraspinal muscles, the facet joints, the nerve roots and their dural coverings, and the interspinous ligaments.[4] It is possible that patients with pain arising from these structures will have radicular symptoms on an intermittent basis. The periodic nature of the symptoms and the likelihood of routine laboratory studies being negative or showing only a disk bulge will discourage most surgeons from considering an operation. Ten percent of back "injuries" are not resolved in 2 months and become chronic, unlike other sprains or ligament-tendon-muscle-joint capsule injuries.[3] Low back pain secondary to changes in posture is far more common than that due to herniated disks and is the result of a shift of the weight-bearing function from the strong column of vertebral bodies with interposing disks to the more delicate posterior elements— the lamina, pedicles, and facet joints that form the vertebral arch around the spinal cord.[4] Subsequent symptoms will be similar to some of those in our case— pain that is diffuse and aching in quality, nonradiating in distribution, and frequently associated with back stiffness, itself a manifestation of reflex muscle spasm related to the pain.

Common mechanisms for acute low back injury include: (1) lifting an excessively heavy object; (2) lifting any load in a mechanically disadvantageous position; (3) direct trauma to the back, or (4) falls that directly cause muscular strain and sprain.[5] These mechanisms of injury must be searched for and a careful history taken from the patient. New work by McCarron et al., has shown that nucleus pulposus material is fully capable of provoking an inflammatory reaction of the nerve roots.[6] One can then logically speculate that a bulging lumbar disk may have microruptures in the annulus of the disk that allow the escape of nucleus pulposus into the epidural space. This results in a clinical picture of radiculopathy that is secondary to nerve root inflammation, but occurs without laboratory studies being positive, such that surgery would be considered. Additionally, Mooney suggests that some radicular pain may be secondary to abnormal chemical events in the nerve roots relating to matters of nerve root blood flow or nutrition.[3]

MANAGEMENT

The primary goal of treatment in acute pain is to eliminate the pain as soon as possible and restore the patient to full function.[2] As suggested above, effective therapy for acute low back pain is crucial because of the socioeconomic and physical/psychological devastation of chronic disease. Various statistics abound, and it is said that 50% of patients with acute low back pain are better in 1 week, 95% of patients can be better in 4–6 weeks, and about 50% of the patients with sciatica are better in 1 month.[2] These results have prompted some to say that the natural history of the disease of low back pain has helped many treatments look effective!

The appropriate goal in the first 4 weeks of symptoms is to rule out specific disease processes in the differential diagnosis of low back pain and to provide conservative therapy. If the pain problem continues more than 4 weeks in spite of treatment, the patient should be reevaluated, as was done in our case, and appropriate therapy, including the continuation of conservative therapy, be recommended.[2] Even conservative therapy generates expense, results in time lost from work, and carries the risk of side effects, so the significance of all of this nonsurgical treatment should not be questioned.[7]

Medications are a most common therapeutic intervention for patients with acute low back pain. Narcotic analgesics should be prescribed if the severity of pain warrants them, and in doses that achieve the desired effect. If these potent drugs are provided *liberally* for a *short* period of time, a good clinical effect will be manifest that is consistent with the primary goal of pain treatment. Inadequate doses used over a long period of time have no place in modern day practice.

It is very common to prescribe NSAIDs as effective co-analgesics that are readily available, reasonably inexpensive, and exert no chemical depressant effects. The practitioner may choose to utilize one of the "muscle relaxant" drugs for a short period of time if muscle spasm is a dominant feature in the patient's presentation. As these generally provide relaxant effects by CNS sedation, they will not be useful on a long-term basis. Combinations of these medications will enhance the physical and emotional rest that the patient with acute pain needs to be ready to comply with the rest of the treatment scheme. The contemporary management of acute pain demands an active patient.

Other common techniques for providing pain relief include sensory modulation therapies, such as massage, heat and cold application, transcutaneous electrical nerve stimulation (TENS), and various injections with local anesthetics and steroids. The sensory modulation therapies are recommended by their ease and simplicity, but are not supported by voluminous scientific literature. Injections can provide prompt, temporary relief, but will be most successful when employed as but one component in a *program* of treatments. In nonsurgical patients with radiating low back pain, a neurosensory deficit, and for whom routine conservative measures have not been helpful, it is popular to inject combinations of local anesthetics and depo-steroids into the epidural space to decrease the symptoms from inflammatory neuropathology and hasten the patient's cooperation with progressive physical therapy and activity restoration.[8] The infiltration of myofascial trigger points in the muscles of the low back area is also a common adjunctive therapy.

Traditional management of acute low back pain used to recommend periods of bed rest of 2–3 weeks. Given the success of rapid mobilization of patients in sports medicine, contemporary dictum would state that patients with acute, nonsurgical low back pain should have limited bed rest, even for periods as brief as 48 hours.[2] Early mobilization therapy is started along with exercise regimens that aim to preserve range of motion, decrease muscle spasm, and help maintain tone and strength of postural and motion-oriented muscles. The patient should avoid sitting, because this markedly increases the intradiscal pressure (more so than standing, which is a position of rest for the back). Once the acute episode has passed, recommendations for daily flexion or extension exercises plus walking are likely, as well as returning the patient to full occupational function. Generally, there will not be any need for the numerous braces and corsets some health-allied practitioners urge.[7]

The patient with acute low back pain does not generally need rehabilitation per se, as might patients with chronic complaints who have been out of the work force and away from his or her usual life style for months at a time. Rather, the generic aim of treatment is a return to work and normal activity as soon as possible. Thus, the physical therapy recommendations must include exercises of a progressive nature, such that all the muscle groups involved in low back function (paraspinal muscles, abdominal wall muscles, hamstring muscles) are toned and conditioned on a regular basis. Motion helps to heal muscles, tendons, ligaments, bones, and disks. Some of one's daily activity should *not* be the physically abusive effort of one's job, but rather that which helps to restore functional integrity and encourages good back health in all aspects of the patient's life. To make the treatment of acute low back pain most effective, some of the therapeutic suggestions must be directed at preventing further trouble. Thus, recommendations such as lifestyle changes, increased fitness, weight loss, and job changes will be beneficial and may minimize future recurrences of low back pain.

REFERENCES

1. National Institute for Disability Rehabilitation and Research: Low back pain. Presented at the Rehabilitation Research and Training Center, Department of Orthopedics, University of Virginia School of Medicine, Charlottesville, Va. September 1987.
2. LeBlanc FE: Scientific approach to the assessment and management of activity-related spinal disorders. *Spine* 1987; 12:S9–S54.
3. Mooney V: Where is the pain coming from? *Spine* 1987; 12:754–759.

4. Cailliet R: *Soft Tissue Pain and Disability.* Philadelphia, FA Davis Co, 1977, pp 41–106.
5. Rowlingson JC: The evaluation and management of acute low back pain. *Curr Concepts Pain* 1983; 1:3–6.
6. McCarron RF, Wimpee MW, Hudkins PG, et al: The inflammatory effect of nucleus pulposus. *Spine* 1987; 12:760–764.
7. Deyo RA: Conservative therapy for low back pain. *JAMA* 1983; 250:1057–1062.
8. Benzon H: Epidural steroid injections for low back pain and lumbosacral radiculopathy. *Pain* 1986; 24:277–295.

30

Lumbar Somatic Nerve Impingement

Verne L. Brechner, M.D.

The patient was a 43-year-old woman who had had multiple surgeries for low back problems, and complained of pain in the right big toe and the second and third toes of the right foot. There was weakness of dorsiflexion of the right foot, and weakness of dorsiflexion of the toes of the right foot. There was also evidence of denervation on electromyographic (EMG) testing. The EMG was felt to be more compatible with an S1 root syndrome than with an L5 root syndrome. A recent myelogram and computed tomographic (CT) scan showed deformity of the right L5 root consistant with a recurrent ruptured disk. However, there had been so much scarring observed about the root during past surgeries that it was felt the deformity could conceivably be that of an old residual scar. The patient was referred for diagnostic somatic nerve blocks in an attempt to differentiate the L5 versus the S1 as a major conduit of the pain.

DISCUSSION

Selective anesthetizing of a single nerve root at the intervertebral foramen is a diagnostic procedure that may identify the nerve root responsible for the conduction of pain. The information may be useful in diagnosing the site generating pain in a complex pain problem.

For the procedure to have diagnostic significance, the injection of local anesthetic about the nerve root must be precise, and the subjective complaints, as well as physical findings prior to the performance of the nerve block and following the nerve block, must be reported and compared.

The preblock evaluation should describe the location and quality of the pain complaint, as well as factors such as positioning, posturing, and specific activities that aggravate the pain. Neurological findings should be documented; areas of hypalgesia and anesthesia present as a part of the patient's initial pain complaint must be recorded. Gait should be carefully observed. Straight leg raising and other tests of limited motion or function must be noted. Deep tendon reflexes should also be tested and noted.

When the procedure is performed, fluoroscopy is a mandatory guide for needle placement. There are a variety of techniques for performing the block. The author's preference is to use fluoroscopy and, initially, identify the infralateral margin of the transverse process of the vertebral body of the root to be blocked. A skin wheal is placed over this area, and the needle is advanced under direct fluoroscopic guidance through the skin wheal to the intervertebral foramen. Proper placement of the needle is confirmed by cross-lateral view, which should identify the needle point in the central area of the foramen. It must be recognized that the dural sheath is present in this area and may be punctured by the needle. In this case, injection of local anesthesia would produce spinal anesthesia. Also, it must be recognized that the needle is in close proximity to the nerve root and that paresthesias characteristic of the specific nerve root can be expected. If such paresthesias occur, the further advance of the needle is discontinued and the paresthesia is used as a landmark.

The patient should describe precisely the location of the paresthesia; this is recorded as information to be compared with the distribution of the patient's pain complaint. After the usual precautions, such as the aspiration of the needle in four planes, 3–4 mL of anesthetic agent are injected. During the injection, there frequently is a paresthesia and again, the distribution of the paresthesia is recorded. Following the nerve block, the patient should be observed for a period of an hour or so. Alterations in the pain complaint are recorded. The patient is then tested in various postures that previously provoked pain. The dermatomal distribution of the anesthesia resulting from the injection is recorded to confirm the validity of the block.

A sequence of events that would indicate high specificity of the blocked root as the major source of the patient's pain complaint would be as follows:

1. Paresthesia provoked during performance of the procedure is identical in distribution to that of the pain complaint.
2. The pain analogue scale would fall from a relatively high preblock value to a value approximating zero, and the pain analog scale would again escalate somewhat after the block wears off.
3. There would be a dermatomal anesthesia consistant with a single nerve root block.

4. The patient would be able to posture herself pain-free in a variety of positions that previously provoked pain.
5. Straight leg raising would significantly improve.

PROCEDURE

Prior to doing any block procedure, there was a dense anesthesia involving the right big toe. However, there was no anesthesia observed in the lateral aspect of the right calf. The patient was capable of weak dorsiflexion of her right foot, and the pain analog scale was estimated at 50 on a scale of 100.

The patient then received a right paravertebral L5 somatic nerve block with the injection of 5 mL of 1.5% lidocaine (Xylocaine) at the L5–S1 intervertebral foramen. During the injection of local anesthesia, the patient described an intense ache in the medial dorsal aspect of the right foot and the right big toe. She stated that the distribution of the ache was identical to that of the pain she had complained of. Following this, the patient developed an anesthesia along the lateral aspect of the right calf, as well as increased weakness on dorsiflexion of the right big toe and right foot. The previously observed anesthesia of the right big toe persisted. With the development of anesthesia as described above, the patient also stated there had been complete pain relief. Pain analogue scale fell from 50 to 0.

On a subsequent day, a transacral S1 block was performed with injection of 5 mL of 1.5% Xylocaine. Paresthesias occurred along the lateral aspect of the right foot, and subsequently the patient developed anesthesia along the lateral aspect of the right foot. However, there was no relief of the pain with the development of this S1 anesthesia. These findings were reported to the surgeon with the diagnosis of L5 being the major conduit of her pain.

The patient was subsequently explored and was found to have "a small extruded fragment under the right L5 root." Recovery was uneventful and pain relief has been persistent for the 9 months that have elapsed since the surgical procedure and the writing of this chapter.

BIBLIOGRAPHY

Brechner T, Brechner V: Accuracy of needle placement during diagnostic and therapeutic nerve block, in Bonica JS, Albe-Fessard D, (eds): *Advances in Pain Research—Research and Therapy,* Vol 1. New York, Raven Press, 1976, pp 679–683.

Brechner T, Brechner VL: Accuracy of needle placement during diagnostic and therapeutic nerve block, abstract Presented at the First World Congress on Pain, 1975, International Association for the Study of Pain. New York, Raven Press, p 169.

Brechner VL: Management of pain by conduction anesthesia techniques, In Youmans JR (ed): *Neurological Surgery,* ed 3. Philadelphia, WB Saunders Co, 1990, pp 4007–4010.

Brechner VL: Pain syndromes—the use of nerve block in diagnosis and treatment. *California Med* 1967; 106:290–302.

Bridenbaugh PO: The lower extremity: Somatic blockade, in Cousins MJ, Bridenbaugh PO, (eds): *Neural Blockade in Clinical Anesthesia and Management of Pain.* Philadelphia, JB Lippincott, 1980, pp 321–324.

31

Arachnoiditis: Treatment by Brain Stimulation

Ronald F Young, M.D.

A 49-year-old man presented with back and bilateral lower extremity pain. The patient's problem dated back to approximately 10 years when he had fallen 6 feet from a scaffold, and struck the buttocks. He developed back and lower extremity pain subsequently, and after prolonged conservative treatment, radiological studies disclosed a herniated intervertebral disk at the L5–S1 level. The patient underwent laminectomy and disk excision, and had excellent immediate relief of his leg pain. For about 3 years, the patient had minimal back and leg pain, and was able to work, although he was restricted in his ability to lift and bend. Subsequently, he developed recurrent back and left leg pain, and further studies revealed evidence of intervertebral disk herniation at L4–5. The patient underwent an L4–5 laminectomy and disk excision. This time, he showed slow resolution of left leg pain over a period of about 3 months. His leg pain never completely resolved, and one year after the second operation, the patient noted the onset of pain in the right leg and increasing pain in the left leg, as well as in the lower back. Repeat studies at this time did not show evidence of intervertebral disk herniation. The patient was continued on a program of physical therapy and transcutaneous electrical nerve stimulation. The pain progressed to the point where the patient was unable to continue employment. Examination 8 years following the patient's original injury showed scattered loss of sensation in the L5–S1 dermatomes bilaterally, absent ankle reflexes bilaterally, and mild weakness in dorsi and plantar flexion of both feet. The patient subsequently developed difficulty with urinary hesitancy, and neurologic studies disclosed evidence of a mild neurogenic bladder. In an attempt to identify the cause of the patient's continued pain and neurologic dysfunction, magnetic resonance imaging studies, along with CT scanning and myelography were carried out. These studies showed evidence of clumping of the nerve roots of the cauda equina, from approximately L4 to the caudal end of the subarachnoid space, which is consistent with the diagnosis of arachnoiditis. The patient was treated in a comprehensive, multidisciplinary pain program that involved physical therapy, transcutaneous electrical nerve stimulation, local anesthetic nerve blocks and epidural blocks, biofeedback, and psychological treatment. He had difficulty on several occasions with excessive use of narcotic analgesics, but was eventually successfully weaned from analgesics and treated with nonnarcotic analgesics, as well as tricyclic antidepressants. The patient continued to complain of severe back and bilateral leg pain, was unable to work, and had extremely limited physical activities. He was referred for consideration of neurosurgical treatment.

DISCUSSION

The patient presented with a distressing, but unfortunately relatively common syndrome of intractable back and lower extremity pain following previous operations on the lumbar spine. The radiological studies confirmed the diagnosis of arachnoiditis for which, at present, no satisfactory direct surgical or medical solution exists. He was treated comprehensively in a multidisciplinary pain program and all nonsurgical avenues for therapy of his chronic pain were thoroughly explored.

Experience has shown that ablative neurosurgical procedures such as dorsal root ganglionectomy, dorsal rhizotomy, and cordotomy are unlikely to produce long-term relief of pain due to arachnoiditis. When pain is present bilaterally, cordotomy, if carried out on a bilateral basis, leads to a high degree of sphincter dysfunction and leg weakness, resulting in paraparesis and inability to walk. In general, ablative neurosurgical procedures are not suited to the treatment of chronic pain related to conditions other than malignancies. The patient was considered for treatment by the placement of chronic stimulating electrodes in the periaqueductal gray region of the brain stem.

In 1969, it was demonstrated that electrical stimulation in the brain stem in animal experiments could produce profound analgesia. Subsequently, a variety of confirmatory studies identified the presence of a descending pathway beginning in the region of the gray matter surrounding the upper end of the cerebral aqueduct and extending through the midportion of the brain stem, down the dorsolateral quadrant of the spinal cord to the region of the dorsal horn of the spinal cord. At this region, inhibition of pain-related activity was identified. Pharmacological studies indicated that this pathway was activated by endogenous opioid substances generally termed the "endorphins."

Other brain targets also appear to relieve pain when they are electrically stimulated. The most common target for stimulation other than the periaqueductal gray has been the somatosensory relay nuclei of the thalamus. These nuclei are the ventralis posterolateralis (VPL) for the trunk and extremities, and the ventralis posteromedialis (VPM) for the face. Stimulation of VPL and VPM appears to be most effective for the relief of pain associated with deafferentation following injuries or for diseases that affect peripheral nerves, nerve roots, the spinal cord, or the brain. The neurotransmitters that may be involved in pain relief by VPL or VPM stimulation are unknown.

Electrical stimulation of the brain to treat chronic pain in man actually began prior to discovery of this basic information concerning pain modulation by the brain. It appears that the first attempts to electrically stimulate the brain to control pain were carried out in approximately 1954. The technique did not gain popularity or interest, however, until the above described research information seemed to provide a solid, anatomical, and physiological foundation for treating chronic pain in humans by electrical stimulation. In the 1970s, Adams and Hosobuchi, from the University of California, San Francisco, and Richardson, from Tulane University, published their experience in the treatment of chronic pain by electrical stimulation of the brain.

In this technique, often called deep brain stimulation (DBS), electrodes are stereotactically implanted into selected brain targets and connected to a device for chronic electrical stimulation. Formerly, stimulation was carried out when an external battery-powered stimulating system with an attached antenna was placed on the skin, overlying an implanted radio frequency receiver connected to the stimulating electrode. The system was thus externally activated. Recent developments, however, provide for a fully implanted stimulating system, which is comparable to that used for cardiac pacemaking. Such "total implants" are externally programmable, and once programmed, will carry out stimulation at desired stimulus strength, rate, and timing by an internal time control device. A drawback of such systems is the need to replace batteries when they become exhausted. Battery life depends on usage, but with stimulation parameters normally used for DBS, at least 3–5 years of effective stimulation may be anticipated before battery output ceases.

Electrical stimulation via chronically implanted electrodes produces no alteration in the patient's normal sensory function. In fact, it produces no alteration in any aspect of neurological function in the absence of complications. Stimulation of VPL or VPM elicits a sensation of "tingling" in the body region, which corresponds somatotopically to the area stimulated.

The brain-stimulating electrodes are implanted stereotactically through a small burr hole under local anesthesia. Intraoperative stimulation is essential to confirm correct placement of the electrodes in the desired brain target. Percutaneous extension leads from the electrodes are allowed to exit from the scalp through tiny stab wounds. Over a period of several days to several weeks following electrode implantation, stimulation is carried out via an external stimulator connected to the percutaneous extension leads. The purpose of the trial period is to ascertain the most desirable stimulation parameters, and to confirm that the patient's pain is actually relieved by stimulation. In about 10%–15% of patients, initial pain relief does not occur and the electrodes are removed. If pain relief occurs during the trial stimulation period, then the electrodes are internalized and connected, either to the radio frequency stimulation system, or to the fully implanted stimulated system at a second brief operation. The presence of the stimulating system does not interfere with normal activities of daily living, and the system is flexible and strong enough to tolerate vigorous physical exercise of all types. In a rare instance, a direct blow delivered to the head, neck, or upper chest may result in malfunction of the system and the need for replacement.

The author has had experience, beginning in 1978, with implantation of chronic stimulating electrodes for treatment of chronic pain in over 200 patients. The incidence of pain relief is related to the type of pain problem that the patient experiences. Patients presenting with arachnoiditis and other forms of chronic back and leg pain, following previous lumbar spine surgery, experience pain relief in about 65% of cases. For other types of pain of peripheral origin, a similar high rate of pain relief is experienced. A lower rate of approximately 45%–50% of patients with pain related to deafferentation experience pain relief. Examples of the latter type of pain syndromes include pain following peripheral nerve injury, causalgia, spinal cord injury, postherpetic neuralgia, anesthesia dolorosa, postcordotomy dysesthesias, and the thalamic syndrome.

Complications of the brain electrode procedure include brain injury, intracranial hemorrhage, and infection. Injury to the brain from the mere placement of the electrodes is extremely uncommon. The author has experienced contralateral hemiparesis in two patients after electrode placement, both of which cleared subsequently. Abnormalities in eye movements, mainly diplopia, may occur with placement of electrodes in the periaqueductal gray region of the brain stem. Such double vision is usually transient, but in a rare patient, may be persistent. Electrode infection occurs in approximately 5% of patients. In about half of the infections, suitable treatment with antibiotics will clear the infection; however, if an infection is not resolved with antibiotics, removal of the hardware is required. The author has experienced no deaths with the electrode implant procedure, although rare deaths have been reported by other neurosurgeons.

The most distressing problem related to brain stimulation is the so-called "tolerance" phenomenon. Tolerance refers to patients who receive excellent pain relief at the time of electrode placement, but who, with the passage of time, experience progressively less effective pain relief from stimulation, and progressive return of their original pain. In patients with arachnoiditis, about 30%–35% of patients experience such tolerance phenomena, and in patients with central or deafferentation pain, the tolerance phenomenon occurs in up to 50% of patients. Some investigtors have felt that tolerance, which occurs with stimulation, is similar to that which occurs with the use of exogenous opiate substances. The author's investigations, however, indicate that such is rarely the case in the human situation. Recent animal studies indicate that a variety of other neurotransmitter substances, other than opiates, are involved in the modulation and regulation of pain appreciation. These include catecholamines, serotonin, and acetylcholine, among others. In addition, recent animal studies have indicated that a large number of other targets within the brain may produce analgesia when electrically stimulated. Such targets are located in the hypothalamus, the brain stem, and the parabrachial nucleus of the pons. Electrical stimulation of the brain offers a means of treating chronic pain in selected patients without impairment of normal neurological function. The procedure is limited by the development of tolerance in a significant proportion of patients, but the possibility of electrical stimulation in other targets may obviate this problem in the future.

BIBLIOGRAPHY

Hosobuchi Y: Subcortical electrical stimulation for control of intractable pain in humans. *J Neurosurg* 1986; 64:543–553.

Richardson DE: Pain reduction by electrical stimulation in man. Part 2: Chronic self-administration in the periventricular gray matter. *J Neurosurg* 1977; 47:184–189.

Turnbull IM, Shulman R, Woodhurst WB: Thalamic stimulation for neuropathic pain. *J Neurosurg* 1980; 52:486–493.

Young RF, Kroening R, Fulton W, et al: Electrical stimulation of the brain in treatment of chronic pain: Experience over 5 years. *J Neurosurg* 1985; 62:389–396.

Young RF, Chambi VI: Pain relief by electrical stimulation of the periaqueductal and periventricular gray matter: Evidence for a non-opioid mechanism. *J Neurosurg* 1987; 66:346–371.

32

Coccygodynia

Verne L. Brechner, M.D.

The patient is a 24-year-old athletic woman who is nulliparous and recently experienced a fall in which she struck her buttocks firmly across a hard object. Subsequent to this, she developed pain in the low paracoccygeal area, mainly on the left. The pain had persisted for a period of 2 months. The pain was increased by lifting and straining, particularly when resuming a standing position from a squatting position. The pain did not, in itself, interfere with sexual intercourse. There was some mild discomfort with defecation, but the pain had become severe enough that it was interfering with her work activities as a secretary. She was unable to sit for any prolonged period of time. Examination revealed that the coccyx itself was not painful. A finger inserted through the rectum could approach the coccyx ventrally while the thumb on the exterior of the perineum could grasp the dorsal portion of the coccyx. The coccyx could then be moved from side to side to some degree and ventrally dorsally to some degree without provoking any pain. There was no evidence of a pilonidal cyst. Pelvic examination was entirely negative. However, on bimanual rectal examination, there was an area of exquisite tenderness in the soft tissue just lateral to the left of the sacral cornu. Nothing could be palpated in this area and magnetic resonance imaging (MRI) did not reveal any structural defect. However, this tenderness was quite exquisite and was quite localized. It was also felt that the paracoccygeal muscles were, to some extent, more tense on the left than on the right. On several occasions, the paracoccygeal muscles were stroked gently. The area of point tenderness was injected with local anesthesia and the patient was instructed to take sitz baths twice a day, and was also given instruction concerning proper posture while sitting (i.e., to sit upright in a straight-backed chair and distribute the weight equally on the tuberosities of the ischium), to avoid entirely sitting in a slouched position or leaning back on a couch. Over a period of 6 weeks, the symptoms progressively decreased until they were absent.

DISCUSSION

Coccygodynia is a term describing pain in or about the coccyx. It is a symptom and not a diagnosis. The first reference to surgical excision of a coccyx for a painful condition was in 1726, when a coccygectomy was done by Jean Louis Petit. Considering that this operation was accomplished more than 100 years prior to the discovery of anesthesia, it is awesome to contemplate the intensity of pain preoperatively that would induce a patient to endure such an operation, and the stubborn determination of the surgeon to heal a patient by performing the procedure.

In 1859, J.Y. Simpson published a lecture on coccygodynia and defined the condition as "pain in the coccyx and neighboring regions."[1] It should be emphasized that at this early date, a separation was made between pain generated within the coccyx itself and pain arising from the "neighboring regions," all encompassed by the term "coccygodynia." It was recognized early on that coccygodynia is a condition primarily affecting females, the ratio between male and female being approximately 1:5. It was also recognized that it involved mainly young adults to middle-aged individuals, that is ages 20–50 years. A high incidence of trauma involving the buttocks, whether by a fall or by vaginal delivery, was also recognized.

The higher incidence of this condition in females is possibly explained by anatomical differences that make the coccyx more vulnerable to trauma in the female than in the male. The female possesses a wider pelvis and shorter sacrum, which is less curved than in the male. The sciatic notches in the female are of wider diameter. Also, the ischial tuberosities are more widely separated in the female and are somewhat everted. Therefore, the coccyx is in a more exposed condition and, therefore, more vulnerable when compared to the male coccyx, which is more "tucked in" than in the female. The coccyx consists of 3–5 segments that are joined to the sacrum with a synarthrosis. Mobility at this synarthrosis increases during pregnancy, thus enhancing its vulnerability to injury. Anteriorly and laterally, the coccyx attaches to the sacrococcygeal ligaments and muscles, as well as to the ligament of the levator ani muscle. S4 and S5 roots supply the coccygeus muscle and S4 supplies the levator ani. Although conditions involving the coccyx itself have been emphasized by orthopedists as being a major cause of coccygeal pain, proctologists, such as Thiele, have emphasized the importance of spasm of the sacrococcygeal and levator ani muscles, as well as the associated structures, such as the piriformis.[2]

A pragmatic classification of coccygodynia is divided into two groups: (1) coccygodynia associated with conditions involving the coccyx itself; and (2) coccygeal pain involving the structures related to the coccyx. In the first group, trauma is the major cause. This trauma may be acute, as following a fall, or may be chronic as related to poor posture in sitting. Although it is frequently emphasized that the coccyx should be studied for evidence of fracture, such fractures are rarely seen. An extensive review by Duncan of 262 patients with painful coccyx in which the x-rays were compared with 100 male and 100 female patients with no coccygeal problems resulted in the statement, "almost any variation of a coccyx except a fracture or dislocation that is noted in a patient with painful coccyx can be matched in a roentgenogram of the coccyx of a patient who has never complained of pain in the coccygeal region."[3] Actual pathological conditions involving the coccyx that have been identified include avascular necrosis resulting from median sacral artery occlusion, coccygeal body tumor, chordoma, giant cell tumor, interosseous lipoma, metastatic tumor, ependymoma, reticular cell sarcoma, neurofibroma, meningocele, and subfascial fat deposits. Each of these conditions are described in the literature as rare observations.

Of the conditions in the second group, which have been identified as provoking coccygodynia, teratoma, cauda equina tumor, hydatid disease, Ewings' presacral tumor, and pelvic tension have been described. In the male, such inflammatory conditions as urethritis, seminal vesiculitis, prostatitis, cystitis, anal fistulae, pylonidal cysts, and anorectal abscess have been described, while cervicitis, endometriosis, salpingitis, cystitis, vaginitis, anal fissure, proctitis and, again, pylonidal cyst have been described in the female. It is interesting to note that although the obstetrician Simpson was the first to coin the name "coccygodynia," in our present demographics only 3% of patients with coccygodynia are identified in the immediate postpartum period. It seems that the most common association of coccygodynia is with that of muscular spasm of the sacrococcygeal muscles and levator ani as described by Thiele. Rarely is a glomus tumor in the paracoccygeal area identified.

Treatment of coccygodynia vary from the original coccygectomy described in the 16th century, through a variety of less invasive procedures such as injections of alcohol in and about the coccyx and involving the parasacral nerves, to the more subdued conservative approaches such as improving sitting posture, local injections of anesthetics and steroid, manual massage of the coccygeal and levator ani muscles, judicious use of analgesics, and sitz baths.

The division between a surgical approach and a conservative approach depends upon demonstration of a pain mechanism actually involving the coccyx itself, or the immediately adjacent areas. Obviously, a pilonidal cyst has a surgical solution. Less obvious conditions such as avascular necrosis of the coccyx or fracture and dislocation of the coccyx may be suspected by x-ray or physical examination, but even these conditions should not require immediate surgical intervention. Invasive therapy should be approached only after at least a 6-month trial of conservative therapy has proven ineffective. When patients are carefully selected on the basis of fracture or dislocation of the coccyx, or a pathological condition involving the coccyx itself, the results of coccygectomy are quite encouraging. The most frequently quoted paper concerning coccygectomy is that of Albert Keye, and he is quite specific in stating that the diagnosis of pain arising from the coccyx itself, as the result of trauma or some other pathology, is necessary prior to surgery.[4] He also emphasized careful reconstruction of the pelvic floor after removal of the coccyx, thus emphasizing the integrity of the paracoccygeal muscles and the pelvic floor. With the exception of patients in whom surgery is obviously indicated, all treatment should be directed along conservative lines. There is throughout the literature, a consistent theme condemning the use of neurolytic agents because the possibility of catastrophic complication far outweighs the possibility of any benefits. Youmans, in 1919, stated very clearly the philosophy of conservative treatment of coccygodynia: "The fact that many methods of treatment have yielded many varying degrees of success is the best evidence of their unreliability."[5] With such a clear statement of prudent approach to therapy, one should eliminate initially all of the therapies that carry with them the possibility of exaggerated side effects or complications.

REFERENCES

1. Simpson JY: Coccygodynia and diseases and deformities of the coccyx. *Medical Times Gazette* 1859; 1:861.
2. Thiele GH: Coccygodynia: Cause & treatment. *Dis Colon Rectum* 1963; 6:422–436.
3. Duncan GA: Painful coccyx. *Arch Surg* 1937; 34:1088–1104.
4. Keye A: Operative treatment of coccygodynia. *J Bone Joint Surg [Am]* 1937; 19:759–764.
5. Youmans FC: Coccygodynia, further experiences with injections of alcohol in its treatment. *Surg Gynecol Obstet* 1919; 29:612–613.

PART VI

Lower Extremity Pain

33

Phantom Limb Pain of the Lower Extremities

John Rowlingson, M.D.

A previously healthy, right-handed, 36-year-old white man was working in a field with a large auger, when the mechanism jammed. He got into the hole in the ground to help redirect the equipment by wrapping his arms around the bit. The machine suddenly re-engaged, resulting in the traumatic amputation of both arms at the shoulder level. Surgical reimplantation attempts failed, and the patient suffered phantom pain bilaterally with the pain greater in the right upper extremity than the left. He was referred for evaluation 1 1/2 years after his accident secondary to his persistent phantom pain. He reported a constant tingling, which became worse at the end of the day. He also had nearly intolerable constant, burning pain in the right hand and wrist and occasional episodes of excruciating, lancinating pain in the right distal arm. His self-designed treatment for this was to slam his foot into the ground until it hurt him. His pain could also be elicited by discussion of other's pain or seeing a knife cut meat. Physical examination revealed a male with bilateral upper extremity amputations and well-healed scars. There were no neuromas found in the stumps. Treatment with a TENS unit with the electrodes placed at the distal ends of the stumps, turned on for 60 minutes and then turned off for 60 minutes during waking hours produced an encouraging decrease in his phantom limb pain. He was also placed on amitriptyline, 50 mg orally for every hour of sleep (QHS), with additional benefit. Follow-up at 3 months after the initiation of this treatment showed a persistent achievement of 60% reduction in his phantom pain. He needs continued follow-up and is receiving prosthesis training.

DISCUSSION

It is critical that patients who will become amputees understand that the occurrence of phantom sensations is nearly universal (80%–90% of cases).[1] The opportunity to explain this to J.P. was nonexistent given the acute nature of his injury and the subsequent life-saving surgery. These sensations usually begin immediately after the loss of the limb, with tingling that is neither pleasant nor unpleasant being the most common one reported.[1-2] The phantom limb is more likely to be in a position of rest than an abnormal posture, with upper extremity amputees having symptoms more frequently and for longer periods than lower extremity amputees. Over time the phantom sensations decrease in intensity and the limb seems to telescope partially or wholly back into the trunk. This may take 2–3 years.[1] Factors that seem to favor a longer duration of the symptoms include upper extremity amputation more than lower extremity limb loss, old age, shorter stumps vs. longer ones, sudden loss vs. that secondary to chronic disease, and being male.[1] Our patient had all these factors except old age.

The incidence of phantom pain is reported to vary between 1–85%.[1, 3, 4] This is a problem of no small magnitude. It demands treatment because of the devastating effect this chronic pain problem has on the patient and his family, the allocation of health care resources, and the socioeconomics of society. The wide variation in incidence probably relates in part to the study of different populations of patients with amputations, i.e., aged, civilians versus military personnel, as well as the circumstances under which the amputation occurred, the definition of phantom pain used in the study, the time after the amputation, and the psychosocial status of the patient. Jensen et al., studied the incidence of phantom pain in 58 patients at various intervals after amputation occurred and reported the incidence of pain at 8 days, 6 months, and 2 years to be 72%, 65%, and 59%, respectively.[4]

The pain may begin immediately after limb loss or it may manifest itself days, weeks, or months later. It may be intermittent or constant, spontaneous, or precipitated by such varied events as visceral functions, physical activity, emotional upset, or weather change.[1] The pain may be described as cramping, shooting, burning, crushing, sharp, stabbing, pricking, lancinating, aching, squeezing, or as if the digits are twisted or the fingernails digging into the palm with the fist tightly clenched.[1, 2, 4] Greater phantom pain has been associated with being male, being older, with upper extremity loss, with patients who feel that they cannot voluntarily move the phantom limbs and with those patients who had pain in the limb preamputation.

The mechanisms for phantom pain must be stated so that the treatment options can be better understood. In the review of available therapeutic modalities by Sherman et al., patients reported at least an avoidance by their doctors to talk about treatment for phantom pain, if not the implication that they were crazy or that the phantom pain was all psychological.[5] Given the contemporary understanding of chronic pain, pure psychological causation is highly unlikely. That psychological consequences can result in a patient having to endure chronic, intractable pain is now common knowledge, and patients with phantom pain deserve unending emotional support.[1]

Just as phantom sensations must be distinguished from phantom pain, so must reasons for pain that relate to the stump.[1] The stump must have a well-healed scar and be free of redundant skin and subcutaneous tissue that can become irritated by the prosthesis. Pain in the bony component of the stump is usually secondary to osteomyelitis, but can also result from osteomas or spurs. The vascular supply to the stump must be adequate for tissue viability. Signs of inadequate blood flow might include edema, blanching, ulceration, and colder temperature. A most commonly identified source of stump pain is the presence of neuromas. These represent sprouts from the cut nerves that become twisted and matted together and are exceedingly sensitive to mechanical pressure, irritation, and stretching of the tissue (muscles, fascia, skin, subcutaneous tissue) in which they are located.

A most popular theory to explain phantom limb pain involves changes that occur in the nervous system itself when nerves are cut. It is well known that when peripheral nerves are severed, retrograde changes occur up the axon, even to the level of the dorsal horn cell body. This results in changes in neural transmission patterns and modified input to the CNS. That there can be an imprinting phenomenon on the nervous system because of pain prior to amputation has been proposed by a number of authors.[1, 4, 6] Jensen et al., cites the fact that 57 of 58 patients they studied had pain in the limb prior to amputation, and the incidence of phantom pain being less in patients with no preamputation pain or those having shorter duration of pain, as reasons that phantom pain in some patients may represent "surviving" preamputation pain.[4]

Melzack has proposed that phantom pain results from a combination of events.[6] The gate control theory states that there is a gating mechanism at the spinal cord level that modifies sensory input from peripheral nerves. With a decrease in fiber diameter and conduction speed in peripheral nerves after amputation comes a biasing of the system to small fiber input, which is associated with pain. Furthermore, there may be a central biasing mechanism (CBM) in the brainstem reticular formation. This normally exerts a tonic inhibitory effect on all synaptic levels of the somatic projection system. Thus, when amputation decreases the number of peripheral sensory fibers, there is a concomitant decrease in input to the reticular formation. This results in less inhibitory influence on synaptic transmission and allows for more self-sustained activity from the synapses of the somatic projection system.

MANAGEMENT

Numerous authors have discouraging comments to make about the success of treatment for phantom limb pain. Katz states that there is " . . . no treatment that is consistently successful in relieving phantom limb pain."[1] Bach et al., imply that phantom pain is difficult to treat and so far no surgical or medical treatment has proven effective.[2] Sherman et al., reviewed the current treatments in the U.S.A. as recently as 1980 and concluded that " . . . there is no widely recognized, highly successful method of treating phantom limb pain."[5] In a further study comparing civilian with military amputees, Sherman et al., found only a 1% treatment effectiveness rate.[3] This may be due, in part, to difficulties in absolutely identifying *the* cause of the pain (i.e., local vs. central mechanisms), and the fact that "pain," especially chronic pain, can have such varied significance and meaning. The favorable results from small studies with few patients and short-term follow-up have not been confirmed when large studies with longer follow-ups are done.[5]

As in any patient with impending treatment, the diagnosis must be explained and the rationale for the chosen therapy discussed. Medications are a common first choice for decreasing pain. But one must question whether phantom pain warrants a mild analgesic, such as acetaminophen, an anti-inflammatory drug, or chronic narcotics. Urban et al., have recently reported on the safe use of 10–20 mg of methadone a day in five patients with chronic, intractable phantom pain.[7] These investigators also had their patients on doxepin or amitriptyline 25–150 mg qd. It is common practice in the management of chronic pain to use such drugs to increase CNS serotonin and enhance endogenous pain suppression circuits. The chronic use of sedatives and tranquilizers would not encourage the patient to participate in pain-distracting activity and may impair central mechanisms for modifying pain input.[1] Anticonvulsants are used in the management of neuralgic pain and can be tried in patients with phantom pain.

The list of surgical procedures tried in the management of phantom limb pain is incredible.[1, 5] Many carry a high risk to the patient since they are neurodestructive, so great caution is advised. Naturally, meticulous surgical technique is expected at the time of the amputation procedure, and allowing the cut nerves to retract back into the protection of normal tissues may do as much as anything to minimize the likelihood of phantom pain. One may logically consider surgical procedures for the removal of stump neuromas or even sympathectomy if such procedures have been shown to be effective in decreasing pain after injections with local anesthetics or steroids. Trigger point injections and peripheral somatic nerve, sympathetic, epidural, and differential spinal blocks have all been used for diagnostic and therapeutic purposes in patients.[1] Bach et al., have recently reported on the benefit of lumbar epidural blocks in 25 patients.[2] They reasoned that, because phantom pain is similar to the pain experienced preoperatively, modifying the pain preoperatively could influence phantom pain. In a study of 25 patients with painful limbs, 11 were given lumbar epidural blocks with bupivicaine hydrochloride (Marcaine), with or without epidural morphine to make them pain-free for 3 days prior to the amputation surgery. The remaining 14 patients were given only routine analgesics. All were evaluated by standard interview at 7 days, 6 months, and 1 year, and the results showed that the incidence of phantom limb pain was decreased in the first year by lumbar epidural block. Decreasing both sensory input and possible abnormal reflex activity, and decreasing sympathetic nervous system overactivity were cited as explanations for the positive benefit. The incidence of phantom pain in the control group was not unlike that of other studies.

Therapies that stimulate the nervous system and could influence spinal gates or the CMB have been reported.[1] Percussion therapy of the stump has historical interest and similar, modern day therapies could include TENS, acupuncture, ultrasound, whirlpool, and massage. Physical therapy is important because it provides access to many of these therapies and aids the patients with prosthesis fitting, gait training, and extremity use. As stated before, all patients with phantom limb pain deserve emotional support and reassurance. Obviously, formal psychotherapy in the form of biofeedback, relaxation training, or hypnosis will have additive effects by helping with pain control or at least aiding the patient to cope with chronic pain. Active rehabilitation will help the patient resume *productive* activity and restore self-esteem.

In summary (combining the recommendations of Sherman et al., and Sherman and Tippins), the comprehensive recommendations for the management of phantom limb pain are: (1) begin therapy by discussing with the patient prior to amputation that phantom sensations are normal and that phantom pain is less common and influenced by anxiety, tension, and chronic stress; (2) provide appropriate therapy for areas that are referring pain into the phantom limb; (3) use EMG biofeedback from the stump and injection of neuromas to decrease the stump pain-spasm cycle; (4) use sympathetic nerve blocks, temperature biofeedback, and chemical-sympathetic depressant drugs to decrease peripheral sympathetic arousal; (5) obtain maximal functional use of the limb with an appropriate, well-fitted prosthesis and gait correction; (6) consider chemical, behavioral, and relaxation techniques to decrease stress, anxiety, and depression that amplify chronic pain; (7) use TENS, ultrasound, acupuncture, and hypnosis to disrupt self-sustaining pain cycles; (8) assess the patient's "need" for the pain and, if great, refer to a pain management center or a pain clinic.[5, 8]

REFERENCES

1. Katz RL: Postamputation pain. *Semin Anesth* 1985; 4:332–345.
2. Bach S, Noreng MF, Tjellden NU: Phantom limb pain in amputees during the first 12 months following limb amputation, after preoperative lumbar epidural blockade. *Pain* 1988; 33:297–301.
3. Sherman RA, Sherman CJ: A comparison of phantom sensations among amputees whose amputations were of civilian and military origin. *Pain* 1985; 21:91–97.
4. Jensen TS, Krebs B, Nielsen J, et al: Immediate and long-term phantom limb pain in amputees: Incidence, clinical characteristics and relationship to pre-amputation limb pain. *Pain* 1985; 21:267–278.
5. Sherman RA, Sherman CJ, Gall NG: A surgery of current phantom limb pain treatment in the United States. *Pain* 1980; 9:85–89.
6. Melzack R: Phantom limb pain: Indications for treatment of pathologic pain. *Anesthesiology* 1971; 35:409–419.
7. Urban BJ, France RD, Steinberger EK, et al: Long-term use of narcotic-antidepressant medication in the management of phantom limb pain. *Pain* 1986; 24:191–196.
8. Sherman RA, Tippins JK: Suggest guidelines for treatment of phantom limb pain. *Orthopedics* 1982; 5:1595–1600.

34

Reflex Sympathetic Dystrophy of the Lower Extremity

Steven D. Waldman, M.D.

Kathy Waldman, B.S., O.T.R.

A 32-year-old woman sustained a contusion to the dorsum of her right foot when she dropped a brake shoe on her foot while working on an assembly line. Over the ensuing 3 weeks, the patient experienced burning pain and swelling involving the entire foot and distal lower extremity (Fig. 34–1). The patient found it increasingly difficult to bear weight on the affected extremity and it soon became impossible to wear a shoe. Plain radiographs taken by the company physician were reported negative for bony abnormalities. Nonsteroidal anti-inflammatory agents were prescribed without significant amelioration of her pain symptomatology. Physical therapy was prescribed, but had to be discontinued because the patient felt that the treatments were making her pain worse. Oxycodone hydrochloride was prescribed with only mild relief of the patient's ever worsening pain. Additionally, the patient noted significant sleep disturbance because of the pain. She was referred to the pain management center for evaluation of "psychogenic pain" and probable chemical dependence to narcotic analgesics.

DISCUSSION

We are presented with the problem of a healthy 32-year-old female patient who sustained seemingly minor trauma to the dorsum of her right foot while at work.

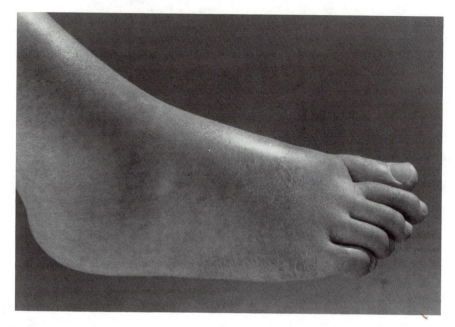

FIG 34–1.
Photograph of reflex sympathetic dystrophy of the distal right lower extremity.

Despite the best efforts of her physician, the pain worsened. She was sent to the pain management center as a last ditch effort for evaluation and treatment of her pain, which her physician had characterized as "psychogenic," and to deal with her increasing demands for narcotic analgesics.

The patient related a history of dropping a brake shoe which weighed less than 2 lbs onto the dorsum of her right foot. The patient further stated that she did not think much about the injury at the time and, in fact, did not seek the attention of the plant nurse. She noticed a small bruised area on the dorsum of the foot that night. The following morning, the foot was more swollen, causing some difficulty in putting on her shoe. Her pain became more severe as the day progressed and she sought the advice of the plant nurse. The nurse informed the patient that in all probability, she simply bruised the top of her foot and suggested that the patient elevate the foot when she finished her shift at work. The next day, the patient was unable to bear weight on her right foot or wear a shoe. When she called in sick for work, the plant nurse advised the patient to continue to elevate her foot and take aspirin for pain. In spite of this treatment regimen, the patient continued to experience more pain. She sought the advice of the company doctor. The doctor evaluated the patient the following day, and concurred with the nurse that the patient had, in all likelihood, bruised her foot. He stated that "in order to be on the safe side," he obtain an x-ray of the foot. The plain radiograph was read and showed no evidence of bony abnormality or fracture. On physical examination, moderate soft tissue swelling was noted over the dorsum of the foot. Ibuprofen 800 mg three times daily was prescribed without benefit. Physical therapy consisting of whirlpool and active-assisted range of motion and gait training was ordered, but was discontinued by the patient because of the marked increase in pain following each session. Oxycodone hydrochloride was then prescribed with only minor improvement in her pain symptomatology. Increasing doses were taken in an effort to obtain pain relief. The patient stated that she was told by the company physician that she was uncooperative because she refused to continue physical therapy, and that the pain was "all in her head." The patient viewed her referral to the pain management center, some 6 months after the initial injury, as punitive and as an effort to prove that, in fact, the patient did not have pain.

PHYSICAL EXAM

The patient's vital signs were as follows: blood pressure 120/80 mm Hg, pulse 88 beats per minute; temperature 98.6°F. The patient walked with an antalgic gait. Her right foot was shoeless, covered only with a loose white stocking. Funduscopic exam was benign, the remainder of her eye, ear, nose, and throat exam being within normal limits. Cranial nerves II through XII were intact. The thyroid was normal and no supraclavicular adenopathy was present. Auscultation of the heart and lungs was unremarkable. Low back examination was normal. Upper extremity motor and sensory exam was within normal limits. Deep tendon reflexes of both the upper and lower extremity were physiologic. Motor and sensory exam, as well as evaluation of the peripheral vasculature of the left lower extremity, were within normal limits. Evaluation of the right lower extremity revealed a grossly swollen and discolored foot and ankle that was moist and cool to touch. The toenails were thickened and untrimmed. Sensory evaluation revealed severe allodynia over the entire affected area with the most sensitive area being the skin overlying the dorsum of the foot. The skin in this area felt indurated to palpation and no dorsalis pedis or posterior tibial pulses could be detected. Hair growth was patchy over the calf and absent distally. Adequate motor testing could not be carried out because of the severe pain the patient experienced with touch or movement of the distal lower extremity. However, it was noted that the patient was unable to fully dorsiflex or plantarflex her ankle and toes.

LABORATORY AND RADIOGRAPHIC EVALUATION

Results of the patient's complete blood count, automated chemistry, and thyroid profile were reported as normal. The erythrocyte sedimentation rate was also reported as normal. Plain radiographs of the bilateral ankles and feet revealed diffuse osteopenia involving the entire right lower extremity, as well as significant soft tissue swelling. No fracture was seen. An electromyogram and nerve conduction velocities of the back and affected extremity were normal, with no evidence of radiculopathy or entrapment neuropathy. A diagnostic procedure was performed.

CLINICAL DESCRIPTION

The salient feature that should stand out when reviewing this patient's care is the history of trauma with resultant pain that felt to be far out of proportion to the degree of injury. This single fact alone should lead the astute clinician to strongly consider the diagnosis of reflex sympathetic dystrophy (RSD).

This syndrome is characterized by constant burning pain, swelling, hyperesthesia, allodynia, and vasomotor and sudomotor changes that, if untreated, may progress to irreversible trophic changes. The pain of RSD is diffuse and does not follow the distribution of radicular segments or peripheral nerves. Local tissue damage involving either central or peripheral nerves appears to initiate a reflex hyperactivity of the sympathetic nervous system, which ultimately results in this symptom complex called RSD. Although the precipitating insults that serve to initiate this reflex response are many (Table 34–1), the common denominator in the vast majority of cases appears to be tissue damage secondary to trauma. Table 34–2 defines some of the more common clinical variants of RSD. As can be readily seen from a review of these definitions, these seemingly separate disease entities have many clinical features in common and, in all likelihood, are the result of the same pathologic process.

In addition to sharing many clinical features, the disease entities also have in common the fact that pain and the attendant vasomotor and sudomotor changes associated with these syndromes are invariably improved and often cured with interruption of the sympathetic nerves subserving the pain.

DIAGNOSIS

The diagnosis of RSD should be considered when: (1) there is a history of trauma, tissue damage, and/or infection; (2) there is constant, burning and/or aching pain that is out of proportion and worsens with physical contact and use,

TABLE 34–1.

Precipitating Factors and Diseases Associated With the Development of Reflex Sympathetic Dystrophy

Soft tissue injury
Operative procedures
Sprains, fractures, and dislocations
Vascular thrombosis
Infection
Radiculopathy
Tendonitis and bursitis
Arthritis
Carpal tunnel syndrome
Malignancy
Immobilization
Myocardial infarction
Cerebral infarction
Brain tumor
Subarachnoid hemorrhage
Cervical cord injury
Head injury
Poliomyelitis
Syringomyelia

but does not follow the distribution of radicular or peripheral nerves; (3) there are vasomotor and/or sudomotor abnormalities; and (4) there are trophic changes.

Winnie has stated that "RSD is the syphilis of the 20th century," because it can mimic many other disease entities. The ability of RSD to mimic other disease states probably is a reflection of the fact that RSD can present at many different points along the continuum of the RSD symptom complex. Because of

TABLE 34–2.

Clinical Variants of Reflex Sympathetic Dystrophy

Syndrome	Description
Causalgia major	RSD symptom complex that occurs with peripheral nerve injury
Causalgia minor	RSD symptom complex that occurs after trauma but in the absence of peripheral nerve injury
Reflex sympathetic dystrophy	RSD symptom complex
Sudek's atrophy	RSD symptom complex with osteopenia that occurs after soft tissue trauma
Shoulder-hand syndrome	RSD symptom complex with frozen shoulder that occurs after myocardial infarction, stroke, or cervical radiculopathy
Algoneurodystrophy	RSD symptom complex that occurs after minor trauma

the nonspecific nature of the symptoms within the complex, i.e., swelling, pain, decreased range of motion, hypersensitivity, care must be taken to rule out other diseases that may be mistakenly diagnosed as RSD. For this reason, the diagnosis of RSD must be one of exclusion.

Radiographic studies are useful in helping to support the clinical diagnosis of RSD. Plain radiographs will reveal patchy demineralization early in the disease as well as soft tissue swelling. If the disease remains untreated, diffuse demineralization will appear, followed by subchondral crumbling erosions. As the disease progresses, ankylosis may appear. Radionucleotide scanning will generally reveal findings consistent with increased blood flow to the affected part, and increased periarticular uptake. It should be noted that the findings of both plain radiographs and radionucleotide studies, while suggestive of RSD, have a low specificity and other conditions that increase bone turnover, such as infection, hyperparathyroidism, and thyrotoxicosis may mimic these findings.

Routine laboratory testing is usually normal in RSD. Complete blood count should be done to rule out an increased white count that may suggest infection and to identify the presence of anemia that may be associated with collagen vascular disease or chronic illness.

A normal erythrocyte sedimentation rate helps rule out occult infection or unsuspected collagen vascular diseases, such as scleroderma, that may mimic RSD. Thyroid profile to rule out hyper/hypothyroidism, as well as serum calcium determination to rule out parathyroid abnormalities are also indicated.

Electromyography and nerve conduction studies are indicated in patients with RSD to rule out somatic nerve injury and to rule out syndromes causing neural compromise, such as carpal tunnel syndrome, that may serve as the triggering factor for RSD.

Since trauma is invariably present, when considering a diagnosis of RSD the clinician must be careful to rule out occult infection or injury to the vasculature that may result in a symptom complex that mimics RSD. When trauma resulting in laceration or crush injury with loss of skin integrity occurs, osteomyelitis should always be ruled out prior to attributing all symptoms present to RSD (although the two diseases certainly may coexist together). Failure to appropriately diagnose and treat osteomyelitis may lead to significant morbidity. Diabetics, immunocompromised patients, and those suffering from sickle cell anemia, are particularly susceptible to osteomyelitis. The bone loss associated with such infections may be incorrectly attributed to RSD. The normal temperature, white blood cell count, and sedimentation rate, coupled with intact skin integrity, made occult osteomyelitis unlikely in the patient presented above.

Superficial thrombophlebitis, alone or in combination with deep thrombophlebitis, must also be ruled out prior to attributing all symptoms present to RSD (although again, the two may coexist together). Venography and plethysmography, is indicated if thrombophlebitis is suspected.

TABLE 34–3.

Treatments Advocated for Reflex Sympathetic Dystrophy

Sympathetic nerve block with local anesthetic with or without steroid
Somatic nerve block with local anesthetic with or without steroid
Intravenous regional anesthesia with local anesthetic and steroid
Intravenous regional technique with guanethedine sulfate
Intravenous regional technique with reserpine
Intravenous regional technique with bretyllium
Physical therapy
Transcutaneous nerve stimulation (TENS)
Immobilization with casting
Corticosteroids
Beta blockers
Calcium channel blockers
Alpha blockers
Intra-arterial reserpine
Surgical sympathectomy
Hypnosis

The best diagnostic test to confirm the clinical suspicions of RSD is the use of differential neural blockade. By utilizing this technique on either a pharmacologic or anatomic basis as the clinical situation dictates, one may confirm, with a high degree of certainty, the diagnosis of RSD. In view of the devastating consequences of missing the diagnosis of RSD, coupled with the high incidence of this diagnoses being missed in patients suffering from unexplained pain, differential neural blockade must be considered as a sine qua non of the diagnostic workup. The diagnostic procedure performed on this patient was a lumbar sympathetic nerve block. The patient experienced no relief when preservative-free saline was injected, but experienced almost immediate relief of pain when 0.5% lidocaine was administered.

TREATMENT

Although many treatments have been advocated to treat RSD (Table 34–3), the mainstay of treatment is the interruption of the sympathetic nerves subserving the reflex cycle, utilizing neural blockade with local anesthetics. The choice of technique of sympathetic blockade is based on the anatomic part affected, the risk-to-benefit ratio of one nerve block technique versus another (as with the use of lumbar sympathetic block versus lumbar epidural block), and the experience of the anesthesiologist administering the block.

For upper extremity or facial RSD, stellate ganglion block with local anesthetic, either alone or in combination with steroid, may be carried out on a daily basis. Brachial plexus block or intravenous regional anesthesia with local anesthetic and steroid may be used as an alternative method to produce sympathetic blockade for upper extremity RSD. Since these techniques produce somatic blockade in addition to sympathetic blockade, they may be beneficial in settings where somatic neural blockade is needed to allow manipulation or therapy of the affected part. For lower extremity RSD, lumbar sympathetic neural blockade may be carried out on a daily basis. In this setting, many authors feel that after the diagnosis of lower extremity RSD is established, therapeutic lumbar epidural blocks may be substituted as the procedure of choice, since they are less painful for the patient, and have a more favorable risk-to-benefit ratio when compared to lumbar sympathetic block in the hands of most anesthesiologists. Intravenous regional anesthesia with local anesthetic and steroid may also be utilized as an alternative treatment for these patients. The frequency and number of nerve blocks should be based on the individual response of the patient. Aggressive daily neural blockade over a period of weeks may be required to obtain complete and permanent relief of symptoms. Should symptoms recur after complete relief has been obtained, neural blockade should immediately be reimplemented.

Intravenous regional administration of reserpine, guanethedine and bretylium have been advocated as an effective treatment for RSD of the extremities. Our results with this approach have been disappointing when compared with the previously mentioned therapeutic modalities, and cannot be recommended as a first-line treatment. Results with intra-arterial reserpine have been equally disappointing.

In patients who cannot tolerate or refuse neural blockade, a trial of systemic corticosteroids may be indicated. Prednisone may be administered orally in dosage ranges of 80–100 mg on a daily basis for 2 weeks, and then tapered by 5 mg per day. Obviously, the administration of high dose corticosteroids is not without risk; however, in view of the poor long-term outcome of untreated RSD, the risk is probably justified.

Physical and occupational therapy should be included in the treatment of RSD as soon as symptoms allow. Early implementation of physical and occupational therapy will facilitate recovery from the physical disability and pain associated with RSD. Initial treatment should focus on tactile desensitization using graded coarse cloth, and hydrotherapy consisting of contrast baths and gentle whirlpool. As tactile sensitivity decreases, the addition of gentle exercises directed toward mobility and functional use should be introduced. If therapy repeatedly causes an exacerbation of RSD symptomatology, somatic neural blockade should be utilized so function can be preserved. Transcutaneous nerve stimulation may also be used as an adjunctive treatment. Monitored relaxation training and hypnosis may be of particular value in the patient in whom anxiety causes exacerbation of symptoms or hinders implementation of therapeutic neural blockade.

Surgical sympathectomy or destruction of sympathetic pathways with neurolytic agents such as alcohol and phenol is reserved for patients who experience consistent but transient relief with neural blockade utilizing local anesthetics and who have also failed to respond to high dose systemic corticosteroids. It should be noted that, should symptoms recur after surgical sympathectomy, reinitiation of sympathetic neural blockade with local anesthetic is often of value.

In the case presented, the diagnosis of RSD was confirmed with a lumbar sympathetic nerve block. Daily lumbar epidural blocks with local anesthetic were performed, resulting in a longer period of pain relief with each successive epidural block. Amitriptyline 50 mg was prescribed with marked improvement in the patient's sleep disturbance. Occupational therapy consisting of tactile desensitization and monitored relaxation techniques was implemented as the patient's pain improved. Physical therapy consisting of gentle, active-assisted range of motion exercises and progressive weight bearing was introduced. The patient required a total of 18 lumbar epidural blocks to achieve complete and permanent pain relief. Physical therapy was continued for an additional 6 weeks to allow complete recovery of function. The patient was then able to return to her employment and remains pain free.

It has been said that one must first think of the diagnosis before one can make it. The diagnostic challenge of RSD certainly fits this dictum. Since delay in diagnosis and treatment often results in devastating pain and disability, early diagnosis and treatment of reflex sympathetic dystrophy is mandatory.

BIBLIOGRAPHY

Duncan KH, Lewis RC, Racz G, et al: Treatment of upper extremity reflex sympathetic dystrophy with joint stiffness using sympatholytic bier block and manipulation. *Orthopedics* 1988; 11:883–886.

Mockus M, Rutherford R, Rosales C, et al: Sympathectomy for causalgia. Patient selection and long-term results. *Arch Surg* 1987; 122:668–672.

Schwartzman RJ, McLellan TL: Reflex sympathetic dystrophy—A review. *Arch Neurol* 1987; 44:556–561.

Waldman SD, Waldman K: Reflex sympathetic dystrophy of the face and neck. *Reg Anaesth* 1987; 12:16–18.

Winnie AP: Reflex sympathetic dystrophy, in Dannemiller Foundation: *Dannemiller Pain Management Review Course Proceedings,* San Antonio, 1988, pp 1–22.

Winnie AP, Collins JJ: The pain clinic: I. Differential neural blockade in pain syndromes of questionable etiology. *Med Clin North Am* 1968; 52:123–129.

35

Deafferentation Pain: Lower Extremities

Allan Nutkiewicz, M.D.

A 25-year-old man was involved in a motorcycle accident 5 years earlier. He was left with a T7 level complete paraplegia. He presented with a 4-year history of severe burning and tingling in both legs with an occasional overlay of electric shooting pain.

DISCUSSION

Deafferentation, as the name implies, is the loss of the afferent or sensory input to the brain. The problem lies, however, in the abnormal behavior of these disconnected central spinal sensory neurons that is experienced as pain.

It is proposed that the deafferented neuron becomes hypersensitive and fires spontaneously or with a reduced electrical threshold—a seizure-like phenomenon. This hypersensitivity is thought to occur from not only the physical damage to the neurons, but from abnormal levels of endorphins and substance P. Whatever hypersensitivity exists, these partially damaged neurons are no longer under the influence of the moderating central inhibitory pathways. The two major causes of lower limb deafferentation pain are sacral nerve root avulsion and traumatic paraplegia.

Lumbosacral roots can be avulsed from the conus due to severe trauma. Typically, these patients have had severe pelvic fracture dislocations from motor vehicle accidents. However, gunshot wounds involving the cauda equina can also result in the same syndrome. These patients present with partially deafferented and paralyzed leg. The diagnostic test of choice is still myelography to demonstrate traumatic meningoceles.

Ten percent of traumatic paraplegic patients with injuries to their spinal cord or cauda equina eventually present with intractable central deafferentation pain. The pain is described classically as burning and tingling, with electric, lighteninglike shooting pains into the paralyzed trunk and lower limbs. Conus lesions have a higher incidence of pain than do cord injuries.

Two major types of injuries occur. Compression to the spinal cord from dislocated vertebral fractures results in total loss of sensation below the injury, but there is a small transitional sensory zone in which pain can be elicited by any type of stimulation.

Paraplegia induced by gunshot wounds to the spinal cord results in asymmetrical neurological deficits, leaving areas of intact sensation that can act as trigger areas for the deafferentation pain.

The diagnostic test of choice in paraplegic patients is magnetic resonance imaging (MRI). Computed tomography scanning, often done initially at the time of injury, will document the level of the lesion but is inferior, even with a preinjection of water-soluble contrast material, to MRI when demonstrating the spinal cord.

This is particularly important in patients who present with pain several years after their accident. These patients must be suspected of harboring a traumatic syrinx. The MRI is the best modality for making this diagnosis.

MEDICAL MANAGEMENT

Many of these patients can be managed conservatively using standard chronic pain management techniques. Tricyclic antidepressants, nonsteroidal anti-inflammatories, and phenothiazines can be titrated to induce significant pain relief, sometimes for considerable lengths of time. Ultimately, almost all of these patients will find the pharmacological treatment of their pain unacceptable, and will demand other treatment.

SURGICAL MANAGEMENT

Fortunately for these patients, there is a procedure that has an excellent record of pain relief with an extremely low morbidity—Dorsal root entry zone rhizotomy (DREZ).

Dorsal root fibers that bring sensory data from the periphery make their synaptic connections with secondary neurons in the dorsal root entry zone of the spinal cord. From here they form ascending somatosensory tracts, such as the spinothalamic tract. This dorsal root entry zone extends the entire length of the spinal cord.

The procedure involves performing a laminectomy over the extent of the spinal cord that will eventually be rhizotomized. Typically, the lesions are performed two to three dermatomal segments above and below the level of injury. This is done to include all the afferent fibers that can ascend or descend several levels before synapsing.

Once the cord is exposed, the dorsal root entry zone is identified under the operating microscope. With either thermocoagulation electrodes or, more recently, the carbon dioxide laser, 2-mm deep lesions are made every 2 or 3 mm along the length of cord previously exposed.

Major complications have included transient loss of hip motion and temporary loss of bladder reflex function. Long-term results over 5 years where patients no longer use analgesics and have a 75% reduction in pain range from 55%–80%.

BIBLIOGRAPHY

Levy WJ, Nutkiewicz A: Laser induced dorsal root entry zone lesions for pain control: A report of three cases. *J Neurosurg* 1983; 59:884–886.

Nashold BS, Bullitt E: Dorsal root entry zone lesion to control central pain in paraplegics. *J Neurosurg* 1981; 55:414–419.

Nashold BS, Ostdahl RH: Dorsal root entry zone lesions for pain relief. *J Neurosurg* 1979; 51:59–69.

PART VII

Cancer Pain

36

Multiple Rib Metastases

Theresa Ferrer-Brechner, M.D.

A 60-year-old white man was complaining of severe pain in the right anterior chest wall, aggravated by movement, deep breathing, and coughing. He had been diagnosed two years earlier with cancer of the prostate and underwent radical prostatectomy and chemotherapy. Ten months ago he started to experience pain in the right anterior chest wall, and repeated radiologic studies demonstrated the presence of metastatic bone lesions at the sixth to ninth ribs, close to their insertion to the vertebrae. A course of radiation therapy was immediately started. However, after radiation was completed, the patient continued to have pain, aggravated by movement and deep breathing. Percocet 2 tablets as needed every 3–4 hours only relieved the pain 30%–40%.

DISCUSSION

The most common cause of pain in patients with cancer is bone invasion either by primary or metastatic tumors.[1] In patients with prostate or breast cancer, pain in the ribs may be the first sign of metastatic disease.

Metastasis to ribs is usually characterized by localized pain, constant and progressive in severity and possibly caused by peripheral mechanisms, especially sensitization of nociceptors by prostaglandins. Osteolytic tumors have been shown to secrete prostaglandins (including PGE_2) exacerbating the pain from tumor growth and accelerating bone resorption due to osteoclastic activity. In some patients, localized bone pain occurs long before positive radiologic findings are seen, indicating that some painful process occurs before the lesion is extensive enough to produce an identifiable change in bone structure or isotope absorption.

235

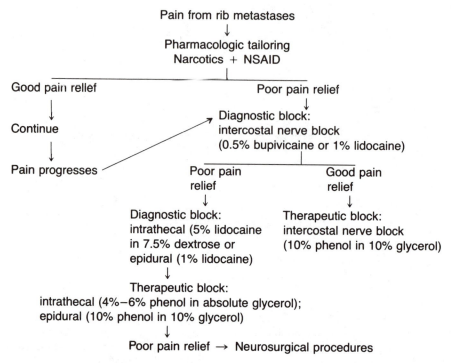

FIG 36–1.
Decision tree, incorporating different modalities for relief of cancer-related pain.

This further supports the theory that PGE_2 release may be an important factor in the occurrence of pain in metastatic bone disease.

Besides cancer-directed therapy, several methods have been tried previously for alleviating this type of cancer-related pain: (1) pharmacologic tailoring; (2) anesthetic regional techniques; and (3) neurosurgical techniques. A decision tree is proposed incorporating these different modalities (Fig 36–1).

Pharmacologic tailoring is best handled with the combination of narcotic and a nonsteroidal anti-inflammatory drug (NSAID), especially with tumors that increase secretion of PGE_2. In a double-blind complete crossover study comparing cancer patients receiving narcotics and placebo vs. narcotic and the NSAID (ibuprofen, 600 mg) patients received significantly higher and longer pain relief with the narcotic-ibuprofen combination, especially those with pain due to bone metastasis.[2] This combination also reduced the CNS side effects associated with increasing doses of narcotic while it provided better analgesia. Ventafredda et al. also reported that 55% of 763 cancer patients had significant relief with administration of NSAID.[3]

Anesthetic regional techniques include intercostal nerve blocking and segmental epidural or intrathecal neurolyses. Before undertaking these procedures, it is important to document how many ribs are involved. If more than three to four ribs are involved it is more comfortable for the patient to undergo an epidural or intrathecal neurolysis.

Intercostal nerve blocking procedure is easily done on an outpatient basis. The patient is placed in a semiprone position with the painful side up. The upper arm is raised above and anterior to the head to lift the scapula away from the midline. A 25 gauge needle is used to infiltrate skin and gauge the depth of the rib. After the rib is stabilized between the thumb and index finger of one hand, a 25 gauge 5 mm, or 22 gauge (for obese or muscular patients), the needle is then slowly "walked" downward to the edge of the rib by pulling the needle skin downward until it falls off the rib. It is important at this point to prevent lunging and penetrating the lung. After the needle is under the rib, it is directed about 20 to 25° cephalad and advanced 2 to 3 mm to lie at the front of the lower part of the rib, where the intercostal nerve is located. For a prognostic/diagnostic block, 3 to 4 mL of 1% lidocaine or 0.5% bupivacaine is injected after negative aspiration for blood or air. Due to dermatome overlap, a minimum of three intercostal nerves should be blocked to produce analgesia in one segment. If the patient has at least 75% pain relief with the diagnostic intercostal block, the procedure can be repeated with 10% phenol in 15% glycerol for longer relief. Although associated with a higher incidence of neuritis and lower success rate than with intrathecal neurolysis, this can be the first block done since it is simple and can be performed on an outpatient basis.

If pain recurs or progression of the disease requires a more profound and widespread analgesic block, a thoracic epidural neurolysis can be planned. With the patient lying on the painful side down, an epidural catheter is inserted as close to the dermatomal distribution of pain as possible. After negative aspiration and negative intravascular injection, increments of 3 mL of 1% lidocaine are injected until the area of pain is analgesic to pinprick sensation. If the patient experiences at least 75% reduction of pain, the catheter is left in place and the local anesthetic effect is allowed to completely wear off. Then, 75% of the volume of local anesthetic that produced analgesia in the dermatomal pain distribution is injected in the form of 10% phenol in 10%–15% glycerol through the same catheter.[4] It is important to make sure the epidural local anesthetic has worn off totally to ensure that some local anesthetic agent is no longer present in the epidural space to act as a spreading vehicle for the 10% phenol in 10% glycerol. This could cause a temporarily wide spread of the phenol block, which could be disconcerting for both the patient and anesthesiologist. The epidural catheter can be left in until the next day, or sometimes over a period of 2 or 3 days, to reinforce the phenol block with further injections of the same.

If a more profound block is indicated, intrathecal neurolysis with phenol or alcohol can be the treatment of choice. Phenol 6% in absolute glycerol is hyperbaric and 100% alcohol is hypobaric to the cerebrospinal fluid. Therefore, if phenol is used, the patient is positioned so that the painful area is placed in the most dependent position. The operating table is flexed and tilted 45° back to maximize layering of the solution at the sensory root. In contrast, with intrathecal alcohol, the patient is positioned so that the targeted dorsal roots are in the highest position.[5] The effect with alcohol is usually immediate, while the effect with phenol might take 15–20 minutes to complete. It is important that the patient be kept in the same position at least 15–20 minutes after injection with alcohol, and 30–45 minutes with phenol, to prevent unintended movement of the neurolytic solution to other dermatomes. Demonstration of a dermatomal block should be documented and correlated with reported absence or presence of pain relief.

Neurosurgical procedures, including preganglionic rhizotomy and median myelotomy, may be included in the armamentarium, especially if the patient does not respond to the anesthetic techniques.

Pharmacologic tailoring in this patient was started with MS-Contin (controlled-release morphine sulfate), 30 mg at 8:00 A.M. and 8:00 P.M., combined with ibuprofen, 600 mg every 4 hours around the clock. The patient's pain immediately decreased to 3–4 from 8–9 on the pain visual analogue scale. The patient was satisfied with this pain relief until 2 months later, when the pain escalated because of disease progression. The MS-Contin was increased to 60 mg twice daily, but this resulted in increased drowsiness and nausea. Intercostal nerve block relieved the pain for the following $2^1/_2$ months, after which the patient underwent intrathecal phenol neurolysis; this provided pain relief until he died 4 months later.

REFERENCES

1. Foley KM: Pain syndromes in patients with cancer, in Bonica JJ, Ventafridda V (eds): *Advances in Pain Research.* New York, Raven Press, 1979, pp 59–78.
2. Ferrer-Brechner T, Ganz P: Ibuprofen (Motrin) as an analgesic potentrator of Methadone [Dolophen] in cancer patients. *Am J Med* 1984; 77(1A):78–83.
3. Ventrafridda V, Fochi C, Conno D, et al: Use of nonsteroidal anti-inflammatory drugs in the treatment of pain in cancer. *Br J Clin Pharmacol* 1980; 10:3435–3465.
4. Ferrer-Brechner T: Epidural and intrathecal phenol neurolysis for cancer pain. *Anesthesiol Rev* 1981; 8:14–19.
5. Swerdlow M: Intrathecal and extradural block in pain relief, in Swerdlow M (ed): *Relief of Intractable Pain.* Amsterdam, Elsevier Scientific, 1983, pp 177–188.

37

The Management of Pain in Pancreatic Carcinoma

Mark Greenberg, M.D.

A 56-year-old man was referred to the pain management center for control of intractable abdominal pain secondary to inoperable pancreatic carcinoma. Two months ago he had presented to his physicians with painless jaundice. A computed tomographic (CT) scan revealed a mass in the head of the pancreas. He underwent an exploratory laparotomy and extensive spread of tumor was found. At surgery, palliative biliary and intestinal bypass procedure were done. The early postoperative course was complicated by peritonitis, pulmonary embolus, and poor wound healing. These problems eventually were managed and he was discharged from the hospital. After several weeks, severe epigastric pain radiating into the back developed and the patient was referred for treatment of this problem.

DISCUSSION

During the past 20 years, the incidence of pancreatic carcinoma has increased dramatically. It now accounts for 3% of all cancers, and 5% of all cancer deaths in the United States. Approximately 25,000 new cases of pancreatic cancer are diagnosed each year. While the peak incidence of the disease is in the fifth and sixth decades, pancreatic carcinoma is the third leading cause of death due to cancer in men between the ages of 35 and 54 years.

The clinical presentation of pancreatic carcinoma depends upon the location of the tumor. Two-thirds of the cancers are in the head of the gland; the remainder are found in the body or tail. Most are poorly differentiated, ductile adenocarcinoma. However, tumors of the endocrine pancreas with their characteristic endocrine adenopathy are becoming more frequently recognized.

Typically, the tumors become clinically evident when ductile obstruction leads to jaundice. At this stage the disease is usually painless. As progression occurs, local extension to contiguous structures and metastatic spread to regional lymph nodes, peritoneum, and abdominal viscera, especially the liver, will often cause pain. The pain is usually epigastric, often radiating into the back. Usually an exploratory laparotomy will be required for a definitive diagnosis, as well as palliation. Due to the anatomic proximity of the head of the pancreas with vital structures and the propensity of the tumor for local spread, only about 15% of tumors diagnosed during exploratory laparotomy are resectable. These require a pancreatico-duodenectomy (Whipple's procedure). For inoperable tumors, a cholecystojejunostomy or choledocojejunostomy with gastrojejunostomy can palliate jaundice, pruritus, and intestinal obstruction.

The prognosis for these patients is dismal. In the small percentage of patients who are candidates for Whipple's procedure, the operative mortality is high and quality of life postoperatively is poor. Most of the other patients are dead within a year of diagnosis. The overall 5-year survival rate for pancreatic carcinoma is less than 10%. Various regimens of chemotherapy and radiation therapy have proved ineffective in modifying these grim statistics.

Between 75%–90% of patients with unresectable pancreatic carcinoma will experience pain directly due to their disease. Pain can occur from tumor invasion of the retroperitoneal, gastric, and/or perineural structures, or from metastases to the liver, to the peritoneum, lymphatics, vascular structures, or epidural space. In addition, pain can be secondary to the performance of diagnostic studies, or to various treatments themselves. The pain syndrome can be either acute or chronic. Therefore, it is imperative to make a careful clinical assessment of the patient with pancreatic cancer pain in order to delineate its cause and devise an effective management strategy. A complete history and physical exam must be done in order to assess the duration of the pain, exacerbating and relieving factors, and to define the role played by associated symptoms such as nausea, vomiting, or anorexia in the overall pain syndrome. The psychosocial status of the patient must be evaluated, with particular attention paid to the presence of depression. The appropriate diagnosis studies must be ordered and reviewed to assure proper treatment. The complexity of the pancreatic cancer pain and its causes often will require a multidisciplinary team approach that utilizes the abilities and specialized interests of clinical psychologists, anesthesiologists, medical oncologists or internists, and surgeons. Whoever has primary care responsibility should oversee the overall management of the patient and provide continuity of care. For the dying patient, a relatively pain-free course will dramatically affect their ability to find meaning and dignity in the terminal phase of their life.

MANAGEMENT

The management of the pancreatic cancer pain syndrome follows the broad general principles of managing all forms of cancer pain. Surgical, tumor destructive, pharmacological, and neuroablative techniques must be considered and utilized where appropriate. These will be discussed in detail.

Surgical approaches for pain relief include: (1) individual section of the greater, lesser, and least splanchnic nerves; (2) celiac and superior mesenteric ganglionectomy; and (3) division of the postganglionic celiac plexus from T5 to T10 or T12. Any of these can be done during the initial exploratory laparotomy. However, since most patients do not have pain prior to exploration, this approach is rarely undertaken. In addition, biliary drainage procedures done palliatively can also provide pain relief. Unfortunately, the pain relief obtained from these techniques is almost always transient.

While various chemotherapeutic regimens have been utilized for pancreatic carcinoma, the overall results have been disappointing. The majority of patients receiving chemotherapy have pain. Perhaps 10% of these patients experience some relief attributable to the therapy. It is important to keep in mind that the chemotherapeutic agents utilized have appreciable painful side effects, such as mucositis, which will contribute to the overall pain experience of the patient.

The most common radiotherapeutic treatment of pancreatic carcinoma is external beam radiation. While several studies show some beneficial response to pain from conventional external beam radiation, none of the studies was blind or well-controlled, prospectively designed to look specifically at this question. Several small studies utilizing intraoperative radiation therapy with electrons or combinations of various radiotherapeutic modalities have been inconclusive in regard to pain relief.[1]

Oral analgesic drug regimens are the cornerstone of therapy for pancreatic cancer pain. In general, the same principles followed for all types of cancer pain are appropriate and applicable to the management of pain due to pancreatic carcinoma. Nonnarcotic, mild narcotic, and finally, potent long-acting narcotic agents should be utilized in a stepwise fashion until pain control is achieved. Often, combinations of drugs will be required to maximize analgesic potency and minimize side effects. Adjuvant agents can be used to control gastrointestinal symptoms or unwanted sedation and drowsiness. In addition, psychotropic medications play an important role as well.

This stepwise, or ladder approach to cancer pain management was developed by a panel of experts brought together under the auspices of the World Health Organization to address this problem.[2] There are three rungs to the ladder that can be summarized as: Step 1—nonnarcotic analgesics administered for mild pain; Step 2—the weak narcotic agents for moderate pain; and Step 3—the potent narcotics reserved for the treatment of severe pain (Table 37–1). Patients

TABLE 37–1.

Stepwise Approach to Analgesic Therapy for Pancreatic Carcinoma Pain

Class	Prototype	Examples	Comments
Nonnarcotics	Nonsteroidal anti-inflammatory agents	Aspirin, ibuprofen (Motrin), diflunisol (Nalfon), piroxicam (Feldene)	Chronic excessive use may lead to renal failure Avoid use in hemostatic disorders Watch for gastrointestinal bleeding
	Acetaminophen	Tylenol, Panadol	Toxicity mainly hepatic in overdosage
Weak morphinelike agonists	Codeine	Oxycodone, hydrocodone, propoxyphene	Usually combined with Step 1 agents, Percocet, Darvocet, i.e., Tylenol #3
Potent narcotics Short half-life	Morphine	Agonists— hydromorphone (Dilaudid), oxymorphone, (Numorphan), meperidine (Demerol)	Dilaudid available both for p.o. and parenteral use; Numorphan available in parenteral form and in rectal suppository only
		Mixed agonist/antagonist—pentazocine (Talwin), butorphanol (Stadol)	Avoid Demerol in patients with renal disease
Long half-life	Methadone Levorphanol		Mixed agonist/antagonists have limited utility in treating cancer pain; may precipitate withdrawal in physically dependent patients

with pancreatic carcinoma most often either fail treatment with step 1 agents, or present with moderate to severe pain requiring a step 2 or step 3 agent early on. Adjuvant agents should be utilized when specific indications exist and will be discussed in detail.

The step 1 agents are either the nonsteroidal anti-inflammatory drugs (NSAIDs), or acetaminophen. Doses should be started low and titrated up as needed, usually on a weekly basis. When using NSAIDs, care must be taken with elderly patients or those with hemostatic problems or renal insufficiency.

Gastrointestinal side effects can be managed with the concomitant use of antacids.

Patients failing step 1 agents or those presenting with moderate pain will require a step 2 drug. The most useful agents in this category are codeine, oxycodone, and hydrocodone. These drugs can be used in combination with aspirin or acetaminophen; however, they are available without the coanalgesic when higher doses are required. These drugs can be highly effective in controlling pain, especially when combined with adjuvants to control side effects (see later discussion). Again, doses should start low and be gradually increased until efficacy is attained or intolerable side effects occur.

For the most severe or refractory pain, step 3 agents should be utilized. These are the morphinelike drugs that include morphine, hydromorphone, methadone, and levorphanol. While all these agents have similar analgesic properties, methadone and levorphanol have significantly longer half-lives and may provide a longer duration of action than morphine. When given in an every 4–6 hour dosing interval, these long-acting potent narcotics can provide continuous pain relief.

All analgesics for cancer pain should be prescribed on an "around the clock" rather than as needed schedule. If as needed dosing is utilized, an unacceptable cycle of under-medication and pain, alternating with periods of over-medication and drug toxicity will occur. The optimal 24-hour drug requirement should be established by carefully titrating the dose. This is especially important when the potent, long-acting agents such as methadone, with elimination half-lives greater than 24 hours, are used. Too rapid an increase in dose will invariably lead to drug accumulation and overdose. Keep in mind that the elimination half-life and the analgesic half-life are different, and an appropriate dosing interval for even the longest acting agents is 4–8 hours. During the period of dose titration, shorter acting agents can be prescribed as needed for "breakthrough" pain.

The most important side effects of opioid agents are sedation, constipation, nausea, vomiting, and respiratory depression. The sedation can usually be managed by decreasing the dose and increasing the frequency of administration. If this proves ineffective, dextroamphetamine (2.5 to 7.5 mg orally, twice daily) can be added. All patients placed on narcotics chronically should also receive stool softeners and laxatives prophylactically. Nausea and vomiting are a difficult problem, but can be managed with prochlorperazine (Compazine), hydroxyzine (Vistaril), or metoclopramide (Reglan). The new onset of vomiting in a patient who had been tolerating narcotics well should raise the suspicion of gastrointestinal obstruction. Clinically important respiratory depression rarely occurs when narcotic agents are carefully prescribed orally, since the threshold for such depression is well above the sedative threshold, which should limit intake. If analgesic-induced respiratory depression does occur, it should be treated with naloxone (Narcan) given I.M. or I.V. However, this may precipitate emergence of previously well-controlled pain and/or a narcotic withdrawal syndrome. Keep in mind that the half-life of Narcan is only 20–30 minutes, and repeated and prolonged therapy will be required in severe cases of narcotic overdose, especially with long-acting agents.

The anticipation and treatment of narcotic tolerance is crucial to successful pharmacological management. Tolerance usually occurs along with physical dependence, but both are distinct from psychological dependence or addiction. Tolerance means that a larger dose of narcotic is required to maintain the original effect; it is a function of the dose and frequency of administration and will develop predictably in patients taking narcotic analgesics on a chronic basis.

Tolerance can be managed by: (1) combining narcotics with nonnarcotic analgesics; (2) switching agents and using less than the predicted equianalgesic dose since cross-tolerance amongst the agents is not complete; (3) switching routes of administration. Physical dependence will become evident if a patient taking chronic opioid narcotics is abruptly taken off the drug. Symptoms will include anxiety, chills, irritability, rhinorrhea, lacrimation, diapheresis, pylo-erection, salivation, nausea, vomiting, abdominal cramps, and rarely, multifocus myoclonus. This syndrome may also occur if a patient taking a narcotic agent is switched to a partial agonist/antagonist agent such as pentazocine (Talwin). The withdrawal syndrome may be prevented by stopping narcotics gradually; usually only 25% of the previous daily dose is required to prevent withdrawal. The syndrome can be attentuated as well, by use of an alpha$_2$-adrenergic agonist agent, such as clonidine.

Psychological dependence or addiction can be viewed as "a pattern of compulsive drug use characterized by a continuous craving for a narcotic and the need to use the narcotic for effects other than pain relief."[3] These patients exhibit drug-seeking behavior. It is a complex problem that will only develop in a specific psychosocial milieu. In cancer patients, the risk of iatrogenic addiction is extremely low; fear of this should not inhibit the physician from prescribing, or the patient from taking, adequate narcotic analgesics.

The use of tricyclic antidepressants as an analgesic adjuvant in the treatment of pancreatic carcinoma is well established. These agents provide direct analgesic effects by blocking synaptic serotonin and norepinephrine reuptake. They exhibit this effect at doses much lower than their usual antidepressant dose. In addition, they are effective in ameliorating insomnia and, in higher doses, will attenuate the depression that often accompanies pancreatic cancer.

Route of administration has become a significant consideration as new modalities have emerged. Patients with pancreatic cancer pain often are unable to take oral medications. Rectal administration might provide an acceptable alternative. In the last several years, patient-controlled analgesia (PCA) devices have become available for use via the subcutaneous, intravenous, or intraspinal route. These pumps are designed for ambulatory use and are highly effective when used in appropriate patients. Moreover, the intraspinal (either intrathecal or epidural) administration of narcotics in ambulatory patients via implantable pumps and tunneled catheters is a highly efficacious route of delivery associated with few side effects and complications.[4] It is often effective even in those patients on very high doses of narcotics with seemingly intractable pain. In addition to opioids, local anesthetics can be administered via various routes to provide pain relief. Epidural or intrathecal local anesthetic infusions are effective for acute pain exacerbations, or during the immediately postoperative period. An exciting new approach, utilizing the installation of local anesthetics into the interpleural space (located between the parietal and visceral pleura), has been reported to provide profound and long-lasting analgesia in several patients with pain of pancreatic origin. This approach will require further study before becoming an accepted modality in the pain control armamentarium.

Finally, the role of invasive neuroablative procedures must be addressed. The most common of these for pancreatic carcinoma pain is the celiac plexus block. The celiac plexus is formed from pre- and post-ganglionic sympathetic efferent fibers, parasympathetic fibers, and visceral sensory efferent fibers. Pain transmitted via the celiac plexus arises primarily from the upper abdomen, including the pancreas, stomach, upper duodenum, liver, and spleen. Anatomically, the plexus is located anterolateral to the aorta immediately caudad to the origin of the celiac artery at the cephalad border of the first lumbar vertebra. Typically, the procedure is performed using a posterior retrocrural approach, with the patient prone. Needles are placed into the plexus bilaterally, and neurolysis is achieved with either alcohol or phenol. Needle placement can be confirmed either fluoroscopically or under CT guidance.

Recently, Brown et al., from the Virginia Mascon Clinic, published their experience with neurolytic celiac plexus blocks for pancreatic cancer pain.[5] Good pain relief was obtained in 85% of 136 patients with pancreatic cancer who underwent the procedure. Procedure-related morbidity was limited; two patients developed a pneumothorax, and eight experienced orthostatic hypotension. In some patients, gastrointestinal side effects (either constipation or diarrhea) will occur. Occasionally, a patient will outlive the duration of neurolysis and require a repeat procedure.

In summary, the management of the pancreatic cancer pain syndrome is a therapeutic challenge requiring thorough evaluation and implementation of an array of treatment modalities. Often, the involvement of a physician specially trained in pain management techniques will be necessary.

REFERENCES

1. Minsky BD, Hibris B, Fuks Z: The role of radiation therapy in the control of pain from pancreatic carcinoma. *J Pain Sympt Mgmt* 1988; 3:199–205.

2. Walker VA, Hoskin PJ, Hanks GW, et al: Evaluation of WHO analgesic guidelines for cancer pain in a hospital-based palliative care unit. *J Pain Sympt Mgmt* 1988; 3:145–149.
3. Payne R, Mitchell M, Inturrisi, C, et al: Principles of analgesic use in the treatment of acute pain and chronic cancer pain. *American Pain Society Syllabus.* Washington, DC, 1987.
4. Coombs DW, Maurer LH, Saunders RL, et al: Outcomes and complications of continuous intraspinal narcotic analgeia for cancer pain control. *J Clin Oncol* 1984; 2:1414–1420.
5. Brown DL, Bulley CK, Quiel EL: Neurolytic celiac plexus block for pancreatic cancer pain. *Anesth Analg* 1987; 66:869–873.

38

Pain Due to Liver Capsular Distension*

Dennis W. Coombs, M.D.

A 34-year-old, red-haired, white woman was referred to the pain management service approximately 2 years after undergoing right modified radical mastectomy for primary angiosarcoma with negative axillary node dissection. She presented with a history of about 6 months of sharp right lower chest wall pains, with intermittent stabbing and cramping, that was progressively increasing in frequency. She had a nearly constant aching pain in the right subscapular area and right flank that responded somewhat to heat, massage, chiropractic manipulation, local applications of dimethyl sulfoxide (DMSO), and ibuprofen, though these had no apparent effect on the sharp stabbing pain. A local physician had prescribed oxycodone 10 mg four times daily a month earlier with little effect on the pain. She had experienced about an 8-lb weight loss, anorexia, metallic taste to her food, and periods of nausea since her last breast clinic follow-up. Her liver function profile had yielded nothing initially, but her most recent studies revealed an elevated aspartate aminotransferase (AST). Several myofascial trigger point injections relieved the aching muscular pain preparatory to a liver scan and further GI workup. Over the next few weeks, however, the visceral symptoms and right upper quadrant pain became greatly magnified. She was unable to eat consistently due to nausea and emesis, and couldn't keep her analgesics down. She was admitted for pain control and further workup. She was experiencing sweats and an unstable fever chart with daily peaks to 38.5°C. Chest x-ray revealed a moderate sympathetic effusion and a question of right lower lobe

* This work was supported in part by grants from PHS CA-33865-05 (DWC); the Robert Osgood, Jr., Memorial Fund; the Kingsbury Fund; and the Hitchcock Clinic Anesthesia Research Fund.

atelectasis or consolidation. Liver spleen scan and CT abdominal scan both documented a large right hepatic mass with questionable filling defects in the left lobe
on technitium scan. She was seen perioperatively by the pain team to consider
analgesic therapy before and after exploratory laparotomy.

DISCUSSION

Among many types of viscerally generated pain, the pain of liver capsular
distension is unique, often presenting peculiar differential diagnostic challenges.
The liver capsule is a restrictive barrier to enlargement of the hepatic parenchyma.
The parenchyma is capable of rapid volume changes in contrast to the limited
distensibility of the capsule.[1] The sensory innervation is carried through the
vagus, thoracic sympathetic, and celiac plexus. Not surprisingly, therefore, a
variety of visceroaffective responses are observed in association with hepatic
capsular distension. These include nausea, emesis, hypo- or hypertension, and
perspiration. The pain may be acute, sharp and localizing, or referred and poorly
localized, with or without muscular spasm or hypertonus distant to the organ.
Not infrequently, depending upon the underlying etiology, other metastases or
organs emit nociceptive signals that further confuse the situation. The first issue
at hand is, therefore, to separate those processes that are associated with acute
processes of a more fulminating type from subacute processes perhaps superimposed upon chronic passive congestion.

CLASSIFICATION

A variety of processes may result in an increase in intrahepatic pressure with
consequent capsular distension. These include inflammatory infective processes
of a subacute or fulminate nature (i.e., gonococcus, parasitic infection), in which
case antimicrobial therapy with oral or I.V. analgesic therapy is sufficient. In
contrast, rapidly enlarging tumors with or without capsular invasion, especially
vascular lesions such as angiosarcoma, may yield such pain.[1] Some liver tumors
may be accessible to debulking with or without attempt at primary cure, especially
with the introduction of newer instruments for operating on the liver. Palliative
radiation may be very effective.[2] When a remediable situation exists, such as
with infection, leukemic capsulitis prechemotherapy, or a resectable tumor, pain
management need only be sufficient and not permanent. In contrast, when a
nonresectable hepatic metastasis exists in a terminal case, an aggressive neurodestructive or continuous deafferenting local anesthetic-based therapy is easily
rationalized. The choice must be commensurate to the duration of need. The
goals are clearly somewhat different in the acute setting compared to the chronic.

ACUTE CAPSULAR DISTENSION

Acute capsular pain can result in several types of physiological compromise despite rather aggressive parenteral narcotic therapy. The patient's overall condition may become compromised through deleterious effects on organs other than the liver. Principal of these is the reduced functional residual capacity (FRC), vital capacity, and cough consequent to severe splinting from inadequately controlled pain, perhaps aggravated by diaphragmatic pressure when ascites and passive congestion coexist. Despite titration of analgesics per continuous infusion or patient-controlled analgesic delivery systems, rapid shallow respiration with poor sigh or cough may predominate. Coexistent nausea and/or emesis from the visceral syndrome may further complicate the milieu.

Regardless, if narcotic therapy is complicating the situation without yielding either adequate pain control or control of the physiologic compromise associated with the pain, several strategies should be considered to obtain and sustain pain control until the underlying etiology is rectified or no longer practically at issue.

THERAPEUTIC ALTERNATIVES FOR ACUTE HEPATIC CAPSULE PAIN

In this setting, a variety of alternatives will no doubt improve pain control. This patient's systemic morphine intake escalated rapidly, while the patient's overall condition declined. This was due to a combination of visceroaffective symptomatology, poor pulmonary effort, pleural effusion, and the constitutional effects of the liver malignancy. What is needed is an alternative therapy to block the visceral pain syndrome, as well as the sharp distention pain. This can be accomplished with one of three continuous local anesthetic approaches without resort to permanent blocking techniques: (1) continuous epidural analgesia with local anesthetic with or without narcotic combination;[3] (2) continuous intrapleural local anesthetic infusion;[4] (3) continuous celiac plexus infusion of local anesthetic. Epidural and intrapleural methods can be adapted to control all or part of the visceral symptoms and inhibit, to a greater or lesser extent, the postoperative incision pain. Celiac plexus block is an exception, effecting predominately the visceral symptomatology.

Continuous epidural analgesia is perhaps preferable, since this will offer the best control of a midline incision while clearly reducing sympathetically mediated pain. To accomplish this most efficiently, thoracic epidural catheter placement should be accomplished at the T6–T8 level assuming facility exists with the technique. Coadministration of 6–10 mL/hr of 0.25%–0.1% bupivacaine with epidural fentanyl 1–2 mcg/kg/hr and appropriate local anesthetic level monitoring will yield combined control of visceral pain and incision pain while permitting outstanding recovery of pulmonary function.[3] We have found in a series of studies employing a duodenal distention stimulus in the rat, that both mu agonists like morphine, and alpha$_2$-adrenergic agonists like clonidine, when given intrathecally, potently block the initiation of the mechanical visceral pain syndrome.[5]

In the absence of facility with thoracic epidural catheter placement, continuous intrapleural bupivacaine infusion may be advised. This technique requires only an understanding of the use of continuous peridural catheters and needles and reasonable attention to detail. A further plus in this case is the absence of a chest tube drainage that, in our experience, increases the volume and dose to maintain analgesia. As applied originally by Reistad and colleagues, an 18-gauge epidural needle is placed aseptically in the mid-axillary line at the T6 level and an epidural catheter is threaded gently posteriorly, much as "intracath" pleurocentesis was performed in the past.[4] We employ a loading dose of 15–20 mL of 0.5% bupivacaine followed by a continuous infusion of 6–10 mL/hr adjusted with intermittent bolus as needed to reestablish analgesia. Periodic attempts to taper the infusion rate are recommended, especially in cases with impaired metabolic and elimination systems. Serial bupivacaine levels, if available, may be helpful in complicated cases.

As applied to this case, a pleural effusion may have some dilutionary effect upon the analgesia. Additionally, there may be a tendency for a leak to develop along the catheter with the potential for sepsis over time. Thus, more frequent dressing changes may be required. Clearly, gravitational effects may alter the distribution of analgesia, necessitating positioning for best results. Another disadvantage is the potential unilaterality of the effect, thus yielding somewhat reduced midline wound pain control. However, this may be offset by the impedence of the sympathetic and vagal transmission, initiating the visceral pain syndrome. Both epidural and intrapleural analgesia have the potential to disguise serious undiagnosed pathology. We recently observed a case wherein this technique obscured the presentation of a right hepatic ischemic thrombosis, with acute liver infarct and related parenchymal swelling and pain. In a second case, intrapleural infusion was pushed to control progressive left upper quadrant and midline pain in a multiple trauma patient with severe rib fracture pain on the same side. The origin of much of the pain was a ruptured spleen with delayed (7 days) mesenteric and intraperitoneal hemorrhage, and related pain that finally presented with severe hypotension. Bupivacaine overdose was initially mistakenly considered as the culprit for hypotension. Vigilance is thus necessary to safely apply this technique.

Evolution of Case

Exploration and biopsy revealed an unresectable angiosarcoma involving the liver capsule with extension to the diaphragm and lateral abdominal wall. An attempt to embolize and shrink the mass had little secondary impact on the pain with her epidural infusion turned off. A decision was made as to which chronic pain control option to pursue: chronic epidural narcotics, systemic narcotics, or a neurolytic alternative. On the one hand, some control of visceral symptoms was afforded by the spinal narcotics, but the sharp pain was only affected significantly by coadministration of the local anesthetic. Further, the patient was not able to consistently keep food down. Placement of a Hickman or chronic indwelling I.V. access system for narcotic administration, chronic subcutaneous morphine, or a chronic program of suppository administration, were all considered. However, given scant likelihood of survival past a few months, a neuro-destructive alternative was considered the best approach.

TREATMENT OF CHRONIC VISCERAL PAIN AND CAPSULAR DISTENSION

In the absence of clear chest wall pain or extension to yield other distant somatic sites of pain, celiac plexus neurolysis alone will control both the capsular and visceral pain in most cases. The presence of these other factors may require additional measures. For instance, limited epidural or cryoneurolysis may be required to deal with rib pain. A number of techniques and agents are promoted for the neurolysis of the celiac plexus. This subject has recently been reviewed by Lebovits and Lefkowitz as it applies to pancreatic cancer.[6] Brown and colleagues called attention to the utility of this procedure as it applies to peripancreatic and upper abdominal metastatic syndromes.[7] The most poignant conclusions are that the procedure (celiac neurolysis) is frequently applied too late and that both the pain and visceral symptoms are prominently ameliorated until the patient dies often with near elimination of adjunctive analgesics.

Choice of technique is largely a function of training with proponents of both "classical" bilateral needle positioning posterior to the diaphragm or alternatively transcural in placement, versus more recent transaortic and ventral transabdominal approaches.[6] It should be emphasized that most techniques (though details of outcome are sketchy) report about 70%–95% success with variations probably accounted for, in part, by differences in the magnitude of metastasis. Since the posterior and periaortic injection probably achieves both celiac and splanchnic block, better effect might occur upon the vagal and splanchnically mediated syndromes associated with disease outside the pancreatic bed, including the liver capsule. A second important point is that the location of midline structures in the presence of tumor or inflammatory masses in the abdomen is unpredictable. For this reason, we routinely perform celiac neurolysis under fluoroscopic, or preferably, CT-guided imaging. As a further point, it is important, if at all feasible, to perform a diagnostic celiac block with local anesthetic first in order to assay the likelihood of success. Unrelieved pain may point to the need for either adjunctive blocks previously outlined, or an entirely different approach.

Our agent of choice is 70% alcohol in a volume of 50 mL divided between two needles. This is diluted in local anesthetic (bupivacaine) to attenuate the significant discomfort and occasional respiratory difficulty that patients would otherwise suffer. Further, the patients are significantly sedated in the prone position. A small amount of radiographic water-soluble contrast is injected prior to the alcohol to verify placement of the needle tips. The most common side effects are the following: orthostatic hypotension occurs in about 60% of cases, and thus an I.V. should be in place. Hypotension often persists for 3–5 days and will often require that the patient make provisions for dealing with this chronically; transient tachypnea and chest pain; weakness or anesthesia in a thigh/groin distribution; a variable period of diarrhea; failure of ejaculation in males; pneumothorax rarely; and even more rarely, paraplegia. Though various concentrations (5%–6%), and volumes of phenol are also used, there is a distinct risk of seizures if an unrecognized intravascular phenol injection occurs.

In summary, the techniques exist to address the control of both acute and chronic hepatic capsular pain. In some cases, both issues will need to be addressed and coordinated in the same patient. The appropriate application of continuous epidural, intrapleural, or celiac local analgesics is predicated upon a careful evaluation of the patient and the disease. For the more chronic applications, celiac plexus neurolysis should be considered early to reduce the need for systemic narcotics, control visceral pain syndromes, and improve overall quality of life. This can be safely accomplished by appropriate preneurolysis testing with local anesthetic and the utilization of radiographically guided techniques.

REFERENCES

1. Hill K: Pathologic Anatomy of Cancer Pain, in *Pain in the Cancer Patient,* in Zimmermann M, Drings P, Wagner G (eds): *Recent Results in Cancer Research,* vol 89. Heidelberg, Springer Verlag, 1984, pp 33–44.
2. Randall ME: Radiation therapy and pain management, pain classification and treatment efficacy. *J Pain Mgmt* 1989; 2:21–27.
3. Coombs DW: Management of Postoperative Pain: Medical and Administrative Aspects. Regional Refresher Course Lectures, Copywrite, ASA. Philadelphia, Lippincott, 1988; 234:1–7.
4. Riestad F, Stromskag KE: Intrapleural Catheter in the Management of Postoperative Pain. *Reg Anaesth* 1986; 11:89–92.
5. Colburn R, Coombs DW, Degnan C, et al: Mechanical visceral pain model: Chronic intermittent intestinal distention in the rat. *Physiol Behav* 1989; 45:191–197.

6. Lebovits AH, Lefkowitz M: Pain management of pancreatic carcinoma: A review. *Pain* 1989; 36:1–11.
7. Brown DL, Bully CK, Quiel EL: Neurolytic celiac plexus block for pancreatic cancer pain. *Anesth Analg* 1987; 66:869–873.

39

Pain From Colorectal Cancer*

Dennis W. Coombs, M.D.

A 52-year-old man was referred by a local physician because of uncontrolled pain in the legs, buttocks, and sacrum. A previously healthy executive, 4 years prior to admission he had undergone a colorectal resection without intraoperative radiation. Aside from his colostomy care, he had few complaints until 1 year ago, when he had the onset of pain in the sacrum and left buttock. Bone scans and CT exams had revealed a midline mass anterior to the sacrum extending toward the left sciatic notch. This was irradiated with 6,000 rads and he was followed up with a series of narcotic prescriptions. He refused chemotherapy after considering the likely complications and poor response rates quoted him. His pain improved for about 2 months and then gradually returned to its original level. He developed early bladder dysfunction and required intermittent catheterization. Two months prior to admission, substantially greater pain became manifest in the sacrum and buttocks. This pain was bothersome when he was on his feet for any period of time and was greatly exacerbated by sitting. His regimen included 75 mg of amitriptyline at bedtime, ibuprofen 300 mg four times daily, intermittent oxycodone up to 10 per day, and MS Contin (controlled-release morphine sulfate), 600 mg, in divided doses. He complained of dry mouth, periods of inattentiveness, foggy memory, and occasional bad dreams day or night. Chest x-ray now revealed several ill-defined densities in both right upper and lower lobes, suggestive of metastases. Liver function tests were essentially normal, as was a liver spleen scan.

---

* This work was supported in part by grants from PHS CA-33865-05 (DWC); the Robert Osgood, Jr., Memorial Fund; the Kingsbury Fund; and the Hitchcock Clinic Anesthesia Research Fund.

DISCUSSION

Resistance to systemic analgesic therapy is common in cancer patients with tumor-associated plexopathy. The situation is most difficult when there is a slow-growing malignancy and the patient has good functional capabilities but for the limitation due to pain. This scenario is commonly associated with colorectal carcinoma and pelvic reproductive malignancies uncontrolled by local surgical extirpation with or without radiation. In this setting, intraspinal narcotics may greatly improve the quality of life for such patients. To simplify greatly, spinal narcotic administration leads to inhibition of sensory transmission arriving primarily via small unmyelinated C fibers. This is accomplished at the level of the dorsal horn in the spinal cord through pre- and postsynaptic opioid receptor activation.[1]

This case presentation, or one similar to it, repeats itself several times a year in most referral oncology practices. This malignancy is much like cervical carcinoma in that recurrences tend to spread by local extension first. Complaints of pain in such patients are overwhelmingly likely to presage identification of local recurrence. Frequently the coccyx, sacrum, and lumbosacral plexus are involved early. Pain thus may occur unilaterally with involvement of the sciatic nerve by external invasion or compression. Alternatively, the sacrum may be invaded with ascending involvement of the sacral nerves. Often after aggressive radiation to such tumors, some degree of radiation neuritis results, with related burning pain and dysesthesias. This radiation neuritic pain is usually not sustained beyond a few months. Review of new pelvic pains occurring in the course of malignant disease almost always predicts further activity of the cancer process. Pain may occur due to bony invasion or related fractures with or without nervous compression. The key features in our minds are as follows:

What Can Be Done to Clinically Treat or Arrest the Disease?

Comment.—Assuming that no further chemotherapy is to be given and the maximum radiation therapy has been administered (limited to about 6,500 rads due to the risk of radiation neuritis and intestinal injury), then only palliative treatment is indicated.

What Is the Functional Status of the Patient and, Relatedly, What Approach Will Sustain the Best Quality of Existence for the Patient's Remaining Time?

Comment.—Clearly, as the objecting attorney might say, this calls for a conclusion from the witness [doctor]. Though it is difficult to reliably estimate survival, we are forced to attempt this to avoid aggressive therapy when it is either too late to have any real meaning or so early that complications or later failure might be equally disappointing. The dynamic and unpredictable nature of metastatic disease obviously makes this difficult. However, pain, in association with colorectal and cervical carcinoma with these presenting features, usually has been tracked long enough to help render such a survival prediction. Further, even with metastatic involvement, such patients will survive for extended periods of time, often 1 to 2 years. Also, the patient who initially rejects chemotherapy may be heartened by family support, encouraging medical news in the lay press, or a positive shift in overall attitude. It is thus helpful to have an alternative to offer such patients that is not destructive and irreversible on the one hand, and is relatively less likely to depress intellectual or cognitive spheres on the other. In this situation, one of several approaches to chronic delivery of spinal analgesics has been very helpful. In the case presented, it may be that this patient will remain fully mobile and self-caring for 6 months to a year or more, despite the presence of metastasis, given the slow rate of disease progression seen in many such patients.

Is the Patient's Analgesic Regimen Adequate?

Comment.—This patient has progressed through the cancer pain analgesic ladder proposed by the World Health Organization and promoted by the International Association for the Study of Pain. We would consider this to be a reasonable program, since a nonsteroidal, anti-inflammatory agent is in place to treat inflammation-related pain. A modest dose of a tricyclic antidepressant is used to facilitate sleep and for its analgesic properties, especially against deafferentation pain. Finally, an effective, sustained duration and potent narcotic is being used in reasonable doses. Unfortunately, the patient is unable to tolerate the agent despite inadequate pain control. Several manipulations might be tried, including changes in the agent, coadministration of a stimulant such as amphetamine, altering the dose and timing of the antidepressant (buspirone or other less sedative agents) or narcotic (levodromoran or methadone). However, many patients will develop psychomotor depression and sedative-inattention syndromes on high dose narcotics. For such patients, only neurolysis or spinal analgesic infusion seem to offer relief. Thus, assuming that the patient does not have a reactive depression driving pain report, the issue reduces itself to whether or not there is a viable and acceptable neurodestructive alternative to control pain.

Is There a Neurodestructive Alternative and Will the Patient Accept This?

Comment.—If the patient has bilateral lower extremity pain, then cordotomy or neurolytic therapies are a late alternative applied best to the patient who has lost mobility, bowel, and bladder control. In contrast, it is the opinion of many that a cordotomy is the best single alternative for patients with unilateral lower extremity/sciatic pain. It must be realized that something in excess of one-third of such patients will develop bilateral symptoms and require further procedures such as neurolysis, notwithstanding complications associated with cordotomy. In the absence of all potential mitigating features, spinal narcotic infusion may be a miracle for mobile patients responsive to spinal narcotics, whether pain is unilateral or bilateral.

A Corollary Question Is, to What Extent Is the Pain Neurogenic or Incident Related?

Comment.—Incident and neurogenic pain is relatively resistant to narcotics regardless of dose, short of significant blunting of the cognitive sphere. If this is an issue, it must be defined preoperatively before embarking upon a course of spinal analgesics. In the absence of a significant response to spinal narcotic, a neurodestructive alternative might better suffice.

What Is the Patient's Response to a Test Dose of Spinal Narcotic?

Comment.—In most cases we perform a test injection of spinal narcotic to first establish that the patient will be functionally improved, and secondly, to define the starting dose range for chronic administration. The choice of a test dose is made empirically based upon our experience estimating the comparative CSF partitioning of systemic morphine relative to spinal injection of morphine where the ratio is about 10–25:1 for epidural morphine, and at least 100–200:1 for intrathecal morphine, based upon comparative CSF levels. First, convert the patient's systemic narcotic intake into I.M. morphine equivalents based upon bioavailability data with the respective agents. Houde and colleagues at Memorial Sloan-Kettering have published conversion tables for this purpose. The patient in question might have substantially reduced bioavailability of oral morphine or neurogenic pain that would predict widely divergent morphine equivalents. Be conservative, therefore, and assume a bioavailability of 25% based upon the MS Contin (controlled-release morphine sulfate) alone. This translates in the case presented to about 150 mg of morphine per day. We would choose a spinal morphine test dose 0.5%–1% or 5%–10% of this morphine equivalency as an intrathecal (0.75–1.5 mg) or epidural (7.5–15 mg) test dose, respectively. An adequate response is presumed if at least a 50% reduction of pain intensity is reported, lasting at least 8–12 hours with a significant reduction in pain with ambulation and movement.

INITIATION OF CHRONIC SPINAL MORPHINE

Assuming there is a positive response, the patient is offered an appropriate chronic delivery system to permit sustained delivery of spinal narcotic. The choice and application of these systems are beyond the scope of this discussion, but have been reviewed elsewhere recently.[2] Similarly, an overview of experience with implanted infusion systems has been compiled recently for the interested reader, including the relative risks of complications and side effects.[3–4] The decision to use an implanted infusion pump is usually made when the duration of narcotic delivery will exceed 4–6 months; when the pain is bilateral and midline in a patient with pelvic malignancy; when systemic narcotics have been poorly tolerated; when the resources of the patient, family, or local medical community are such that percutaneous or transcutaneous injection systems are not viable options; and when the support system is in place to provide intermittent recharging of the implanted system. Finally, the integument and receptor sites must be adequate to permit implantation and intermittent percutaneous access, and there must be free communication of spinal fluid along the spinal neuraxis. Intractable pain at the spinal level is often a premonitory sign of epidural tumor compressing the spinal cord.[5] Obstruction of the spinal fluid column by an epidural tumor process leads to failure of the spinal narcotic approach. It may be that such patients will respond to infusion of narcotic either above the level of the obstruction or intracerebroventricularly.

The simplest system is an intrathecal catheter anchored to the supraspinous ligament and wedded to a subcutaneously tunneled pump/catheter. Alternatively, the epidural route may be chosen with the caveat that the initial doses will be higher, and there is some real risk that epidural fibrosis will occur with eventual attenuation of CSF morphine levels at a given rate of morphine infusion. Both routes may lead to meningitis if ascending trans/pericatheter bacterial contamination occurs, though this result is certain with the intrathecal route.

A variety of implantable devices exists; most are either in development or are yet unapproved for intrathecal infusion. The reader is referred to a recent review by Waldman and Coombs.[2] The simplest chronic delivery pump is the continuous flow device driven by a fluorocarbon-compressed bellows. Until recently, we have principally used the Shiley Infusaid model 400 pump with 50 mL reservoir and constant flow rates of about 2.5–3.5 mL per day. We are now using the Therex implantable continuous pump, with a slightly smaller 30 mL reservoir and about 1.0–2.2 mL/day flow rates, and a central septum that is much easier to palpate and access. Figure 39–1 shows a Therex implanted pump in a typical patient with colorectal carcinoma and intractable lower extremity pain. Once implanted, continuous flow pumps are essentially maintenance free except for refills.

With continuous infusion of intraspinal narcotic, the patient may be able to

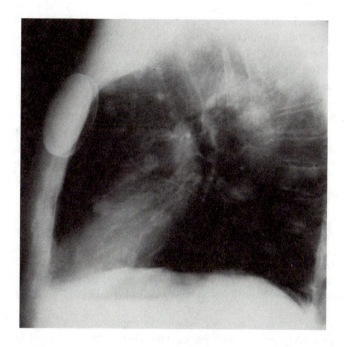

FIG 39–1.
Myelogram taken in a patient with colorectal carcinoma to document the intrathecal placement site of lumbar silicone conduit attached to an implanted Therex continuous infusion pump.

discontinue much of the oral or systemic narcotic intake. We keep most patients on nonsteroidal, anti-inflammatory drugs, as well as a tricyclic antidepressant. Adjunctive medications, regional blocks, and various other supportive therapies are introduced or added as needed. The general experience has been that the majority of such patients are controlled for 3–6 months or even longer, though at the expense of progressive narcotic escalation.[5] This increase in spinal narcotic dose is usually 3- to 4-fold over the starting dose in most cases, though quite variable across reported series.[3] Since the maximum solubility of morphine in saline is about 65 mg/mL, this factor limits the maximum dose that can be delivered per 24 hours by this approach. The reader is referred to other sources for a discussion of the alternatives available to deal with uncontrolled pain in the setting of massive spinal narcotic resistance.[4]

SUMMARY

Spinal narcotic infusion may provide a convenient method for control of pelvic malignancy associated pain. The principal advantages are the reduced cognitive impact of this mode of narcotic delivery and the stable levels of spinal narcotic acting upon opioid-dependent, sensory modulatory systems in the dorsal horn. This has the further advantage of minimizing the risk of respiratory depression vis-à-vis the risk of this complication during bolus spinal narcotic injections. The inconvenience of the surgical procedure and the relatively small, but real risk of infection, reinforce the need to consider all other alternative approaches. Lastly, since intractable narcotic-resistant pain may later emerge, occasionally, it is still necessary to employ neurodestructive procedures in such cases.

REFERENCES

1. Yaksh TL: Multiple opioid receptors systems in brain and spinal cord: Part II. *Eur J Anaesthesia* 1984; I–II:171–245.
2. Waldman S, Coombs DW: Selection of implantable narcotic delivery systems. *Anesth Analg,* in press.
3. Yaksh TL, Onofrio BO: Retrospective consideration of the doses of morphine given intrathecally by continuous infusion in 163 patients by 19 physicians. *Pain* 1987; 31:211–223.
4. Coombs DW: Intraspinal analgesic infusion by implanted pump, in Penn R (ed): Neurological applications of implanted pumps. *Ann NY Acad Sci* 1988; 531:108–122.
5. Coombs DW, Maurer LH, Saunders RL, et al: Outcomes and complications of continuous intraspinal narcotic analgesia for cancer pain control. *J Clin Oncol* 1984; 2:1414–1420.

40

Diagnosis and Treatment of Pathological Compression Fractures

David H. Clements, M.D.
Narayan Sundaresan, M.D.

A 53-year-old man presented with a 3-month history of unremitting interscapular pain without radiation. He was initially treated for musculoskeletal or arthritic pain for 6 weeks. When the pain did not subside, radiographs of the cervicothoracic region were obtained, which revealed an abnormality (Fig 40–1). He was then referred for further evaluation. On neurological examination, no focal findings were noted except for mild triceps weakness on the left side. Computed tomography (CT) scan and MRI (magnetic resonance imaging) revealed a tumor involving the C7, T1 vertebra with anterior soft tissue extension, as well as epidural cord compression (Figs 40–2 and 40–3). A radionuclide bone scan revealed no other sites of bony abnormalities. A CT scan of the chest and abdomen showed a possible primary site in the kidney (Fig 40–4). The tentative diagnosis of a metastatic tumor from the kidney was therefore made, and the patient was placed on high dose corticosteroid therapy (dexamethasone [Decadron] 4 mg I.V. every 6 hrs.) with resulting pain relief. Needle biopsy of the kidney was nondiagnostic due to inadequate sampling. In view of the known hypervascularity of metastatic kidney tumors, spinal angiography of the cervicothoracic lesion was performed. A highly vascular tumor mass was noted, and embolization was performed with both polyvinyl alcohol (Ivanlon), and absolute alcohol. Following embolization, the patient noted transient numbness in his right lower extremity. Three days following embolization, the patient underwent surgery through an anterior transternal route, at which time a highly vascular

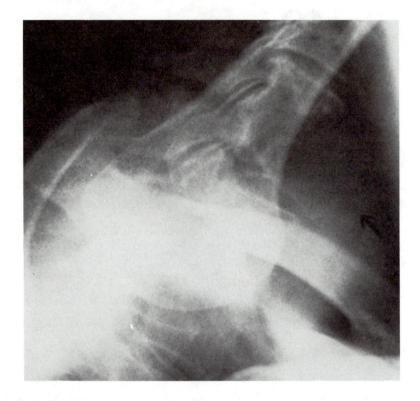

FIG 40–1.
Lateral, cervicothoracic spine, swimmer's view. Note destruction of the C7 vertebra (shown by arrow).

tumor involving the C7–T1 vertebra was resected. The resected segment was reconstructed with methyl methracrylate and Steinmann's pins (Fig 40–5). Two weeks following this procedure, a radical nephrectomy was performed through a right thoraco-abdominal approach. Postoperative radiation therapy (3,000 rads) was then administered to the cervical spine. Since that time, the patient has been closely followed with bone scans, flexion-extension views of the spine, as well as chest CT scans. He continues to be active, fully functional, and free of pain more than two years past surgery, with no known clinical evidence of his cancer.

DISCUSSION

Accurate diagnosis and evaluation of the patient presenting with spinal pain is a common problem for the clinician. The vast majority of spinal pain is benign, reflecting musculoskeletal or ligamentous injury, and it is estimated that approximately 5% of all Americans will suffer from such pain due to ligamentous or disk disease. The life-time prevalence of discogenic pain is approximately 60%–90%, and it disables approximately 5 million people in the United States annually, with an overall economic cost of $16 billion dollars. This enormous clinical problem is probably attributable to complex psychological, societal, and legal factors.

In the majority of such pain syndromes, treatment with analgesics, rest, immobilization with a soft prosthesis, and a program of physical therapy will result in complete relief. When spinal pain persists for more than 6 weeks, more vigorous evaluation is necessary. While 10% of patients with benign musculo-skeletal pain will remain symptomatic for such prolonged periods, that differential diagnosis of pain *not* responding to therapy includes both infectious, tumor-related causes, or other anatomical features of the vertebral column, causing mechanical deformity in the spinal cord. Additional radiologic studies such as

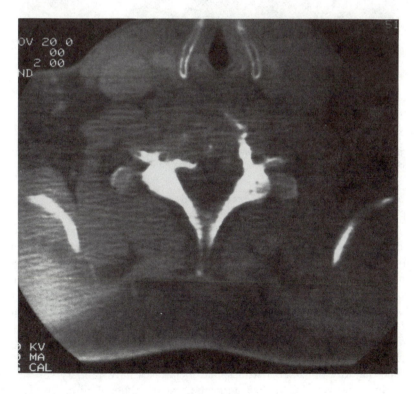

FIG 40–2.
Axial CT scan showing destruction of C7 vertebral body.

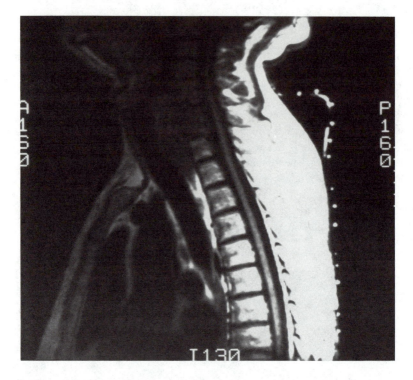

FIG 40–3.
MRI scan, sagittal view, T1 weighted image. Note abnormal signal in the C7 body with tumor extension anteriorly over T1 vertebra, as well as posteriorly toward thecal sac.

radionucleide scanning, or more recently, MRI should be performed to evaluate pain that persists despite conservative therapy.

Persistent pain is also the most common manifestation of metastasis to bone, and the axial skeleton is the most common site of osseous involvement.[1–2] Spinal pain of malignant origin is generally gradual in onset, and frequently worse at night. Metastatic foci frequently involve the vertebral body first, but they may not be detectable on plain radiography because 30%–50% of the bone must be destroyed before changes are visible on plain films. With the introduction of MRI, early involvement of the marrow can be detected by changes in signal intensity on T1- and T2-weighted images. Therefore, this imaging modality is the test of choice for evaluation of tumors involving the spine.

The majority of patients with spinal metastases have primary sites in the breast, lung, prostate, or the hematopoietic system, although virtually any neoplasm may metastasize to the spine. Such vertebral metastases may be asymptomatic until the tumor breaks through the cortex to compress the neural elements, or else replace the vertebra to a sufficient extent that pathologic fractures and instability develop.[3] It is only recently that the role of spinal instability as an important factor in the genesis of pain from tumors involving the vertebral column has been recognized.[3-5] The recognition of spinal instability has been greatly aided by the MRI scan, which provides a multiplanar view of the spinal cord and the bony elements. The presence of localized kyphosis, collapse of the body greater than 50%, involvement of all three columns in the spine, and translational deformities all indicate instability of the spine.

Apart from *known* cancers that metastasize to the spine, the vertebral column is sometimes affected by occult metastatic tumors from unknown primary sites.[6] It is estimated that such cancers account for 7%–10% of all solid tumors seen in major oncology centers. The management of this common and important problem is frequently vexing and frustrating. At present, data on bone presentation of occult primary cancers are scant. Symptoms are generally caused by pathological compression fractures, and this may result in spinal cord compression when the spine is involved. The differential diagnosis of a pathological fracture of the spine should include a metastatic tumor, primary spine tumor, or

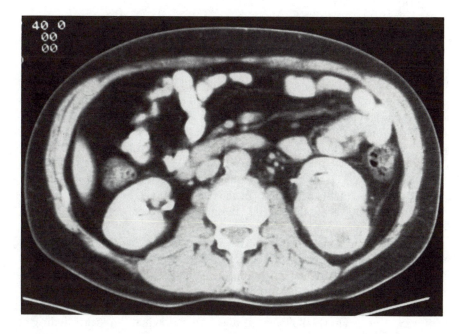

FIG 40–4.
Abdominal CT scan shows large kidney lesion, compatible with a primary hypernephroma.

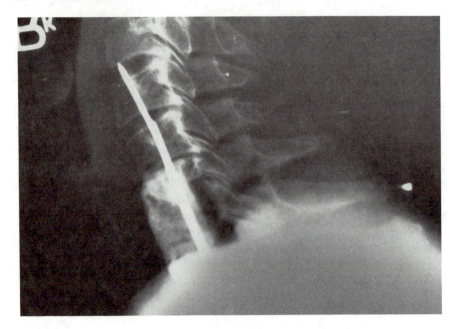

FIG 40–5.
Lateral cervicothoracic x-ray. One year following resection and stabilization, no recurrence of tumor or loss of alignment has been noted.

plasmacytoma (myeloma). In addition, spinal infections such as osteomyelitis and Pott's disease may frequently mimic a neoplasm. Skeletal metastases may present with simultaneous involvement of other sites such as lymph nodes or liver, which may help the physician establish a tissue diagnosis by biopsy of an accessible site other than the spine. Simon reported 14 patients who presented with bone pain, in whom bone scans or x-ray revealed metastases.[7] Of these, three were diagnosed with renal cell carcinoma, two with lung cancer, two with myeloma, and one with hepatoma. In the remaining six patients, the primary tumor was never detected during life. In one patient, renal cell carcinoma was found at postmortem.

In our series of approximately 300 patients who have undergone surgery for various neoplasms involving the spine, approximately 40% have had spinal involvement as the initial manifestation of malignancy.[2, 8] Frequently, the primary site may be obvious on a routine chest x-ray. If abnormalities are not detected on careful physical history and physical examination, a routine screening profile and hemogram should be performed. An abdominal CT scan is indicated in all these patients to rule out an occult kidney neoplasm. Although relatively uncommon, kidney cancer is an important diagnostic consideration in the patient presenting with pathologic compression fractures.[9] Approximately 20%–50% of the patients with renal cell carcinoma present with metastatic disease at the time of initial diagnosis. Of these, osseous metastases account for 15% of single organ sites and up to 40% when more than one site is involved. The prognosis of patients who present with metastatic disease is generally poor, with medial survival rates of approximately 6 months, with less than 10% surviving 2 years. A small subset of patients, however, benefit from more aggressive therapy. In such patients, resection of both the metastatic focus and the primary tumor should be performed, as in our patient.

The importance of identifying a possible kidney tumor is also related to the extreme hypervascularity of such tumors metastatic to bone. Angiography should, therefore, be performed to determine the vascularity of the spinal lesion if a kidney tumor is suspected. Frequently, the diagnosis of kidney cancer can be established by a CT-guided needle biopsy of the kidney mass. Spinal angiography is also used to decrease tumor neovascularity in bone by embolization with a variety of agents, such as Ivalon (polyvinyl alcohol), or absolute alcohol. With the use of such selective angiography and embolization, blood loss during surgery can be minimized to an acceptable level.

Although radiation therapy (RT) is generally recommended as palliative treatment for spinal metastases from solid tumors, there is increasing recognition that such therapy only provides short-term palliation of pain and is beneficial in less than 50% of patients with radioresistant tumors. Our data, and those of others, suggest that a more vigorous approach including tumor resection and stabilization provides better long-term palliation and improvement in neurological function. In patients with malignancies, the use of methyl methacrylate for reconstruction is recommended because its strength is not affected by the use of postoperative RT. To prevent the methyl methacrylate construct from dislocating, additional reinforcement with instrumentation is required. The use of Knodt or Harrington rods, and various forms of distraction devices has been advocated, but the simplest technique that is effective is the use of Steinmann's pins, which are fixed to the vertebra above and below the level of resection. Careful positioning of Steinmann's pins in the midportion of the vertebral body is important to prevent injury of vascular structures anterior to the spine. If additional involvement of the posterior elements is present, a second-stage posterior stabilization following anterior reconstruction may be required.

At present, concepts of posterior stabilization have evolved from the use of distraction rods such as Harrington rods to segmental spinal instrumentation. The major advantages of segmental fixation (which includes the Luque Rod System, and the Pedicle Fixation Systems, such as the Codrel-Dubousset Universal Systems) include a more rigid fixation in which the stresses are transmitted throughout the columns and more evenly across the spine. These forms of instrumentation are complex, time-consuming, and require considerable technical expertise.

The second major advantage of resecting pathologically diseased vertebra is the possibility of obtaining sufficient tissue to make a more accurate histologic diagnosis. With the recent development of immune-histochemistry using immunoperoxidase techniques, a variety of treatable malignancies can be identified. Clinicians may not often realize the limitations of needle biopsy for spinal tumors, and the potential scope of specialized techniques in correctly identifying a possible primary site of cancer. In these complex cases, proper consultation with the surgical pathologist is important, and a clear understanding of the techniques and limitations is essential. In many cases, fresh tissue needs to be stained for optimum results. Immunoperoxidase techniques are helpful in the diagnosis of metastatic prostate cancer, which frequently presents with bony metastases. Thus, the detection of prostate specific acid phosphatase (PSAP) is a simple way of establishing the prostatic origin of a metastatic carcinoma. Similarly, the detection of carcinoembryonic antigen (CEA) excludes a prostate cancer, but shifts the diagnosis toward the colon, lung, pancreas, breast, or biliary tract. Similarly, tumors of the lymphoid and hematopoietic system can be evaluated by immunocytochemical techniques. A major application of the frozen section immunoperoxidase technique is to distinguish between reactive and neoplastic B-cell lymphocyte proliferation. The demonstration of monotypic staining patterns facilitates the distinction between lymphoma and a reactive proliferation. A number of normal cellular components are confined to certain tissues, and can be detected using antibodies. These include Factor VIII-related antigens for endothelial tumors, keratin for carcinomas, vimentin and desmin for sarcomas, and neurofilaments for neural tumors. Endocrine products such as thyroglobulin can also be detected. In addition to providing a more precise diagnosis, it is also possible to evaluate the potential chemosensitivity of the tumor using a variety of commercial kits that may aid in the proper choice of chemotherapy, or to detect the p-glycoprotein associated with multiple drug resistance. Although such testing is still in its infancy, our experience indicates that potentially useful agents can be identified, and these techniques hold considerable promise for the future.

In conclusion, the identification of a pathological compression fracture as a cause of spinal pain should no longer arouse a feeling of complete pessimism if malignant diagnosis is suspected. Current methods of tumor diagnosis and surgical stabilization of the spine have considerably improved the prognosis for pain relief in the management of these patients, and have also improved survival, providing a tumor that is responsive to therapy can be identified.

REFERENCES

1. Harrington KD: Metastatic disease of the spine. *J Bone Joint Surg [Am]* 1986; 68:1110–1115.
2. Sundaresan N, Digiacinto GVD, Hughes JEO: Surgical treatment of spinal metastases. *Chin Neurosurgery* 1986; 33:503–522.
3. Sundaresan N, Galicich JH, Lane JM, et al: Stabilization of the Spine Involved by Cancer, in Dunsker SB, Schmidek HH, Frymoyer J, et al: *The Unstable Spine.* Orlando, Fla., Grune & Stratton, 1986, pp 249–276.
4. Bridwell KH, Jenny AB, Saul T, et al: Posterior segmental spinal instrumentation (PSSI) with postero-lateral decompression and debulking for metastatic thoracic and lumbar spine disease: Limitations of the techniques. *Spine* 1988; 13:1383–1394.
5. Kostuik JP, Errico JJ, Gleason TF, et al: Spinal stabilization of vertebral column tumors. *Spine* 1986; 13:250–256.
6. Fer MF, Greco FA, Oldham RK: *Poorly Differentiated Neoplasms and Tumors of Unknown Origin.* Orlando, Fla., Grune & Stratton, 1987.
7. Simon MA, Katluk MB: Metastases of unknown origin. *Clin Orthop* 1982; 166:96–103.
8. Sundaresan N, Galicich JH, Lane JM, et al: Treatment of neoplastic epidural cord compression by vertebral body resection and stabilization. *J Neurosurg* 1985; 63:676–684.
9. Sundaresan N, Scher H, Yagoda A, et al: Surgical treatment of spinal metastases in kidney cancer. *J Clin Oncol* 1986; 4:1851–1856.

41

Superior Sulcus Tumor (Pancoast Tumor) With Spine and Brachial Plexus Invasion

Narayan Sundaresan, M.D.

Ved P. Sachdev, M.D.

George Krol, M.D.

The patient is a 58-year-old woman who presented with pain in her left shoulder and periscapular region approximately 1 year ago. Following initial radiologic evaluation of the shoulder and cervical spine, she was diagnosed as "osteoarthritic" and treated with nonsteroidal anti-inflammatory agents, as well as with cortisone injections into the left shoulder by her local doctor. The pain intensified, and over a 6-month period, was associated with paresthesias down the ulnar aspect of the left arm. Re-evaluation by a neurologist revealed a Horner's syndrome on the left side. Her past history was significant in that she had a 20 pack-year smoking history. A chest x-ray and a computed tomography (CT) scan revealed a large mass involving the left apex of the lung with destruction of the ribs and extension to the spine. A percutaneous needle biopsy confirmed a poorly differentiated carcinoma. In view of the local extent of tumor, she was treated with external radiation therapy, receiving a total dose of 4,500 rads using conventional fractionation. Following this, she was treated with systemic chemotherapy (cisplatin and etoposide) for two courses. After an initial response, in which her pain decreased to less than 50% of the initial level, recurrence of severe pain and paresthesias along the ulnar aspect of the arm was noted 2 months post-therapy. Repeat evaluation by CT scan and magnetic resonance

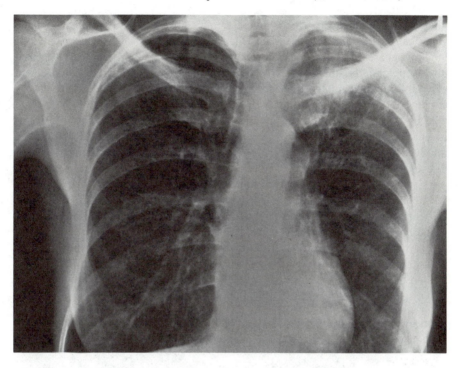

FIG 41–1.
Chest x-ray in patient with brachial plexopathy secondary to recurrent tumor. Note minimal
changes apparent on plain radiography.

imaging (MRI) showed a large tumor with invasion of the upper thoracic vertebra,
ribs, chest wall, and extension into the spine (Figs 41–1 to 41–3). In view of the
radiologic demonstration of spinal invasion, resection was offered to the patient to
prevent spinal cord compression and for pain relief. Through a posterolateral thoracotomy, an en bloc resection of the tumor, chest wall, and spine was performed.
The tumor was also dissected free from the brachial plexus. The tumor bed was
implanted with permanent radioactive iodine-125 seeds, which was estimated to
provide an additional 3,000 rads locally. The postoperative course was uncompli-
cated, and the patient continued to experience marked pain relief with decrease in
narcotic intake. She continued to experience relief of pain from the procedure, but
expired from systemic metastases 5 months after operation.

DISCUSSION

This case exemplifies an important problem in cancer pain resulting from brachial
plexus invasion by tumors. Of the various tumors involving the brachial plexus,

lung and breast cancers are the most frequent primary sites implicated. The American Cancer Society estimates that approximately 150,000 new cases of lung cancer are diagnosed each year, of which less than half present with localized disease potentially amenable to resection. In the majority, regional involvement of vital structures, or the presence of distant metastases precludes surgical attempts at a cure. However, approximately 5% of lung cancers involve the chest wall by local extension. These tend to remain locally invasive without involvement of the mediastinal nodes. In such patients, resection of the tumor and involved chest wall can result in 5-year survival rates of approximately 30%. The most important example of such tumors are those arising from the lung apex, which are called ''superior sulcus tumors,'' or by the familiar eponym, ''Pancoast tumor.''[1-3]

Superior sulcus tumors are distinguished by their frequent neurological presentation, i.e., radiculopathy, as well as by involvement of the brachial plexus and spine. In two classical papers Henry Pancoast described the clinical presentation of tumors located at the thoracic inlet, characterized clinically by pain around the shoulder and down the arm, Horner's syndrome, and atrophy of the

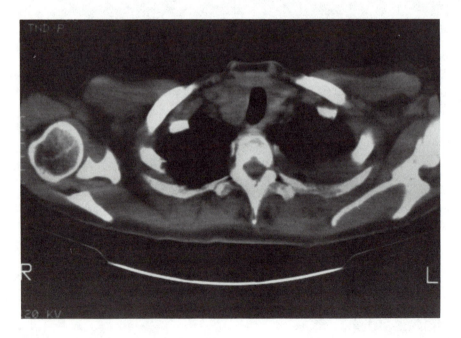

FIG 41–2.
CT scan of upper spine showing paraspinal tumor recurrence. Note that invasion of the spine is not evident, but rib involvement can be appreciated.

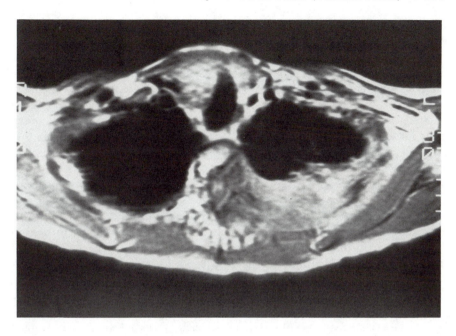

FIG 41-3.
Magnetic resonance image (MRI) at the same level, indicating abnormal signal within the paraspinal region, as well as the spine.

hand muscles.[4-5] This was usually associated with roentgenographic evidence of a small homogeneous shadow at the apex of the lung with local rib destruction and vertebral infiltration. He believed that these tumors arose from embryonic rests within the superior pulmonary sulcus, hence the term ''superior sulcus tumor.'' In the early years, this tumor was considered to be uniformly fatal, and few long-term survivors were noted. In the early 1960s, Shaw and Paulson demonstrated that these tumors could be resected following a course of preoperative radiation therapy.[6] Hilaris et al., further suggested that even if resection was not feasible, palliation and local control could be obtained by the use of local interstitial implants of radioactive iodine-125.[2]

With the advent of computed tomography (CT) and magnetic resonance imaging (MRI), our ability to visualize the true anatomic extent of the tumor has greatly improved; yet it is still not uncommon for a long delay in diagnosis because the clinical presentation is generally one of shoulder or arm pain. Such patients are frequently treated for ''arthritis,'' ''bursitis,'' or other musculoskeletal pain syndromes for several months before the diagnosis is established. In early cases, x-ray evaluation of the chest may be interpreted as normal, or show minimal apical fibrosis. Persistent arthritic-type pain associated with paresthesias down the ulnar aspect of the arm in the C8–T1 distribution in patients with a positive smoking history should alert the clinician to the possibility of a superior sulcus tumor. Paresthesias down the arm imply involvement of the lower cord of the brachial plexus. Horner's syndrome has been reported in 50% of the cases in the literature, but was seen in 90% of our patients because pupillary inequality was carefully looked for.[7] Approximately 20% of patients may present with invasion of the spine or have epidural extension of the tumor at initial presentation. When the diagnosis is suspected, the most important diagnostic evaluation is a CT scan of the brachial plexus and the upper spine. This will outline not only the tumor, but can be used for a CT-guided needle biopsy to confirm the diagnosis. If a supraclavicular mass (indicating node involvement) is present, the diagnosis can also be established by open biopsy. Bronchoscopy is rarely useful because of the peripheral nature of the tumor. In addition, CT scan allows accurate radiologic staging of the tumor because it can be used to scan both the mediastinum for adenopathy, as well as the abdomen for adrenal metastases. Although current experience with MRI is still evolving, our preliminary data indicate that MRI scans may show abnormal signals within the vertebral body in more than 20% of patients at initial evaluation, thus indicating early involvement of the spine.

Once a tissue diagnosis of non-small cell cancer is established, the traditional treatment is to use a course of preoperative radiation. This generally includes a course ranging from 4,000–4,500 rads given to the tumor, supraclavicular region, and mediastinum. Following this treatment, an assessment for thoracotomy is made and offered to the patient if disease is still localized. Relief of pain generally indicates a favorable response to radiation, while escalation of pain indicates a poor response. The standard surgical treatment includes resection of the tumor and involved ribs, an upper lobectomy, and mediastinal node resection. With the addition of a neurosurgical team, resection can often be improved upon because frequently, tongue-like extensions of tumor are present along the brachial plexus which can be dissected free with microtechniques.[8] The T1 nerve root has to be sacrificed as perineural extension along this nerve is common. We believe that resection can be accomplished even when the spine is involved, although many consider such involvement a sign of inoperability. When invasion of the spine is present, this may require removal of the upper two thoracic vertebrae and reconstruction with methyl methacrylate and Steinmann's pins.[9, 10] Unfortunately, when extensive invasion of the brachial plexus or mediastinal vessels is present, total resection is not feasible. In such instances, local control can be enhanced by the use of radioactive implants of iodine-125.

These extended resections are well tolerated by the patient, and provide gratifying pain relief in 75% of treated patients, with mortality rates of less than 3% when performed by experienced hands. However, local treatment failure is the major cause of morbidity within the first year. This is frequently heralded by the return of brachial plexus pain, which generally has a different quality from the original nociceptive pain experienced during the initial onset of the tumor. In all cases, the diagnosis of recurrent tumor should be confirmed by CT. Recurrent brachial plexopathy pain presumably results both from tumor recurrences and deafferentation. Deafferentation pain may be burning, be associated with dysesthesias, and may require frequent escalation of narcotics. The use of oral narcotics in combination with ancillary drugs such as amitriptyline 75–100 mg/day, or fluphenazine 5 mg/day, is recommended. When a deafferentation component is evident, the use of phenytoin (Dilantin) 100–300 mg/day or carbamazepine (Tegretol) 200–400 mg/day, has also been advocated. In addition, when recurrent tumor is documented, the use of parenteral steroids such as prednisone or dexamethasone may be helpful.

When pain continues to escalate despite medical measures, therapeutic options include the use of local neurolytic blocks such as 5%–10% phenol, or the implantation of drug delivery systems for intraspinal morphine. In our experience, the effectiveness of intraspinal-implanted devices is limited because tolerance rapidly develops. The most appropriate surgical procedure is a high percutaneous cordotomy, which can be expected to provide pain relief in more than 50% of patients until death.[11] Recurrent local tumor is also amenable to repeat local resection, since palliative debulking of the tumor has the added advantage of delaying or preventing the onset of paraplegia. We therefore recommend re-exploration and resection of tumor in selected patients, since pain relief is often gratifying and equal to that obtained from pain procedures alone. In view of the potential morbidity, such extensive procedures should be restricted to centers where the necessary expertise is available.

REFERENCES

1. Bonica JJ, Ventafidda V, Pagni CA: Advances in Pain Research and Therapy, in *Management of Superior Pulmonary Sulcus Syndrome,* vol 4. New York, Raven Press, 1981.
2. Hilaris BS, Martini N, Wong GY, et al: Treatment of superior sulcus tumor (Pancoast tumor). *Surg Clin North Am* 1987; 67:965–977.
3. Paulson D: Extended resection of bronchogenic carcinoma in the superior pulmonary sulcus. *Surg Rounds* 1980; 1:10–21.
4. Pancoast HK: Importance of careful Roentgen ray investigation of apical chest tumors. *JAMA* 1924; 83:1407–1411.
5. Pancoast HK: Superior pulmonary sulcus tumors. *JAMA* 1932; 99:1391–1396.
6. Shaw RR, Paulson DL, Kee JL: Treatment of superior sulcus tumor by irradiation followed by resection. *Ann Surg* 1961; 154:229–240.
7. Sundaresan N, Foley KM, Hilaris BS, et al: Neurological complications of superior sulcus tumors. *Proc Am Soc Clin Oncol* 1985; 4:189.

8. Sundaresan N, Hilaris BS, Martini N: The combined neurosurgical-thoracic management of superior sulcus tumors. *J Clin Oncol* 1987; 5:1739–1745.

9. Sundaresan N, Galicich HG, Lane JM, et al: Treatment of neoplastic epidural cord compression by vertebral body resection and stabilization. *J Neurosurg* 1985; 63:676–684.

10. Sundaresan N, Galicich JH, Lane JM, et al: Stabilization of the Spine Involved by Cancer, in Dunsker SB, Schmidek HH, Frymoyer J, et al (eds): *The Unstable Spine*. Orlando, Fla, Grune & Stratton, 1986, pp 249–274.

11. Ischia S, Ischia A, Luzzani A, et al: Results in the treatment of persistent cervicothoracic (Pancoast) and thoracic malignant pain by unilateral percutaneous cordotomy. *Pain* 1985; 211:339–355.

42

Bone Metastasis Pain:
Medical Management

Michael H. Levy, M.D., Ph.D.

A 71-year-old white man presented with progressive bony metastasis from prostatic carcinoma despite initial definitive radiation therapy, subsequent bilateral orchiectomy, diethylstilbestrol, chemotherapy, and multiple courses of palliative radiation therapy. The patient was admitted with overwhelming pain and over-sedation on 15 mg of methadone every 6 hours. The patient's pain was brought under control and his mental status improved on indomethacin (Indocin) 50 mg orally three times daily and increasing doses of hydromorphone (Dilaudid). He was discharged and resumed daily living activities on Dilaudid 14 mg orally every 4 hours and Indocin 50 mg orally three times daily.

DISCUSSION

Bone metastasis is the most common cause of cancer pain.[1-2] It occurs frequently in patients with cancer originating in the lung, breast, prostate, and colon, and accounts for approximately 30% of cancer-induced pain. Bone metastasis pain is often exacerbated by activity or weight bearing, making it one of the most difficult cancer pains to manage. Due to this variable, incident nature, it is difficult to give patients with bone metastasis pain enough narcotics to prevent activity-induced pain exacerbations without producing narcotic-induced toxicity while the patient is at rest. Pathologic fractures cause even more intense exacerbations in bone metastasis pain and require aggressive local therapy. Finally, hypoventilation secondary to painful rib metastases or decreased mental status

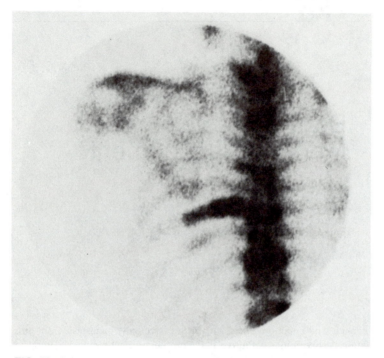

FIG 42–1.
Posterior view of an isotope bone scan of a patient with advanced prostatic cancer showing multiple areas of metastasis to thoracic spine and left seventh rib.

secondary to hypercalcemia further narrow the therapeutic window for safe and effective use of systemic narcotics in patients suffering from pain from bone metastasis.

The pain of bone metastasis can vary from a dull ache to a deep pain. It is occasionally worse at night or with increasing humidity or decreasing barometric pressure. Bone metastasis pain is variable from patient to patient and is often the cause of overlying painful muscle spasm. The most sensitive way to diagnose bone metastasis is with the use of an isotope bone scan. Such bone scans actually detect the bone's osteoclastic reaction to abnormalities within it and are, therefore, less specific than conventional radiographics. Bone scans are diagnostic in approximately 95% of patients with bony metastasis and can detect bone metastasis 3–6 months prior to their appearance as osteolytic or osteoblastic lesions on routine radiographs. A positive bone scan with a negative radiograph is a common finding in early stages of bone metastasis. Later in the disease, the extent of bone metastasis is usually more apparent on bone scan (Fig 42–1), than on a routine radiograph (Fig 42–2), taken at the same time. Patients with painful, bone scan-documented bone metastasis in their spine or extremities should have supplementary routine radiographs to assess the extent of cortical erosion and risk of impending fracture. Other indicators of bone metastasis are progressive anemia and elevations of serum alkaline phosphatase, calcium, lactate dehydrogenase, and acid phosphatase. Computed axial tomography (CT), and magnetic resonance imaging (MRI), are particularly useful in evaluating the base of the skull and vertebral bodies. Computed tomography and MRI scans may also be diagnostic in patients with negative bone scans from metastases that

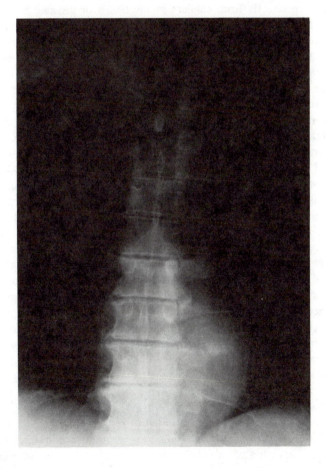

FIG 42–2.
Routine radiograph of the thoracic spine of a patient with advanced prostatic cancer showing osteoblastic bone metastasis, loss of the left facet of the seventh thoracic vertebra, and dissolution of the proximal portion of the left seventh rib.

do not elicit an osteoblastic reaction. Finally, needle biopsy may be necessary to diagnose bone metastasis in some patients with small cell carcinoma of lung, lymphoma, or myeloma, who have bone pain but show negative bone, CT, and MRI scans.

MANAGEMENT

The treatment of bone metastasis pain begins by treating the underlying malignancy. Bone metastasis from cancers of the breast or prostate are exquisitely sensitive to hormonal maneuvers. In the case presented here, the patient underwent a bilateral orchiectomy when his prostatic carcinoma first metastasized to bone, and later received a brief trial of diethylstilbestrol. Luteinizing hormone releasing hormone (LHRH) analogues form a third type of hormone intervention for prostate cancer. In general, however, patients whose metastatic prostate carcinoma progresses through their first hormonal intervention rarely respond to a second hormonal therapy. Patients with bone metastasis from estrogen receptor-positive breast cancer can experience significant objective and subjective control of their cancer with the use of tamoxifen (Nolvadex), or megestrol acetate (Megace). Unlike prostatic cancer patients, breast cancer patients who respond well to a first hormonal maneuver will often respond to second and third hormonal interventions once progression occurs from initial therapy. Cytotoxic chemotherapy can also reduce bone metastasis pain, especially in patients with lymphoma, myeloma, breast cancer, and small cell carcinoma of the lung. Chemotherapy can also help some patients with non-small cell lung cancer, colon cancer, and prostate cancer. Radiation therapy is another anticancer treatment that offers significant benefit for patients with bone metastasis. As many as 86% of patients show some improvement, with 52% showing complete improvement of bone metastasis pain following local palliative radiation therapy. Finally, orthopedic surgery can reduce the pain of bone metastasis by securing damaged bones and preventing impending fractures, or by stabilizing pathologic fractures once they have occurred.

A second approach to controlling bone metastasis pain is treating the body's physiologic reaction to the presence of bone metastasis. Calcitonin (Calcimar), and plicamycin (Mithracin) are effective agents in reducing the hypercalcemia of bone metastasis and have been reported to reduce bone pain as well. More commonly, treating the body's inflammatory reaction to bone metastasis with its attendant production of prostaglandins has been shown to have significant analgesic value.[1-2] Prostaglandins appear to be involved in the destruction of bone and in the sensitization or direct stimulation of pain receptors in the bone and periosteum. Antiprostaglandin, nonsteroidal anti-inflammatory drugs (NSAIDs), have been shown to be more effective than narcotics in the man-

TABLE 42–1.

Recommended NSAIDs for Bone Metastasis Pain

Drug	Dosage
Choline Magnesium Trisalicylate (Trilisate)	1,500 mg p.o. q12h
Ibuprofen (Motrin)	800 mg p.o. q8h
Diflunisal (Dolobid)	500 mg p.o. q12h
Naproxen (Naprosyn)	500 mg p.o. q12h
Indomethacin (Indocin)	50 mg p.o. q8h

agement of early bone metastasis pain and to be narcotic-sparing later in the disease process.[3–4] Of note, prostaglandin synthesis does not appear to be involved in the bony involvement of myeloma and lymphoma, thereby limiting the benefit of NSAIDs in these malignancies. All patients with bone metastasis from solid tumors should be considered for NSAID therapy. Over-the-counter aspirin or ibuprofen are readily available and should be taken in full therapeutic dosages of 1,000 mg every 4 hours and 400 mg every 4 hours, respectively. The use of prescription NSAIDs (Table 42–1) in controlling bone metastasis pain is similar to their use in nonmalignant rheumatologic diseases. Each patient seems to experience idiosyncratic benefits and/or toxicities from different NSAIDs. In any given patient, therefore, it may be necessary to try a series of NSAIDs until the optimal one is found. The most common side-effect of NSAID therapy is gastrointestinal distress, which can usually be diminished with concomitant use of antacids or sucralfate (Carafate). Recent reports have indicated that many nonsteroidal anti-inflammatory drugs can reduce the rate of glomerular filtration, which can be problematic in patients with pre-existing renal failure or those receiving renal-dependent agents such as cisplatin, methotrexate, or gentamicin. Finally, interference with prostaglandin synthesis decreases platelet aggregation, adding to the risk of bleeding in patients whose cancer or cancer therapy causes thrombocytopenia. Aspirin-induced platelet damage is permanent and requires 10–14 days for new platelets to reach the circulation from the bone marrow to normalize prolonged bleeding time. The antiplatelet effect of the other nonsteroidal anti-inflammatory drugs is temporary, with normalization of prolonged bleeding time occurring within 8–24 hours after discontinuation of their usage. To date, sulindac (Clinoril), and choline magnesium trisalicylate (Trilisate) have not been reported to interfere with renal function. Trilisate also does not interfere with platelet function and, therefore, could be considered the NSAID of choice for many cancer patients.[5] Trilisate appears to be equal in efficacy with ibuprofen. Indomethacin (Indocin), and naproxen (Naprosyn) appear to be more potent than ibuprofen, but are often accompanied by a greater incidence of adverse side effects. Due to the severe nature of the patient's pain in the case above, and his attendant narcotic toxicity, the more potent Indocin was chosen as initial NSAID therapy. The patient was able to tolerate its usage and, with the addition of appropriate doses of Dilaudid, experienced significant improvement. Another consideration in the use of nonsteroidal anti-inflammatory drugs is their metabolic half-lives. Drugs such as Trilisate, diflunisal (Dolobid), and Naprosyn can usually be given on a 12-hour basis with improved patient convenience and compliance.

In advanced bone metastasis, nonsteroidal anti-inflammatory drugs can only reduce the pain by 20%–40%.[1, 2] Narcotic therapy must, therefore, be offered to these patients to gain more complete control of their pain.[1, 6] Narcotic therapy should also be offered to patients awaiting the onset of anticancer therapy-induced analgesia. Individually titrated doses of narcotics should be given around the clock, with rescue supplements for breakthrough or incident pain provided on an "as needed" basis. Morphine and hydromorphone are the most commonly used narcotics for patients with advanced cancer, and should be given in dosages and time intervals that achieve maximal pain prevention with minimal narcotic side effects.[6] Patients with a significant activity-induced pain should also be offered anticipatory narcotic supplements 30–60 minutes before planned activities. Patients on around-the-clock, 4-hourly narcotics at doses exceeding 30 mg of morphine or its equivalent should be advised to awaken themselves for their middle-of-the-night dose to avoid awakening in the early morning with recurrent pain. Twelve-hourly, controlled-release morphine (MS Contin) is particularly useful in patients with bone metastasis pain, allowing them to have a full night's sleep and to awaken in the morning without recurrent pain. Finally, patients taking narcotics who undergo anticancer therapy or who are begun on nonsteroidal anti-inflammatory drugs should be monitored for signs of narcotic excess should these interventions reduce the source of their pain and, thereby, reduce their narcotic requirement. In such patients, narcotic therapy should be gradually decreased to a point where they are free of both pain and unwanted narcotic toxicity.

Patients who experience uncontrollable toxicity from systemic analgesic therapy of their bone metastasis pain should be considered for local anesthesiologic or neurosurgical procedures presented elsewhere in this text. Patients with a high-incident component to their pain, leading to intolerable toxicity from NSAID and high-dose narcotic therapy, may benefit significantly from epidural steroids and hypertonic saline, epidural phenol, or intrathecal narcotics. Should these procedures fail, rhizotomy or cordotomy may be helpful.

In summary, the management of bone metastasis pain highlights the value of the interdisciplinary team approach to cancer pain management. The medical oncologist and radiation oncologist must do their best to reduce or slow the progression of the patient's malignancy. The orthopedic surgeon must be considered for impending or actual fractures. The primary physician should begin all patients on nonsteroidal anti-inflammatory drugs, and then later add appropriate systemic narcotics. Finally, in those patients for whom these therapies are ineffective or excessively toxic, local anesthesiologic or neurosurgical interventions should be considered. Throughout this series of interventions, skilled nursing care is essential for frequent patient assessment and patient/family education and support.

REFERENCES

1. Twycross RG, Lack SA: *Symptom Control in Far Advanced Cancer: Pain Relief.* London, Pitman Publishing, Ltd, 1983.
2. Hoskins PJ, Hanks GW: Bone pain, in Bates TD (ed): Contemporary palliation of difficult symptoms. *Baillieres Clin Oncol* 1987; 1:431–441.
3. Pollen JJ, Schmidt JD: Bone pain in metastatic cancer of prostate. *Urology* 1982; 13:129–134.
4. Lomen PL, Samal BA, Lamborn KR, et al: Flurbiprofen for the treatment of bone pain in patients with metastatic breast cancer. *Am J Med* 1986; 80 (suppl 3A):83–87.
5. Zucker MB, Rothwell KG: Differential influences of salicylate compounds on platelet aggregation and serotonin release. *Nebr Symp Motiv* 1978; 23:194–199.
6. Levy MH: Pain management in advanced cancer. *Semin Oncol* 1985; 12:394–410.

43

Spinal Cord Compression Pain

Michael H. Levy, M.D., Ph.D.

A 72-year-old white man with progressive, metastatic renal cell carcinoma status post nephrectomy, chemotherapy, hormone therapy, and palliative radiation therapy was admitted with increasing back pain refractory to increasing doses of hydromorphone (Dilaudid) and doxepin (Sinequan). The patient's pain had recently begun to radiate into his thighs and subsequently down to his ankles, and was associated with bilateral lower extremity weakness for 3 days prior to admission. A magnetic resonance imaging (MRI) scan detected epidural metastases from T12–L1. Because of previous radiation therapy to that area, the patient underwent a decompression laminectomy. Following an increase of his narcotic requirement due to his acute postoperative pain, the patient was able to ambulate with the assistance of a walker and was discharged on Dilaudid 24 mg every 3 hours, Sinequan 100 mg orally at bedtime, and dexamethasone (Decadron) 8 mg orally every 6 hours.

DISCUSSION

Spinal cord compression occurs in approximately 5% of all patients with advanced cancer.[1–2] When suspected, spinal cord compression is an oncologic emergency. Back pain is almost invariably present in patients with spinal cord compression and should alert the clinician to intervene immediately in hopes of preventing irreversible spinal cord damage.[3]

The back pain related to epidural compression of the spinal cord may vary from a dull ache to a sharp, stabbing pain. It may have a radicular component with a bandlike or girdle compression sensation. The pain may be aggravated by coughing, sneezing, weight bearing, or lying down. Spinal cord compression pain may also be accompanied by paresthesias or numbness in the involved dermatomes. Late signs of spinal cord compression include bowel and bladder dysfunction and local motor weakness. High cervical spinal cord compression can progress to respiratory failure from diaphragmatic and intercostal muscle paralysis.

Malignant spinal cord compression is most common in patients with carcinoma of the lung, breast, prostate, kidney, and lymphoma. Approximately 9% of spinal cord compressions are the presenting symptom of cancers of unknown primary origin. Seventy percent of malignant spinal cord compressions occur in the thoracic spine, 20% in the lumbar spine, and 10% in the cervical spine. Physical examination often reveals an area of sensory loss at the level of the epidural tumor. There is often pain with vertebral percussion and with straight leg raise. Early in the course of spinal cord damage, there may be decreased deep tendon reflexes in the affected area due to spinal shock. Later, there may be increased, brisk, deep tendon reflexes and upward-going Babinski reflexes resulting from matured upper motor neuron damage. Routine x-rays of the involved spine show abnormalities such as vertebral body collapse, osteolytic lesions, osteoblastic lesions, or effacement of the vertebral pedicles in 70%–90% of patients with epidural spinal cord compression. Eighty-seven percent of patients with greater than 50% collapse of a vertebral body on a routine radiograph will have a positive myelogram. Thirty-one percent of patients with pedicle effacement will also demonstrate epidural extension on myelogram. The absence of any abnormalities on routine x-ray does not exclude the possibility of spinal cord compression. Approximately 7% of patients with spinal cord compression on myelogram will have normal routine radiographs. Inasmuch as it is imperative to diagnose spinal cord compression before irreversible motor fiber damage occurs, patients with the above-mentioned symptoms and cancers, and negative routine x-rays should still undergo myelographic analysis. Once a block of rostral flow of myelogram dye is noted, a cisternal or cervical myelogram should also be performed to determine the rostral extent of the epidural mass. High-pressure injection of saline through the myelogram needle can often force enough dye above the block to visualize the extent of the epidural tumor (Fig 43–1). As many as 20% of epidural metastases have been noted to involve multiple levels at the time of presentation. More recently, magnetic resonance imaging (MRI) has been shown to be of significant value in the diagnosis of epidural tumors (Fig 43–2). An MRI scan avoids the possible complication of spinal headache following spinal puncture to inject the myelographic dye. In addition, MRI is probably the diagnostic study of choice in patients with documented allergy to iodine or iodine-based contrast materials. It is not yet decided whether a negative MRI scan obviates the need for a myelogram or vice versa. For now, the studies

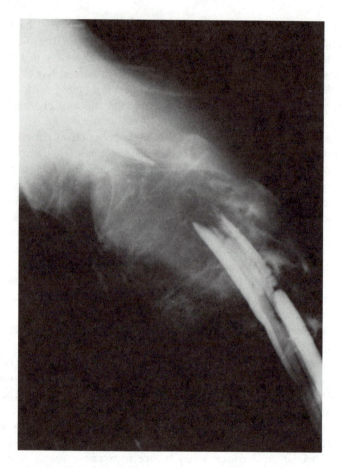

FIG 43–1.
Lateral view of a myelogram of epidural spinal cord compression at T3–4 in a patient with metastatic, non-small cell carcinoma of the lung.

should be considered complementary in those patients who have significant symptoms that elude specific diagnosis by either of these studies.

MANAGEMENT

The management of spinal cord compression pain is integrated into the overall management of the newly diagnosed epidural tumor. Initial therapy consists of high-dose steroids, which, by reducing the inflammatory component of the tumor's mass, reduce the tumor's compression of the spinal cord.[4] Steroid-induced tumor mass reduction relieves pain and often reverses some of the presenting neurologic dysfunction. One treatment protocol calls for 100 mg of dexamethasone to be injected intravenously, followed by 25 mg intravenously every 6 hours until definitive therapy has begun and the patient's symptoms have stabilized or improved.[1, 3] Alternatively, 40 mg of dexamethasone may be given intravenously initially with 10 mg given intravenously every 6 hours thereafter. Once definitive therapy has been initiated, the intravenous dexamethasone may be tapered gradually by reducing each 6-hourly dose by 2–4 mg every 2 or 3 days. Caution should be taken not to taper the steroid therapy too rapidly.

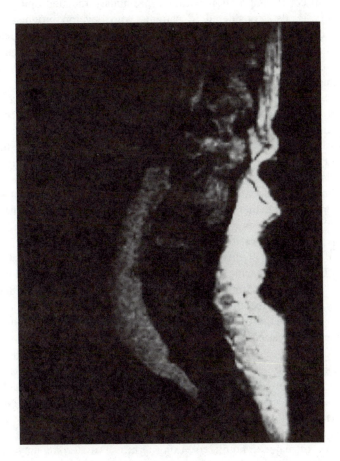

FIG 43–2.
Magnetic resonance imaging (MRI) scan of epidural spinal cord compression at T12–L1 in a patient with metastatic renal cell carcinoma.

Dexamethasone may be converted to oral administration within 1–2 weeks after the initiation of definitive therapy. The dose of dexamethasone may then continue to be tapered with consideration for persistence of active inflammation and resumption of normal pituitary-adrenal interaction.

Definitive therapy of spinal cord compression consists of radiation therapy, neurosurgery, or a combination of the two.[1-3] Radiation therapy should be initiated immediately with port determination based on the already mentioned total spinal myelogram or MRI scan. Neurosurgical decompression is considered initial therapy in patients with epidural tumors of uncertain diagnosis, with compression located in the high cervical cord, with radiation therapy-resistant tumors, or in cord compression within a previously radiated spinal segment. Neurosurgery is also considered in patients who develop progression of the neurologic deficit within 48–72 hours of the initiation of radiation therapy and high dose steroids. Following neurosurgery, patients with radiation therapy-sensitive tumors should receive postoperative radiation therapy for residual macroscopic and/or microscopic disease. Depending on the degree of neurologic deficit at the time of therapy initiation, approximately 25%–50% of patients with spinal cord compressions obtain normal neurologic function after the completion of definitive intervention.

In those patients who are not candidates for definitive radiation therapy or neurosurgery, the use of steroids should still be considered as a highly effective co-analgesic intervention. Steroids have a documented mood elevation and appetite enhancement effect, and are narcotic sparing in patients with acute nerve compression pain, whether at the spinal cord, root, or more peripheral nerve basis.[5] High-dose intravenous steroids are occasionally accompanied by acute perineal irritation and pruritis, which usually pass without specific treatment. The use of benadryl or hydroxyzine (Atarax) may be helpful in such patients. The use of high-dose steroids should probably be avoided in brittle diabetics due to steroids' glucose-elevating side effect. Patients taking nonsteroidal anti-inflammatory drugs at the time of developing nerve compression pain should probably discontinue these drugs prior to the initiation of steroids to avoid additive combined gastrointestinal toxicity. Fluid retention may occur in some patients receiving steroid therapy, and can usually be treated with potassium-sparing diuretics such as hydrochlorthiazide plus triamterine (Dyazide). Another common side effect of prolonged steroid use in patients with advanced cancer is oral candidiasis, which can be effectively treated with ketoconazole (Nizoral) or myconizole (Mycelex). Rarely, patients on high-dose steroids may develop a toxic psychosis, which mandates discontinuation of the steroid therapy and possible addition of major tranquilizers. Long-term use of steroids may be complicated by proximal myopathy, which may produce a therapeutic dilemma. The dose of steroids necessary to maintain neurologic function may cause enough myopathy to decrease muscle function and, thereby, subvert the overall therapeutic intent. Finally, some patients may develop a painful steroid withdrawal or pseudorheumatism syndrome during the tapering of the steroid doses. This syndrome can usually be treated by a more gradual decrease in the steroid dosages.

Spinal cord compression pain may persist in patients who have received definitive therapy, even in the face of regained motor function. Pain may also persist or progress in patients who are not candidates for definitive therapy, despite the use of steroids previously outlined. If the upward titration of systemic narcotics does not control this pain totally, or if the narcotic doses required cause undesirable side effects, the use of antidepressant and antiseizure medications should be considered.[6] Persistent spinal cord compression pain is of presumed nerve damage origin, and often is resistant to narcotic therapy alone. Tricyclic antidepressant (TCA) therapy may be initiated with either nortriptyline (Pamelor) or doxepin (Sinequan), at a dose of 25 mg orally at bedtime. The bedtime TCA can be increased by 25 mg every 2 or 3 days to a tolerable, therapeutic dose between 75–150 mg orally at bedtime. In frail patients, Pamelor may be started at 10 mg orally at bedtime with increments of 10 mg every 2–3 nights, as tolerated, to a total dose of 50–80 mg. For most patients, giving the entire dose of Pamelor at bedtime minimizes daytime sedation and utilizes the sedative side effect of the single higher dose as an effective bedtime hypnotic. In patients who are anxious or agitated during the daytime, the bedtime dose of Pamelor may be divided and given on a twice- or three-time daily schedule. If the patient's pain remains incompletely controlled after 2–3 weeks of full dose TCA therapy, the addition of carbamazepine (Tegretol) can be considered. Tegretol therapy can safely be initiated by starting the patient on 100 mg of Tegretol orally twice a day and increasing by 200 mg per day every 2–3 days, until a total dose of 800 mg per day is achieved. Both Pamelor and Tegretol blood levels are available and should be monitored to assure that the patient is within the therapeutic range. Finally, should all of these systemic therapies prove ineffective, patients with intractable spinal cord compression should be evaluated for spinal narcotic or neurolytic therapy, discussed elsewhere in this text.

REFERENCES

1. Posner JB: Back pain and epidural spinal cord compression. *Med Clin North Am* 1987; 71:185–205.
2. Closs S, Bates TD: The management of malignant spinal cord compression, in Bates TD: Contemporary palliation of difficult symptoms. *Baillieres Clin Oncol* 1987; 431–441.
3. Portenoy RK, Lipton RB, Foley KM: Back pain in the cancer patient: An algorithm for evaluation and management. *Neurology* 1987; 37:134–138.

4. Twycross RG, Lack SA: *Symptom Control in Far Advanced Cancer: Pain Relief.* London, Pitman Publishing Ltd, 1983.
5. Ettinger AB, Portenoy RK: The use of corticosteroids in the treatment of symptoms associated with cancer. *J Pain Sympt Mgmt* 1988; 3:99–103.
6. Levy MH: Pain management in advanced cancer. *Semin Oncol* 1985; 12:394–410.

44

Radiation-Induced Brachial Plexopathy

Russell K. Portenoy, M.D.

A 42-year-old woman discovered a breast mass and underwent a lumpectomy with a lymph node dissection. Carcinoma was identified in the mass and one node. Radiation therapy was then given to a port that included the axilla and supraclavicular fossa. After 2 years without symptoms, the patient noted the insidious onset of pins and needles paresthesias in the first and second fingers of the ipsilateral hand, a dull aching sensation in the shoulder and upper arm, and mild clumsiness of fine motor hand movements. On physical examination, radiation-induced skin changes conforming to the described portals were noted. The arm was diffusely edematous. There was mild weakness in the shoulder girdle and normal strength distally. Minimal sensory loss was demonstrable along the cap of the shoulder, the outer aspect of the arm, and lateral hand. The ipsilateral biceps, brachioradialis, and triceps jerks were depressed. There was no Horner's sign and the rest of the examination was normal. The sensation of heaviness and aching discomfort of the arm gradually increased over the next 2 months. Weakness and atrophy progressed, and 1 year later, the limb was functionally useless. Partial pain relief was obtained with oral opioids.

DISCUSSION

The late development of discomfort and neurologic deficits affecting the arm and shoulder in cancer patients who have undergone irradiation of the brachial plexus region represents both a diagnostic and therapeutic challenge. Brachial plexopathy is suggested clinically by symptoms and signs that localize to a region outside of a single dermatome or peripheral nerve distribution. While many other disorders appear on the differential diagnosis, one of two pathologic processes is likely in this setting: recurrent (or new) neoplasm with invasion of the brachial plexus, or radiation-induced brachial plexopathy.

DIAGNOSIS

Radiation fibrosis of the brachial plexus may begin within months of treatment or may be delayed for many years. In one study, a median of 4 years was reported, with one-third of the patients presenting within one year after treatment.[1] The pathology usually involves postradiation fibrosis in the region of the plexus, which results in compression of neural tissues or secondary vascular compromise. The natural history is one of gradual progression to an ill-defined degree of neurologic deficit, which varies from patient to patient and is generally followed by a period of stabilization. There is no specific therapy and efforts at symptom control are of primary importance in maximizing residual function and maintaining quality of life.

The distinction between radiation fibrosis and neoplastic infiltration is essential to provide the patient with appropriate primary therapy and determine a realistic prognosis. The correct diagnosis is suspected on clinical grounds and supported by ancillary electrophysiologic and radiographic procedures (Table 44–1). Confirmation usually requires repeated assessments and the passage of time; in rare patients, surgical exploration of the brachial plexus is the only approach capable of providing a definitive diagnosis.[2]

The symptoms associated with radiation fibrosis of the brachial plexus include pain, a sense of heaviness of the limb, paresthesias, and ultimately, sensory loss and weakness. Although the same symptomatology can be described by the patient with neoplastic invasion of the brachial plexus, there are usually differences in both quality and degree of the complaint. Virtually all patients with neoplastic invasion of the plexus experience pain as a significant problem. Pain related to tumor infiltration is typically experienced in the shoulder, medial elbow, and medial two fingers. It is usually progressive and characterized by some combination of moderate to severe aching, burning, and lancinating pain. In contrast, a significant degree of pain occurs in less than 20% of patients with radiation fibrosis. When present, the pain is usually more moderate, proximal and diffuse in distribution, and aching in character. Often, heaviness, stiffness, or clumsiness of the limb is the most compelling early complaint.

Findings on physical examination are also useful in distinguishing these entities. In those with radiation fibrosis, radiation changes of the skin and subcutaneous tissues occur in approximately one-third of patients, and lymphedema is noted in three-quarters of the patients.[1] These findings can, of course, exist

TABLE 44–1.

Clinical, Electrophysiologic, and Radiographic Features of Brachial Plexopathy Due to Neoplasm and Radiation Fibrosis*

	Neoplastic Infiltration	Radiation Fibrosis
Incidence of Pain	About 50%	About 20%
Location of Pain	Shoulder, upper arm, elbow, medial hand	Shoulder, wrist, hand
Nature of Pain	Aching in shoulder and elbow; burning or lancinating dysesthesias in elbow and medial hand	Aching in shoulder; often prominent paresthesias
Severity of Pain	Moderate to severe	Mild to moderate
Neurologic Signs	Lower plexopathy (C7–T1 distribution); Horner's syndrome common	Upper plexopathy (C5–6 distribution); Horner's syndrome less common
Course	Progressive	Progressive, then stabilization
CT Findings	Circumscribed mass with infiltration of tissue plane	Diffuse infiltration of tissue planes
Electrodiagnostic Findings	Somatosensory evoked potential abnormal; no myokymia on electromyogram	Somatosensory evoked potential abnormal; myokymia on electromyogram

*Adapted from Foley KM: Brachial plexopathy in patients with breast cancer, in Harris JR, et al (eds): *Breast Diseases.* Philadelphia, JB Lippincott, 1987, pp 532–537.

in previously irradiated patients who develop tumor recurrence or a new primary lesion as well; the absence of these changes, however, renders the diagnosis of radiation fibrosis much less likely.

Neurological examination can be similarly helpful. Patients with radiation injury of the brachial plexus typically present with findings that conform to a lesion affecting the upper plexus, in a distribution consistent with C5–6 root lesions. This is reflected by proximal arm weakness, sensory changes along the cap of the shoulder and anterolateral aspect of the upper arm, and reflex abnormalities of the biceps and brachioradialis before demonstrable involvement of the triceps. In contrast, patients with tumor infiltration of the brachial plexus typically demonstrate signs compatible with a lower plexus injury, conforming to a C7–T1 root distribution. These patients develop weakness and atrophy of the hand, sensory loss affecting the inner aspect of the arm and medial hand, and reflex changes of the triceps, before involvement of the biceps and brachioradialis.

Thus, the history and physical findings can strongly suggest the diagnosis of radiation fibrosis of the brachial plexus. Electrodiagnostic tests and imaging procedures must then be performed to provide confirmatory evidence for this clinical impression. Somatosensory evoked potentials from the median nerve can be used as a sensitive indicator of a brachial plexus lesion, but is nonspecific with respect to the type of lesion. Nerve conduction velocities are similarly nonspecific and may reveal reduced or absent sensory or motor potentials in either radiation-induced or neoplastic plexopathy. More useful is electromyography, which can confirm the specific involvement of the upper versus lower plexus, and may also demonstrate the unusual finding of myokymia, which appears to be a relatively specific sign of radiation-induced damage.[3]

Imaging procedures are needed to define the cross-sectional anatomy of the region of the brachial plexus, assess the paraspinal gutter, and determine the integrity of vertebrae adjacent to this area. Computerized tomography (CT) is the most useful modality. Although the CT is abnormal in both neoplastic infiltration and radiation fibrosis, the finding of a discrete soft tissue mass in the region of the brachial plexus is a highly sensitive indicator of tumor. The value of magnetic resonance imaging (MRI) has not yet been determined empirically, but it is likely that this modality will also be a sensitive indicator of disease in this site; the specificity for either neoplasm or fibrosis remains to be determined, however. Occasionally, plain radiography of the spine or bone scintigraphy can reveal a bony lesion consistent with neoplasm in the spine near the plexus. Such a finding should be viewed as suggestive evidence of recurrent neoplasm with proximal extension.

The results of the clinical evaluation and supporting studies usually confirm the diagnosis of recurrent neoplasm or strongly suggest the alternative diagnosis of radiation fibrosis. The latter diagnosis, however, cannot be made with certainty unless adequate time has elapsed and repeated evaluation continues to be negative for neoplasm. Alternatively, surgical exploration of the plexus can be undertaken to obtain a definitive diagnosis. Surgical exploration is rarely indicated, but must be considered in patients with a progressive and well-localized lesion in the plexus, in whom studies of the plexus and an extent of disease evaluation fail to establish the diagnosis of recurrent cancer.

MANAGEMENT

Similar to other cancer-related pain syndromes, a variety of therapeutic approaches can be explored in the management of pain due to radiation fibrosis of the brachial plexus. Pharmacologic therapy is the most important, but adjunctive anesthetic, physiatric, neurostimulatory, psychological, and surgical therapies should be considered in every case. It is essential that aggressive management of pain should be undertaken during the evaluation progress, as well as after the diagnosis is established.

Pharmacotherapy includes the use of three analgesic classes, the nonsteroidal anti-inflammatory drugs (NSAIDs), the opioid analgesics, and adjuvant medications (drugs with other primary indications that are analgesic in selected circumstances). Since the pain associated with radiation fibrosis is often relatively mild, a therapeutic trial with an NSAID is a reasonable first step. The selection of a specific drug is empirical, but should be guided by a history of favorable prior experience with one or more of these agents, a coexistent bleeding ulcer or ulcer diathesis (consider choline magnesium trisalicylate or salsalate, since these agents have little to no gastrointestinal or platelet toxicity), or known renal insufficiency (consider sulindac, which may have less renal toxicity). Since the response of a patient to different NSAIDs can vary dramatically, a failed trial with one should be followed by an attempt with another. The initial dose of the NSAID should be relatively low, then titrated upward at weekly intervals until favorable effects occur, toxicity supervenes, or an increment fails to provide any additional benefit. Since both a ceiling dose and dose-related toxicity characterize this class of drugs, it is recommended that upward dose titration also be limited to no more than 1.5–2 times the standard recommended doses. Doses in this high range require periodic monitoring of gastrointestinal blood loss, hepatic and renal functions, and blood counts.

Many patients with pain due to brachial plexopathy may benefit from the use of adjuvant analgesics. Although there are no controlled trials to suggest the use of any of these agents in this condition, clinical experience suggests that one or another may be of value in selected patients. A trial with a tricyclic antidepressant, specifically amitriptyline, doxepin, or imipramine, is usually considered in those with continuous dysesthesias, while an anticonvulsant drug, such as carbamazepine, phenytoin, clonazepam, or valproate is typically used in patients with a paroxysmal lancinating quality to the pain. The use of other adjuvants, such as a neuroleptic (most often fluphenazine or haloperidol), or an oral local anesthetic can also be considered for refractory cases, although experience with these agents is limited.

Should other drugs fail to provide adequate relief, or should the patient present with moderate to severe pain, opioid drugs must be considered. Although chronic opioid therapy in patients with pain determined to originate from a nonmalignant cause remains controversial, there is accumulating clinical experience that suggests that this approach may be valuable in some patients.[4]

A small group of anesthetic approaches may be appropriate for the management of pain due to radiation fibrosis of the brachial plexus. Neurolytic procedures should be eschewed due to the functional incapacity they may cause and the long life expectancy of the patient. Nonneurolytic procedures include trigger point injections, which may be extremely useful in patients with coexistent myofascial pain, and neural blockade with local anesthetic. Of the latter procedures, occasional patients may benefit from stellate ganglion blocks, and one or more of these is a reasonable intervention in patients who fail to respond promptly to pharmacologic measures. Somatic nerve blocks are unlikely to provide more than transitory relief to patients with pain in this setting.

Physiatric approaches are extremely important in the management of these patients. Reduction in lymphedema is often highly therapeutic, both in terms of limb function and the common symptoms of pain and heaviness. The use of wraps, pressure stockings, or more sophisticated devices should be considered in every case. Additionally, intensive physical therapy is often useful in forestalling or preventing the secondary painful complications of contractures and ankylosis of the shoulder.

Of the neurostimulatory approaches, transcutaneous electrical nerve stimulation is most commonly employed. Data from surveys suggest that many patients will obtain partial relief initially, but this generally wanes over time. Nonetheless, the technique is extremely safe and a trial is often worthwhile. Invasive neurostimulatory techniques, such as dorsal column stimulation and deep brain stimulation, are unproved in this setting and carry some risk. They should be considered only by practitioners highly experienced in their application.

In addition to formal psychotherapy, psychological approaches to pain control include a variety of modalities designed to diminish pain intensity and improve the function of the patient. Cognitive therapies such as hypnosis, biofeedback, relaxation, and distraction techniques, may be extremely salutary, both in reducing pain and providing a sense of enhanced personal control over the problem. Specific behavioral interventions may reverse many of the destructive concomitants of chronic pain, such as physical inactivity, social isolation, and inability to work or perform avocations. Intensive treatment with these therapies may improve the patient's quality of life even if pain control is incomplete.

Surgical techniques of pain control play no role in the management of pain due to radiation fibrosis of the brachial plexus. These patients may have lengthy survivals and surgical neurolysis is rarely proposed in this situation. Moreover, consideration of any neurolytic procedure has to be tempered by the possibility that the neuropathic pain resulting from damage to the plexus is, in part, due to deafferentation, a type of lesion widely believed to be poorly responsive to neurolytic approaches.

In sum, both accurate diagnosis and intensive efforts at pain management are essential in patients who are eventually determined to have radiation fibrosis of the brachial plexus. Analgesic techniques must be accompanied by rehabilitative efforts designed to reduce lymphedema, prevent secondary myofascial and joint complications, and increase the functional capacity of the patient. Analgesia can usually be provided with one or more analgesic drugs, often combined with adjunctive anesthetic, neurostimulatory, or psychologic approaches.

REFERENCES

1. Kori SF, Foley KM, Posner JB: Brachial plexus lesions in patients with cancer: 100 cases. *Neurology* 1981; 31:45–50.
2. Foley KM: Brachial plexopathy in patients with breast cancer, in Harris JR, Hellman S, Henderson IC, et al (eds): *Breast Diseases*. Philadelphia, JB Lippincott, 1987, pp 532–537.
3. Albers J, Allen AH, Bashow JA, et al: Limb myokymia. *Muscle Nerve* 1981; 4:494–496.
4. Portenoy RK, Foley KM: Chronic use of opioid analgesics in non-malignant pain: Report of 38 cases. *Pain* 1986; 25:171–186.

45

Malignant Lumbosacral Plexopathy

Russell K. Portenoy, M.D.

A 42-year-old woman with locally extensive ovarian carcinoma invading the pelvic side wall presented with the insidious onset of progressive leg pain. The pain was localized to the knee and anterior thigh, and was described as burning and aching in quality, at times associated with paroxysmal, lancinating pain shooting into the inguinal region. After several months of worsening pain, the patient developed ipsilateral leg edema, numbness in the anterolateral thigh, and mild weakness in the proximal leg. Examination at that time revealed positive reverse straight leg raising, weakness in the iliopsoas and hip adductors, sensory loss in the inguinal region and anterior thigh, and an absent knee and ankle jerk. After several opioids had been titrated orally with intolerable side effects and no relief of pain, a trial of spinal opioids was instituted. This, too, was poorly tolerated and percutaneous cordotomy was performed. Pain relief was adequate until the patient's death 3 months later.

DISCUSSION

Neoplastic infiltration of the lumbosacral plexus is a common and challenging neurooncologic problem characterized by progressive pain and neurologic dysfunction. Management of this entity depends on systematic assessment of the pain and the medical status of the patient. This process defines the underlying lesion and determines the availability of primary antineoplastic therapy. Analgesic management with drugs and other modalities is almost always needed, however, and in most cases, primary analgesic therapy is necessary throughout the patient's course.

DIAGNOSIS

Lumbosacral plexopathy secondary to tumor infiltration most often complicates progressive or recurrent tumors of the genitourinary system or colon. The diagnosis is suspected on clinical grounds, then confirmed using electrophysiologic and imaging procedures.

Clinically, patients with this lesion complain of progressive pain, the location of which is determined by the region of the plexus affected.[1] Medially located tumors deep in the true pelvis commonly invade the lower plexus, resulting in pain in the buttock and posterior thigh and leg. Tumors infiltrating the pelvic side wall, in contrast, typically produce dysfunction in the upper plexus. In these patients, pain is usually experienced in the anterolateral or anteromedial thigh, as well as in the knee. In all cases, pain and neurologic signs commonly localize to a distribution outside of a single nerve root.

The pain associated with malignant lumbosacral plexopathy is usually spontaneous and constant, although fluctuation with a change in position or movement is common. The continuous pains are typically described as aching in quality, with or without burning dysesthesias; a superimposed severe paroxysmal pain may also occur.

On physical examination, the leg is often edematous. Straight leg raising is usually negative, but may exacerbate the pain in some cases of lower lumbosacral plexopathy. Reverse straight leg raising is often positive in patients with upper lumbosacral plexopathy. Neurologic examination may be normal or may reveal some combination of weakness, sensory disturbance, or loss of reflexes. Again, the distribution of these findings conform to the pattern of plexus involvement. The sensory disturbances experienced by these patients may include hypesthesia or hyperesthesia, hypalgesia or hyperalgesia, and occasionally, allodynia (pain on light touch) or hyperpathia (exaggerated pain response). After some time, atrophy of the muscles of the leg may be demonstrable, unless obscured by overlying edema.

The clinical diagnosis of plexopathy is usually suspected on the basis of the history and physical examination. Appropriate imaging procedures are selected to confirm this impression. At times, electrophysiologic testing is also useful, distinguishing plexopathy from multiple mononeuropathy, or more commonly, from polyradiculopathy. In the case of plexopathy, electromyography may demonstrate acute and chronic changes consistent with denervation in muscles conforming to multiple myotomes. Paraspinal muscles are often spared, an important indication of plexopathy over radiculopathy. Nerve conduction testing may demonstrate reduced amplitude, consistent with loss of peripheral nerve fibers. This pattern of findings supports the clinical impression and further indicates the need for imaging procedures to evaluate the region of the plexus. Conversely, a pattern of findings consistent with polyradiculopathy suggests the need for evaluation of the intraspinal space as well.

Imaging of the lumbosacral plexus is best accomplished by computed tomography (CT) or magnetic resonance imaging (MRI). Experience with the latter technique is still very limited, but preliminary experience suggests the potential utility of this modality in the evaluation of the pelvis and paraspinal region. Other methods of imaging the retroperitoneal space rarely provide additional clinically significant information than that provided by the CT or MRI. Occasionally, however, sonography and intravenous or retrograde pyelography may provide unique information about the status of the ureters, from which inferences about the integrity of the retroperitoneal space may be drawn.

Ancillary procedures designed to evaluate the spine or intraspinal space may also be useful in those cases in which bony invasion or a paraspinal mass suggests the need to rule out intraspinal extension of the neoplasm. Bone scintigraphy may provide an early indication of this proximal extension, and spine radiographs, CT, or MRI may define it better if necessary. Evaluation of the intraspinal space is best done with myelography, although MRI may be useful in selected cases.

RADIATION-INDUCED VS. MALIGNANT LUMBOSACRAL PLEXOPATHY

A common differential diagnosis with important implications for therapy is encountered in those patients with prior radiation to a pelvic port who subsequently develop progressive pain and neurologic dysfunction in the leg.[1-2] The distinction between a radiation-induced plexopathy and malignant plexopathy due to recurrent tumor is essential to provide adequate treatment and clarify prognosis. Similar to the evaluation of malignant plexopathy in those without previous radiation, the diagnosis in this setting depends on the clinical findings, electrophysiologic features, and the result of imaging procedures.

Severe pain is far more common with malignant plexopathy than radiation-induced plexopathy. Paresthesias occur in both disorders, but are more typical in radiation-induced plexopathy. On examination, edema can occur in malignant plexopathy, the result of impaired venous outflow, but is far less common. On electromyography, the finding of myokymia has been suggested to be a relatively specific concomitant of radiation-induced peripheral nerve damage. Finally, the finding of a discrete mass on axial imaging with CT or MRI, rather than diffuse disruption of tissue planes, is strong evidence of tumor recurrence. Rarely, surgical exploration is needed to make this important diagnosis.

MANAGEMENT

Aggressive analgesic management should be undertaken during the assessment process. After the offending lesion has been identified, consideration must be given first to the possible analgesic effects of primary therapy. Radiotherapy to the plexus can be considered, if not performed previously, and should the patient be a candidate for chemotherapy, the discovery of a progressive neoplastic lesion in the region of the lumbosacral plexus may provide the impetus to implement it.

Primary analgesic therapy for the pain associated with lumbosacral plexopathy is based on the same principles that guide the management of other cancer pain syndromes.[3] Pharmacotherapy is the mainstay, with consideration given to the use of techniques or procedures included under one or more of five ancillary approaches: anesthetic, neurostimulatory, physiatric, surgical, or psychological.

The pharmacological approach to cancer pain management requires expertise in the use of three broad classes of medications—opioid analgesics, nonsteroidal anti-inflammatory drugs (NSAID), and adjuvant medications (drugs that have other primary indications, but are analgesic in selected circumstances). A useful general approach developed by the Cancer Pain Relief Program of the World Health Organization is known as the analgesic ladder. According to these guidelines, patients who present with mild pain are treated first with a nonsteroidal anti-inflammatory drug, with or without the addition of an adjuvant analgesic should a specific indication for one exist. Patients who present with more moderate pain or who fail to achieve relief with the NSAID are then treated with a so-called "weak" opioid, the prototype of which is codeine, in combination with an NSAID and an adjuvant analgesic, should a specific indication for one exist. Finally, patients who develop severe pain or who fail to achieve adequate analgesia by the use of the "weak" opioid are treated with a potent opioid drug, morphine as the prototype, with or without the use of an NSAID or adjuvant analgesic.

Detailed guidelines for the administration of these drugs have been reviewed recently.[3] A standard approach involves upward titration of an oral opioid until desired effects occur or until intolerable and unmanageable side effects supervene. Since the pain syndrome experienced by patients with lumbosacral plexopathy is often neuropathic in quality, usually with some combination of continuous dysesthesias and paroxysmal lancinating pain, early use of adjuvant analgesics, such as tricyclic antidepressants or anticonvulsants, should be considered in targeting these specific complaints.

Another approach to the pharmacologic management of patients with pain from lumbosacral plexopathy is the use of spinal opioids. Generally, this modality is considered in patients with pain in the lower half of the body, who develop intolerable central side effects with systemic opioid drugs. Continuous intrathecal infusion using an implanted pump may be appropriate for those with lengthy life expectancies. Epidural administration is a more economical and flexible approach, however, and can be provided via a percutaneous catheter or totally implanted system. Morphine remains the prototype drug, although others have been utilized in a small series of patients with chronic cancer pain. There have been no controlled studies of the use of spinal opioids in the management of patients with painful lumbosacral plexopathy and a number of clinical controversies persist, including drug selection, timing of the approach, and the relative efficacy of epidural vs. intrathecal administration. Nonetheless, the techniques employed are widely accepted and clearly efficacious in a subgroup of patients, the selection and management of whom remain in the realm of clinical judgment.

Most patients are adequately managed by the use of pharmacologic measures alone. Alternative approaches are sometimes needed as primary therapy in those who fail to respond to drugs, and should be considered as adjunctive measures in patients who show an incomplete response.

Anesthetic approaches have a long history in the management of cancer pain, such as that associated with malignant plexopathy. Regional anesthetic techniques can be broadly classified by neural target into sympathetic and somatic blockade, and by the solution used into temporary blockade with local anesthetic and permanent blockade with a neurolytic substance. Patients with prominent burning dysesthesias of the leg associated with evidence of vasomotor or sudomotor disturbance should be considered for a diagnostic sympathetic block through either a paralumbar or epidural approach. If prolonged relief of pain is observed, a course of repeated blocks can be undertaken, followed at some point by consideration of sympathetic neurolysis, if necessary. Temporary somatic blocks with local anesthetic, usually administered into the epidural space, can sometimes be a useful adjunct in patients undergoing titration of analgesic medications. Repeated epidural instillation of local anesthetic or continuous anesthetic epidural infusion can also be a primary approach for patients with advanced disease and refractory pain. Somatic neurolysis with phenol or alcohol may compromise urinary and motor function, and is generally considered only in those patients in whom bladder function has already been lost.

Neurostimulatory approaches to analgesia include counterirritation (systematic rubbing of the painful part), transcutaneous electrical nerve stimulation, acupuncture, and several invasive approaches, such as percutaneous electrical nerve stimulation, dorsal column stimulation, and deep brain stimulation. Although analgesia in cancer pain syndromes can be observed with these techniques, particularly in those syndromes characterized by neuropathic pain such as lumbosacral plexopathy, the effects are generally modest and unsustained. Nonetheless, the use of a noninvasive technique, such as transcutaneous electrical nerve stimulation, may be useful in providing transitory analgesia during the period of opioid titration.

Physiatric approaches to cancer pain management include physical therapy, occupational therapy, and the use of orthoses or prostheses. The analgesic potential of these modalities in painful lumbosacral plexopathy is generally limited, although physical therapy may be useful in preventing secondary painful complications, such as joint ankylosis or contractures.

A broad spectrum of psychological approaches may also be useful in selected patients to reduce pain intensity and improve function. Cognitive therapies, for example, including biofeedback, hypnosis, relaxation training, and distraction, have achieved wide acceptance. These approaches have the potential to diminish pain and enhance a sense of personal control. Other interventions, including supportive psychotherapy, may improve both the mood and function of those with painful lesions.

Patients refractory to noninvasive modalities of pain control may be candidates for neurolytic surgical procedures, particularly cordotomy. Cordotomy has been used for over 50 years in the management of severe malignant pain, and large surveys suggest efficacy in up to 90% of cases, with a relatively small risk of significant adverse effects. The procedure can now be done percutaneously in the awake patient using a radiofrequency lesion. Traditionally, patients with lumbosacral plexopathy have been considered particularly good candidates for this procedure, since both the pain and its cause are usually unilateral.

In sum, the management of painful malignant lumbosacral plexopathy depends on the definition of the offending lesion, consideration of primary antineoplastic therapy, and the expert application of a multimodal approach to analgesic management, in which pharmacotherapy plays the central role. Comprehensive and ongoing pain assessment by a concerned and knowledgeable clinician, who can aggressively manage pharmacologic therapy and make appropriate referrals for invasive approaches when necessary, is the essential factor in this process. Many of these patients pose extremely challenging pain problems, but most have the potential for adequate analgesia if this outcome is given appropriately high priority.

REFERENCES

1. Jaeckle KA, Young DA, Foley KB: The natural history of lumbosacral plexopathy in cancer. *Neurology* 1985; 35:8–15.
2. Thomas JE, Cascino TE, Earle JD: Differential diagnosis between radiation and tumor plexopathy of the pelvis. *Neurology* 1985; 35:1–7.
3. Foley KM: The treatment of cancer pain. *N Engl J Med* 1985; 313:84–95.

PART VIII

Psychological Issues

46

Drug Detoxification in Nonmalignant Pain

Theresa Ferrer-Brechner, M.D.

A 35-year-old man with a history of job-related back injury was referred to the pain center because of difficulty in medication control. One year prior to referral, the patient sustained an injury while employed as a construction worker, when he slipped and fell on his back while carrying a heavy load. This caused immediate severe pain in his back and buttocks area. Radiologic studies at that time did not reveal any fracture or disk protrusion. The patient was treated with physical therapy and analgesics, initially with nonnarcotic analgesics. However, his pain persisted despite all treatments and he sought help from several physicians. He was given prescriptions of narcotic analgesics by different physicians. On entry to the clinic he was on hydromorphone (Dilaudid) 2 mg every 4 hours as needed, controlled-release morphine sulfate (MS-Contin) 30 mg 2–3 times per day, I.M. shots of meperidene (Demerol) when the pain was severe, and Halcion 0.5 mg at night for sleep. The total average intake per day was 12 mg of Dilaudid, 90 mg MS-Contin, and Demerol 100 mg I.M. When the patient arrived at the clinic, his cognitive dysfunction was obvious as a result of the drug intake. His physicians sent him to us because they no longer wanted to prescribe his narcotics due to the escalating trend in dose necessary to obtain analgesia, especially during the last 2 months prior to referral. Results of the initial physical exam revealed severe myofascial pain involving the lumbar paraspinal muscles, quadratus lumborum, and the piriformis muscles. Neurological exam was negative.

DISCUSSION

This case is a demonstration of what usually happens in a young patient who is started on narcotic analgesics because the patient continues to complain of pain despite negative medical workup. Because of the tendency to seek various medical specialists in search of a definitive diagnosis, each physician prescribed narcotics independently, not knowing of the attempts on the part of the other physicians to reduce the pain by other narcotic analgesics. As a result, many patients referred to a pain center usually present problems with excessive opioid or sedative-hypnotic medications.[1] Obviously, this patient who presented suffering from myofascial pain syndrome will not respond to narcotic analgesics on a long-term basis. Therefore, the first step in this patient's treatment is a systematic drug detoxification before a myofascial pain program even has a chance for any success. Chronic use of opioid and sedative-hypnotic drugs produces dysphoria and other symptoms such as decreased energy, sleep disturbance, and decreased weight. Patients can mislabel withdrawal symptoms as increased pain.[2]

Drug detoxification can be done on an inpatient or outpatient basis, depending on the severity of the problem, presence of family support, and economic condition of the patient. I usually attempt an outpatient detoxification program with a majority of my patients because withdrawal can be done slowly over time, can be integrated with the pain program, and is definitely more cost effective than an inpatient detoxification program.

Before a detoxification program is started, the patient and their significant other are brought in for a conference to emphasize the need for detoxification as an integral part of the pain program. It is important to elicit motivation on the patient's part since, if the patient is not motivated, the detoxification program has a high probability of failing. If the patient shows strong interest in withdrawal, a written treatment contract is drawn up containing the following points of agreement:

1. Patient agrees to obtain all his/her analgesic medications only from you or a designated physician.
2. Patient gives permission to contact and inform all recent physicians that you are the only source of medications and agree that they will not prescribe any analgesics during the detoxification process.
3. Patient agrees to come to your clinic weekly to obtain the pain cocktail.
4. Patient agrees to a "no loss" agreement, i.e., if medications are lost or accidentally spilled, there is no replacement.
5. Patient and family understand fully that withdrawal is being done for the patient's medical benefit.

PROCESS OF WITHDRAWAL

There are essentially four steps to a drug detoxification, as described by Halpern.[3]

1. Establishment of total intake per 24 hours.
2. Changing from pain-contingent to time-contingent intake of medications.
3. Substitution of short-acting to long-acting narcotics and/or sedatives, and mixing ingredients in a masked vehicle, such as cherry syrup.
4. Systematic reduction of active ingredients while keeping the volume of the vehicle constant.

Establishment of total intake in a hospital environment can be done by literally having the patient express freely his first 24–48 hour analgesic and/or sedative needs, and allowing him or her to receive their self-prescribed narcotics or sedatives. On an outpatient basis, this could sometimes be tricky, since patients often give you an underestimated total for an entire week, usually expressed in a frantic call before the week is ended, since they have run out of medications. If this happens, the patient can be given another chance to give their total drug intake for their second week. For example, in this patient, the total daily drug intake is reported as MS-Contin (controlled-release morphine sulfate), 90 mg, and Dilaudid (hydromorphone), 12 mg orally, Demerol (meperidine), 100 mg I.M., and alprazolam 0.5 mg orally at night. This dose was multiplied by 7 and the patient was given a week's supply of his reported intake. However, after 4 days, he frantically called to inform us that he had run out of Demerol 50 mg I.M. shots, and when recalculated, the patient was actually self-administering Demerol 200 mg per day. The patient was then given a chance to express his real total drug intake and the amount readjusted for the second week. In addition, the patient was asked to submit a daily dairy indicating the times when he takes his medications.

The second step is to teach the patient to take his existing medications on a time-contingent instead of pain-contingent regimen in order to obtain a more constant plasma level, preventing "peaks and valleys" that produce drowsiness and "mini" withdrawals in between doses. In addition, switching to a time-contingent regimen removes pain as the trigger to obtain more medications, since the medication is taken at designated times, whether or not pain is present at that time. In the case presented, Dilaudid 4 mg was administered every 4 hours on a time-contingent basis around the clock. Demerol 50 mg I.M. was given with the Dilaudid only during the hours spent awake for 4 doses. The patient actually reported improved pain relief when switched from a pain-contingent to time-contingent regimen.

The third step is substitution from short-acting to long-acting narcotics. Usually, Dolophine (methadone) is given as a cherry syrup suspension. In this

TABLE 46–1.

Narcotic Analgesic Equivalency of Common Narcotics

		IM[†]	Oral	PR[†]
Morphine[‡]	MS			
	MS-Contin	10	30–60*	10–20
	Rexanal			
Codeine	Tylenol w/codeine			
	Phenaphen	120	200	—
	Empirin w/codeine			
Hydromorphone	Dilaudid	1.5	7.5	—
Oxymorphone	Numorphan	1.5	—	10
Hydrocodone	Vicodin			
	Anexia	—	5–10	—
	Hycodan			
Oxycodone	Percodan			
	Percocet	10–15	5–30	—
	Tylox			
Meperidine	Demerol	75	300	—
Methadone	Dolophine	10	20	—
Levorphanol	Levo-Dromoran	2–3	4–5	—
Propoxyphene	Darvon			
	Darvocet	—	300–400	—

*Modified from *Principles of Analgesic Use in the Treatment of Chronic Pain and Chronic Cancer Pain: A Concise Guide to Medical Practice,* ed 2.
[†]*IM = intramuscular; PR = per rectum.*
[‡]Single-dose study shows relative potency of PO/IM morphine as 6:1. In practice, repetitive dosing indicates a ratio of 3:1.

case, daily equipotent doses of morphine (MS-Contin), Demerol, and Dilaudid were calculated as substitutes for methadone (Table 46–1). (Demerol I.M. 200 mg = 30 mg orally methadone; MS-Contin 90 mg = 60 mg methadone; Dilaudid 12 mg orally = 32 mg methadone orally; therefore, total daily equivalent of oral methadone = 122 mg divided into 6 doses = 20 mg methadone every 4 hours.) It is also advisable to include a nonnarcotic analgesic in the pain cocktail, such as acetaminophen at a dose of 3 grams per day maximum. Remember to caution use of acetaminophen in patients with liver dysfunction. Therefore, the "pain cocktail" for the first week will be the following:

- Methadone: 854 mg
- Acetaminophen: 28 gm
- Cherry syrup: 420 cc
- Sig: 10 cc every 4 hrs around the clock

The fourth and final step for detoxification is the systematic reduction of narcotic ingredients in the cocktail without decreasing the volume. Usually, the patient could tolerate a 20% decrease per week. If withdrawal symptoms occur and/or pain increases, the reduction can be suspended for another week and/or a NSAID, such as ibuprofen 600 mg, can be added as an open drug.

Taking the present case as an example of a systemic reduction regimen is reflected in the prescription for the following week after substitution:

- Methadone: 684 mg
- Acetaminophen: 28 gm
- Cherry syrup: 460 cc
- Sig: 10 cc every 4 hrs

The amount of methadone in the cocktail is then decreased 20% per week until it is totally eliminated. Halcion (triazolam) was decreased 10% per week and substituted with amitriptylin 25 mg at bedtime.

It is important to start the pain program the second or third week of withdrawal. In this particular case, the patient started physical therapy, a home exercise program, stimulation-induced analgesia, and relaxation techniques in the second week of systemic reduction. This allows switching of dependency from the medications to programs enhancing activity increase. The patient was totally withdrawn from the narcotics and sedative in 6 weeks and, surprisingly, expressed lower pain reports despite elimination of narcotics. This result coincides with results obtained in drug withdrawal done in inpatient pain programs.[4-5]

REFERENCES

1. Ready LB, Sarkis E, Turner JA: Self reported versus actual use of medications in chronic pain patients. *Pain* 1982; 12:285–294.
2. Brodner RA, Taub A: Chronic pain exacerbated by long-term narcotic use in patients with non-malignant disease: Clinical syndrome and treatment. *Mt Sinai J Med (NY)* 1978; 45:233–237.
3. Halpern LM: Substitution-detoxification and its role in the management of chronic benign pain. *J Clin Psychiatry* 1982; 3:8,10–14.
4. Swanson DW, Maruta T, Swenson WM: Results of behavior modification in the treatment of chronic pain. *Psychosom Med* 1979; 41:55–61.
5. Taylor CB, Zlutnick SI, Corley MJ, et al: The effects of detoxification, relaxation and brief supportive therapy on chronic pain. *Pain* 1980; 8:319–329.

47

Work-Related Injury and Pain

Frederick M. Stampler, Psy.D.

The patient is a 34-year-old woman who worked in a fabric warehouse. Two and one-half years ago, she lifted a large bolt of fabric and experienced a sharp pain in her lower back. She heard a popping sound and felt a radiation of pain down her left leg. She informed her supervisor, but continued to work for the next 3 days in a "light duty" capacity, until the pain was too great to allow her to continue. She has not worked since. After approximately 4 months of conservative treatment, which included bed rest, hot packs, massage, ultrasound, and pain medication, the patient was still completely disabled from work due to back pain and lower extremity weakness. A computed tomography (CT) scan revealed disk herniation at L4–5, and soon thereafter she received a decompressive laminectomy and diskectomy. The patient experienced some relief following the surgery and progressed well enough in physical therapy to begin a vocational rehabilitation computer training program. She enjoyed the training very much, and looked forward to a new career. Three weeks before completing her training, however, she suffered a severe flare-up of her back pain and dropped out. Over the next year, the patient underwent several acute hospitalizations for pain, months of physical therapy, several changes of doctors, and an ill-fated attempt to return to her vocational rehabilitation program. Today, a full $2^1/_2$ years after her work injury, she remains completely disabled from work and most household responsibilities, and is depressed, frustrated, anxious, and angry.

BACKGROUND

The case history described above is not atypical for a work-related back injury that persists beyond the first few months. It is estimated that approximately 85% of workers who injure their backs on the job return to work within 60–80 days postinjury.[1] Those who fail to recover within a 3–6 month time frame are particularly vulnerable to prolonged periods of disability, often associated with inactivity, hostility, mood disturbance, financial hardship, litigation issues, and failed efforts at rehabilitation. This is a health care problem with social, political, and economic dimensions, as more and more resources are channeled toward industrial medical costs and disability benefits. Fordyce has recently cited evidence to suggest that while the incidence and severity of back injury has not increased over the years, the number of individuals receiving compensation or disability status due to back pain is disproportionately on the rise.[2] This has led Fordyce to pass on the caveat of Swedish orthopedist, Alf Nachemson, that "physicians should not treat back pain; nor should psychologists. Politicians should."[2]

In light of such concerns, the conventional wisdom for many in the field of clinical pain management has been that physicians should not treat patients with pain while they are engaged in litigation or a worker's compensation suit.[3] The belief is that pressures to maximize disability in pursuit of financial compensation will inevitably compromise the patient's effort to comply with treatment and improve. This position holds that injured workers should first resolve their cases and pursue pain management treatment afterward. In fact, many of the early studies on pain program efficacy carefully screened out subjects with litigation or worker's compensation suits pending.[4–5]

While it is true that operant (or secondary gain) factors are inherent within the worker's compensation system and must be considered when designing a program for injured workers, it can no longer be accepted that the suit must be resolved before pain management treatment can begin. Many recent empirical studies have shown compensation status not to be predictive of treatment outcome in programs offering multimodal treatment approaches.[6] Additionally, it is neither practical nor wise public policy to deny appropriate chronic pain treatment to such a large and costly segment of the medical population. These patients are rarely not treated, and if specialists abdicate, the alternative is inadequate and often costly treatment by other practitioners not skilled in the management of chronic pain. There is a growing realization that the expertise provided by interdisciplinary pain practitioners, when cost effectively and accountably administered, can actually help facilitate the injured worker's rehabilitation, often by attending to the potentially deleterious influences of the worker's compensation system and addressing them in treatment.

REFERRAL ANALYSIS

The first step in approaching a case such as this patient's is to analyze the nature of the referral. Who made the referral? Was it the insurance company's claims examiner or attorney? The patient's attorney? A physician? If a physician made the referral, was he authorized by the insurance company, self-procured through the patient's attorney, or was he an "agreed medical examiner" who is approved by both sides. The worker's compensation system is, in most states, adversarial. It is incumbent upon any health care provider who becomes involved to have a clear understanding of the dynamics of the system and the expectations of those to whom he may be accountable. The patient's attorney, for example, may desire evaluations of the patient biased in the direction of disability, while the insurance carriers may reward evaluators who downplay disability and need for treatment. One must be aware of any direct or indirect pressures to be "defense minded" or "applicant minded" and maintain integrity in the process.

In this patient's case, the referral was made by her physician of choice, through the office of her attorney. The pain practitioner should make clear to all parties involved that the preeminent goal of the pain management evaluation is for a thorough, honest assessment of *all* factors, medical, psychological, and environmental, that may be contributing to the patient's pain and degree of disabled functioning. Similarly, it should be made clear to all that the objective of pain management treatment is to restore the patient to the highest possible level of behavioral functioning. The prevailing philosophy is that the patient's interests are best served when maximum functioning takes priority over maximum compensation. It is sometimes useful to forewarn the patient explicitly, at the outset of treatment, that successful rehabilitation will necessarily reduce the severity of disability and, therefore, the magnitude of possible financial compensation. Frank discussion of this issue tends to result in the self-selection of some insincere patients out of the program, while diffusing the potential resistance of those patients who elect to participate.

If the patient was referred directly by the insurance company, the same priorities of evaluation and treatment should be made explicit. Additionally, the practitioner should not shy away from being an advocate for the patient with the claims examiner if it is warranted by the facts of the case. For example, if the patient's pain and suffering cannot be explained by the organic findings alone, malingering may incorrectly be assumed automatically; the pain psychologist can clarify factors other than malingering that may account for discrepancies between organic findings and function.

EVALUATION

Once the circumstances of the referral have been considered, the evaluation can proceed. The psychological evaluation of work-injured patients with chronic pain has several objectives, which include assessing: (1) the subjective and objective dimensions of the patient's pain experience (e.g., frequency, intensity, duration, and quality); (2) the impact of pain on the patient's mood, cognition, and behavior; (3) the patient's mental status and general level of psychological functioning; (4) the nature of concurrent environmental antecedents and consequences that may have an effect on the patient's pain behavior and activities; (5) the psychological suitability of the patient for elective invasive procedures; (6) the patient's current disability status; (7) issues pertaining to industrial causation and apportionment; (8) the patient's rehabilitation potential; (9) the patient's appropriateness for various psychological treatments; and (10) specific recommendations on how best to manage the patient behaviorally in the treatment setting.

Much has been written on behavioral pain assessment strategies, and they will not be detailed further here. Additionally, instruction on how to evaluate psychological disability, industrial causation, and apportionment is beyond the scope of this chapter. However, one aspect of the psychological evaluation that bears particular relevance to work-related injury is the delineation of nonorganic factors that may contribute to disability. The severity and duration of disability will quite often exceed that which is expected from the organic findings alone. Individual psychological variables, interpersonal environmental factors, and worker's compensation system-related factors can all have an impact on the "pain behavior" and "disability behavior" exhibited by the patient.

The psychological assessment of the patient found her to be a woman who had endured a difficult early life. As a young child, she had been victimized by physical and sexual abuse perpetrated by her father. Her mother had rheumatoid arthritis and was often bedridden. Consequently, from as early as the age of 9 years, the patient was forced to assume a great deal of responsibility in the household; she virtually raised her seven younger brothers and sisters. These experiences resulted in the patient being an anxious child with low self-esteem, and with little time to devote to the development of normal peer relationships. Nonetheless, she was extremely conscientious in her assumption of the excessive responsibilities foisted on her.

Historical information, as well as the results of the Minnesota Multiphasic Personality Inventory (MMPI), suggested that the patient was an individual who lacked psychological mindedness. She had always been something of a "tomboy," priding herself on her physical prowess and mechanical interests. When the patient was injured, it was difficult for her to cope with the degree of physical compromise she experienced. Reliance upon her physical capacities was fundamental to her identity, and the experience of pain and lower extremity weakness frightened her terribly.

During the months that followed her surgery, the patient's fear and anxiety were joined by growing hostility toward the worker's compensation insurance carrier whom she felt was delaying the payment of her temporary disability benefits. This hostility added to resentment she experienced toward her employer prior to the injury, over what she thought were unfair working conditions. Consequently, the patient felt angry, victimized, passive, and helpless.

Despite these emotions, the patient wanted to complete her vocational rehabilitation computer training, in part, to allay the financial hardship she was experiencing. But, twice as she approached her goal, she developed anticipatory anxiety over the prospect of completing her training; she feared losing the safety net of her disability status, and then not being able to perform physically in the new work role. Injured workers with pain often meet each increment of progress with increased anxiety, fearing that their improvement will cause the expectations that others have of what they can do to escalate beyond their control. The patient was not willfully malingering, but was sabotaged by her own anxiety, of which she had little awareness.

The individual, interpersonal, and systems-related psychological factors that combined to affect the patient's degree of pain and disability behavior can be summarized as follows: (1) depression, anxiety, and anger; (2) poor coping skills for dealing with physical compromise; (3) the existence of an illness-behavior model in her family history (her disabled mother); (4) a life history of excessive responsibilities that increased her susceptibility to develop operant pain behavior; her pain behavior was reinforced by providing her with the only means of escape or "time-out" from undue burdens acceptable to her; (5) additional operant reinforcement accrued from the pain-contingent nurturance supplied by her husband; usually the patient was on the giving, not receiving, end of nuturance; (6) limited psychological awareness of the emotional stress factors that affected her well-being, and a tendency to manifest stress through a somatic focus; (7) her long-standing resentment toward her employer which became accentuated through the adversarial nature of the system; and (8) the sabotaging effects that her anticipatory anxiety had on her ability to complete the vocational rehabilitation program.

TREATMENT

In her $2^{1}/_{2}$ years of prior treatment, the patient had not received any professional psychological or behavioral intervention. It is not surprising that she failed to respond to the many medical treatments attempted. In complex cases such as this, successful rehabilitation requires that behavioral intervention be provided closely in concert with medical treatment.

Appropriate treatment for the patient would consist of an intensive, highly structured program administered by an interdisciplinary team of physicians, psychologists, physical therapists, occupational therapists, and nurses. Treatment should be conducted either in an inpatient program, or in a structured outpatient program with daily involvement. Central to the rehabilitation effort would be a concentration on increasing the patient's strength, endurance, flexibility, and general functioning through a physical activation and exercise program. The musculoskeletal factors contributing to her pain, which have been exacerbated by long-term disuse, should be addressed through activation and the teaching of self-management coping skills, such as stretching exercises, relaxation training, transcutaneous electrical nerve stimulation (TENS), pacing, and proper body mechanics. The activation program should conform to established learning theory principles of "time-contingent" as opposed to "pain-contingent" activity-rest cycles. Pain behaviors should not be reinforced by rest, attention, or medications, and healthy behaviors should be promoted. A more detailed description of the behavioral-rehabilitation model can be found in Fordyce and Steger.[7]

The patient will need psychotherapeutic assistance to address the psychological factors identified in the evaluation. Individual sessions with the pain management psychologist can help her increase her awareness of stress factors and mood states that interfere with her rehabilitation efforts. She must, in some way, come to terms with her anger, and work toward not allowing it to undermine the pursuit of her goals. She must take responsibility for her own improvement, and overcome feelings of victimization and helplessness. Psychotherapy, and possibly psychotropic pharmacotherapy, can address her depression. The patient must learn how to become more aware of her needs for support and nurturance, and how to fulfill those needs assertively rather than through reliance on pain behaviors. It will be necessary to involve her husband in conjoint sessions to modify patterns of reinforcement for pain behavior, and to address any marital stress factors associated with the chronic pain syndrome.

The pain psychologist can become the patient's advocate in the worker's compensation system by having good communication with the insurance company's claim examiner or rehabilitation representative. For example, the psychologist can help the carrier's representative understand how the patient's lack of confidence in her past physical progress, and anxious anticipation of increased demands from others have prevented her from maintaining her gains. A better understanding of this dynamic on the part of both the patient and the vocational rehabilitation team can lead toward problem-solving efforts to prevent this problem from recurring when the patient is ready to resume her training.

The pain program must earn the trust and confidence of the insurance carrier that it is hard-minded in its efforts to work with the patient. If it appears that the patient is not sincere in her attempts to reduce her disability, she should be discharged from the program and the reasons should be documented. The program must stand by the conviction that the interests of all parties are best served when the patient reaches the highest level of functioning possible.

REFERENCES

1. Andersson G, Swensson H, Anders O: The intensity of work recovery in low back pain. *Spine* 1983; 8:880–885.
2. Fordyce WE: Pain and suffering: A reappraisal. *Am Psychol* 1988; 43:276–283.
3. Follick MJ, Zitter RE, Ahern DK: Failures in the Operant Treatment of Chronic Pain, in Foa EB, Emmelkamp PMG (eds): *Failures in Behavior Therapy.* New York, Wiley, 1983, pp 311–334.
4. Abram SE, Anderson RA, and Maitra-D'Cruze AM: Factors predicting short-term outcome of nerve blocks in the management of chronic pain. *Pain* 1981; 10:323–330.
5. Roberts AH, Reinhardt L: The behavioral management of chronic pain: Long-term follow-up with comparison groups. *Pain* 1980; 8:151–162.
6. Dworkin RH, Handlin DS, Richlin DM, et al: Unraveling the effects of compensation, litigation, and employment in treatment response in chronic pain. *Pain* 1985; 23:49–59.
7. Fordyce WE, Steger JC: Chronic Pain, in Pomerleau OF, Brady JP (eds): *Behavioral Medicine: Theory and Practice.* Baltimore, Williams & Wilkins, 1979.

Index